Once Upon a Table

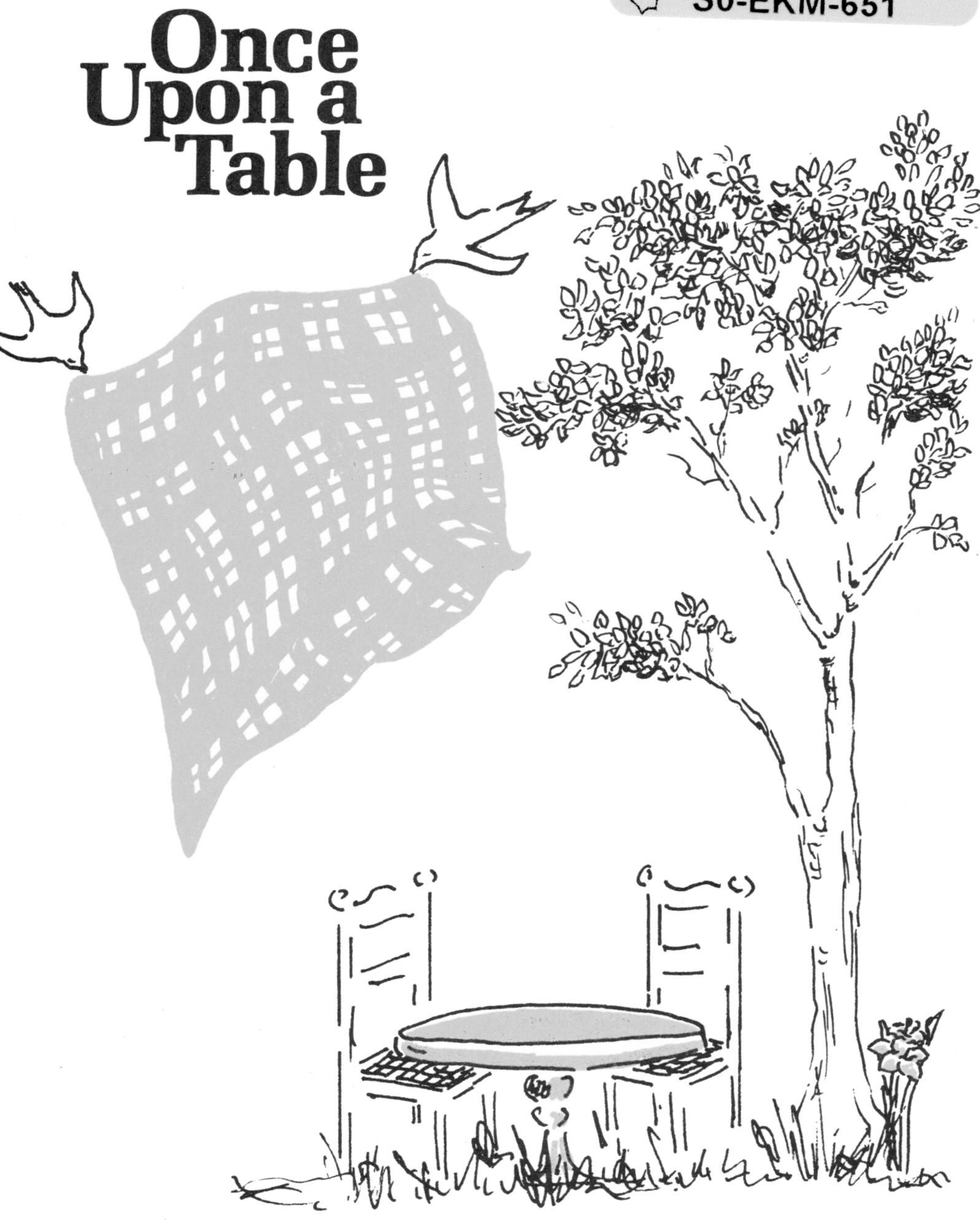

Cover design and illustrations by Honey Rice

WOMEN'S AUXILIARY OF
THE AMERICAN CANCER SOCIETY
Pittsburgh, PA
1981

All proceeds realized from the sale of this book will be given to the American Cancer Society.

The Women's Auxiliary thanks the following for their generous support:
Alcoa Foundation
H.J. Heinz Company Foundation
Rockwell International
First Federal Savings and Loan Association
Cinemette Corporation

For additional copies, use order blanks at the back of the book or write directly to:
ONCE UPON A TABLE
241 Fourth Avenue
Pittsburgh, PA 15222

First Printing — 10,000 — October, 1981
Second Printing — 20,000 — December, 1981

ISBN #0-9607282-0-1
Library of Congress Catalog Card #81-69959

Printed in the United States of America by Albert E. Deeds Associates, Inc.
Pittsburgh, Pennsylvania

THE WOMEN'S AUXILIARY OF THE AMERICAN CANCER SOCIETY

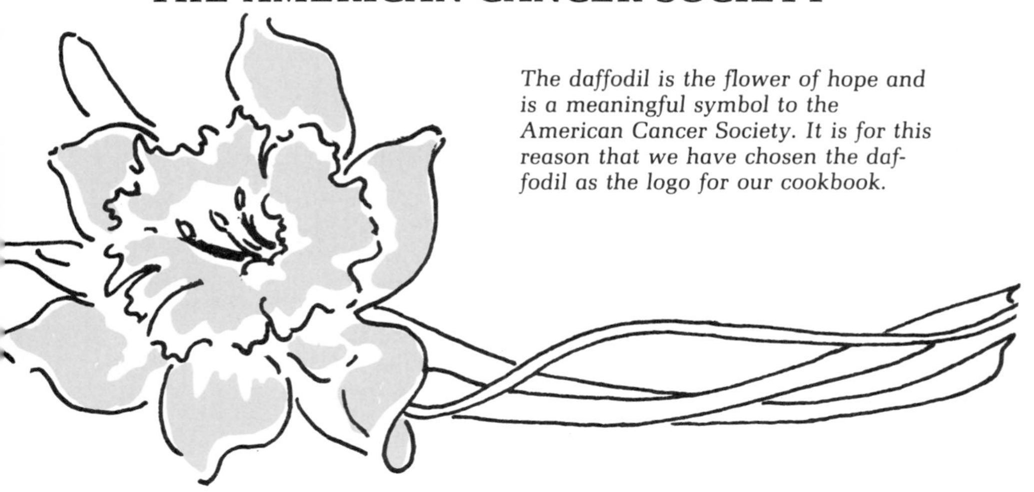

The daffodil is the flower of hope and is a meaningful symbol to the American Cancer Society. It is for this reason that we have chosen the daffodil as the logo for our cookbook.

The Women's Auxiliary of Pittsburgh, Pennsylvania, formed in 1973, was the first of its kind in this country. In eight years, by sponsoring our Cancer Society Ball, by holding an annual luncheon and fashion show and other special events, we have raised nearly one half million dollars, all of which has been given to the American Cancer Society to support their efforts in research, service and education. We are now involved in a new project.

Our cookbook, *Once Upon A Table*, contains the very best of recipes submitted by our membership, their friends and family. We have received recipes from all across the country. Each recipe included has been carefully tested, and every recipe is followed by a comment that either compliments or expands upon it.

Sixteen menus have been thoughtfully compiled to incorporate more than 100 of our recipes. Peter Machamer, noted wine connoisseur, generously agreed to suggest wines for our menus, course by course. We are also pleased to include a "Special Chefs" section in which chefs from some of the world's finest eating establishments have shared a few of their favorite recipes.

We present this book to you with pride and pleasure.

Shirley Losch

Shirley Losch, Chairman

Anita Zebrovious, Co-chairman
WAACS COOKBOOK

WINE UPON A TABLE

Wine belongs with food. Even the simplest luncheon or dinner can attain new aesthetic dimensions by the addition of a properly chosen bottle of wine (or two bottles, or three, or . . .). Wine not only adds new tastes to any meal, but it aids in digestion, helps along conversation and brings with it an aura that turns mere eating into dining.

Choosing the right wine for a meal is not difficult, though it takes some thought. Wines should be chosen so that they compliment the flavors of the foods. Other than this there are no rules. Drink as it pleases (but think about the drink as you do about the food you serve). The very best way to learn to choose properly is through practice and thought. Consider the ingredients that went into the dishes you are serving. What are their characteristic tastes? Then think about the flavors of the various wines at your disposal. Can you find one that seems the best match? One that would act almost like another sauce for the dish? If more than one wine suggests itself, try them both. You can do this in a trial run before the dinner party, or you can just set two glasses at each place and serve both, asking your guests for comments about which compliments better.

In the menus that follow, I have tried to suggest some interesting wines that I feel harmonize well with the recipes. These are only suggestions. If they help you to experiment, to think about wine and, most of all, to enjoy even more the glories of grand gluttony, I shall be rewarded. One final suggestion: a little wine taken lightly as the menu gets planned, and a bit more imbibed as the dishes are cooked, helps the ingenuity and creativity of the planner and the cook. However, it is well to be remembered that there are times (only a few, perhaps) at which moderation is a virtue. One such time is when excess can lead you to miss your own party.

A votre santé!

Peter Machamer

Peter Machamer
Wine Columnist,
Pittsburgh, *Post Gazette*

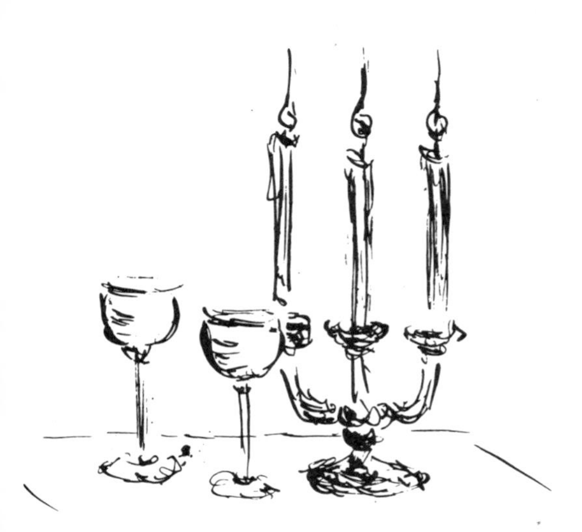

MENUS

DINNERS

Granache Rosé or Gewürztraminer (California)	California Wine and Cheese Spread Mushroom Tarts Chicken Wings Parmesan
	Chilled Zucchini Bisque
Beaujolais (France) or Bardolino (Italy)	Spinach Stuffed Ham Swedish Potatoes Peas with Cointreau Port Wine Cranberry Salad Mold
Late Harvest Riesling (California)	Lemon Cream Pie

Mosel (German) or Riesling (California)	Chicken Liver Paté Asparagus Canapés
	Youghiogheny's Princess Soup
Chianti or Barolo (Italy)	Baked Flank Steak Monterey Potatoes Herb Parmesan Casserole Bread Salad Greens with Russian Dressing
Champagne or Sparkling Wine	Chocolate Sundae Layer Cake

Sancerre (France) or Sauvignon Blanc (California)	Salmon Mousse Gouda Cheese Rolls
	Herbed Potato Soup
St. Emilion (France) or Cabernet Sauvignon (California)	Veal Prince Orloff Broccoli Soufflé Sautéed Cherry Tomatoes Lettuce Wedges with Roquefort Dressing
Port (Portugal or California)	New York Cheese Cake

White Graves (France) or Sauvignon Blanc (California)	Cognac Bleu Cheese Spread Spinach Pie Crisp Bacon Crackers
Red Bordeaux (France) or Cabernet Sauvignon (California)	Broiled Boned Lamb Browned White Rice Broccoli Loaf Tossed Fresh Fruit Salad
Sauternes (France)	Soufflé Glacé Grand Marnier

Macon Blanc (France) or Chardonnay (California)	Mushroom-Artichoke Appetizer Mexican Bean Dip Olive Balls
Soave (Italy)	Flounder Florentine Rice Ring Baked Tomatoes Ginger Ale Salad
Sauternes (France)	Shaker Lemon Pie

Macon Blanc or
Pouilly Fuissé (France)

Anchovy Cheese Spread
Baked Brie
Easy Bacon with Water Chestnuts

Vernaccia di San Gimiango or
Orvieto abbocato (Italy)

Country Style Chicken Kiev
Rice with Pine Nuts
Vegetable Medley
Salad Greens with Celery Seed Dressing

Tokay (Hungary)

Williamsburg Orange Cake

Soave or
Frascati (Italy)

Ceviche
Cheese Cider Cocktail Spread

Zinfandel (California)

Marinated Eye of the Round
Roasted Potatoes
Mushroom Sauce
Spinach Salad
Cornmeal Batter Rolls

Sauternes (France)

Angel Alaska

Chardonnay (California)

Chicken Hors d'Oeuvres
Mushroom Cheese Toast

Zinfandel (California)

Marinated Pork Roast
Potato Salad
Vegetable Salad Vinaigrette
Round Onion Loaves

Late Harvest Gewürztraminer
(California)

Pumpkin Cake Roll

Chardonnay (California) or White Burgundy (France)	Oyster Cheese Roll Chicken Curry Dip
	Tavern Soup
Red Bordeaux (France) or Cabernet Sauvignon (California)	Steak Montrose with Quick Bordelaise Sauce Spinach Souffle Original Caesar Salad
Champagne (France) or Asti Spumante (Italy)	Chocolate Silk

Rhine Riesling (Germany)	Broccoli Beignets Escalloped Oysters
Red Burgundy or Beaujolais (France)	Cornish Hens Mandarin Rice and Mushroom Bake Stuffed Zucchini with Cheese Molded Beet Salad Cornbread
Late Harvest Riesling (California)	Peach-Blueberry Pie

LATE SUPPERS

Rioja (Spain)	Hot Artichoke Spread Chuck Barbecues Celery and Nut Aspic Shoofly Cupcakes

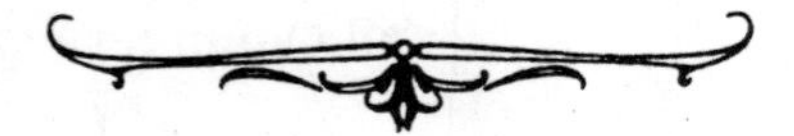

White Burgundy (France) or Chardonnay (California)	Lemon Soup Seafood Casserole Spinach Tossed with Chutney Dressing Pears with Mint Custard Sauce

BRUNCHES

Riesling (Germany or California)	Party Omelet Stuffed Sausage Patties Broiled Mixed Fruit Cinnamon Buns

Gewürztraminer (France or California)	Sausage Brunch Casserole Chili Egg Puff Scalloped Bacon 'n Eggs Minted Fruit Compote Quick Apricot Pastries Swedish Kringler

LUNCHEONS

Zinfandel (California) or Beaujolais (France)	Mushroom Crust Quiche Marinated Broccoli Baked Orange Slices Coconut Cake

Chardonnay (California)	Herb Crêpes Béarnaise Baked Tomatoes Frozen Pea Salad Fudge Pie

Every recipe in this cookbook was tested and approved by committees of 8 to 18 people. Husbands took part in evening testings, and their suggestions, interest and enthusiasm were greatly valued. Thanks beyond measure go to the members of our testing committees:

Jeanne Alexander
Audrey Bailey
Barbara Barry
Shirley Beamon
Barbara Botkin
Barbara Brown
Susan Caesar
Kathy Coco
Margie Cordero
Neva Cunniff
Dorothy Datemasch
Gloria Datillo
Alice DiBella
Ellen Downs
Ann Ferrier
Pat Frank
Chris Griffin
Ann Guffey
Trudy Hannoway
De Hamilton
Ann Hartzell
Doris Hepp
Beverly Howarth
Edna Kane
Gail Lacey
Elima Leoni
Shirley Losch
Cel McCabe
Mary Lou McCurdy
Mary Lou McLaughlin
Alison Moeller
Maryanne Nelson
Mari-Louise Rannow
Barly Rich
Sally Rose
Ginny Rost
Doris Scott
Mary Jo Sinicrope
Lynn Smail
Lily Mae Spehar
Linda Spiker
Mary Struk
Judi Todd
Aggie Wager
Pollyann Wisser
Anita Zebrovious

Marie L. Fork
Val Junker
Lois Kreiger
Dolores W. Smith
TESTING CHAIRMEN

These are the people who made this cookbook possible. We thank them one and all, for each and every recipe.

Terry Abbott
Lois Jean Adam
Jeanne Alexander
Jane W. Allen
Amy Andrews
Barbara Augustine
Jeanne Bacharach
Marge Backus
Audrey Bailey
Ted Barnett
Barbara Barry
Shirley Beamon
Carolyn Benedict
Margaret Bennett
Ruth S. Bierer
Janet Bobincheck
Mrs. E. Jackson Bonney
Lois Botkin
Betty Jane Bower
Madolyn Branham
Suzanne Bress
Marge Brinkworth
Barbara Brown
Ruth Buchanan
B. J. Budday
Mrs. Sharon Burke
Mrs. Porter D. Caesar, II
Joyce Caputo
Rita Carlson
Mrs. Richard Cartun
Mrs. W. P. Cartun
Gail Chambers
Mrs. D. E. Cooper
Margie Cordero
Louise Cox
Elaine Crist
Neva Cunniff
Linda Cuoushare
Dorothy Datemasch
Eleanor Davis
Marcia Deaktor
Mrs. Donald R. Dean
Kathy Dear
Alice DiBella
Terry Dillen
Lindy Dolan
Kay Domurot
Gail Donaldson
Eileen Drake
Mrs. Earle DuBois
Ginny Duncan
Mrs. M. T. Dwyer
Mrs. D. L. Eynon, Jr.
Joyce Elstner
Winnie Engelmeier
Yetta Farber
Phyllis Felman
Judie Ferguson
Ann Ferrier
Lynne Smith Feyk
Mary Fischer
Ruth Fisher
Kathy Fork
Marie L. Fork
Inge Forrest
Grace France

Pat Frank
Bernice Friedlander
Barbara Fuchs
Elizabeth Garvey
Richard Gibala
Florence Glick
Mrs. Milton L. Goldstein
Chris Griffin
Lorraine Wilson Griffin
Phyllis Grimes
Ann Guffey
Mrs. Bernard Halpern
Betty Hamilton
De Hamilton
Marguerite Hannon
Mrs. Stephen Hannon
Mrs. Thomas Hannon
Ann Hansen
Mrs. Casey Harper
Peg Harrison
Ann Hartzell
Mrs. James Hawkins
Jane M. Hawks
M. L. Hedges
Mary Heintzelman
Doris Hepp
Carol Heppner
Mrs. John Herrle
Mary Hideck
Bonnie Hinkle
Betty Hnat
Ethel H. Hollinger
Jane C. Hosey
Beverly Howarth
Kit Ikeler
Mrs. William B. Jackson
Lois Jacob
Shirley James
Blanche Johnson
Mrs. Cecil Jones
Mrs. Joseph M. Joyce
Val Junker
Sue Kadar
Rose Kaiserman
Edna Kane
Natalie Katic
Mrs. H. de S. Kennedy
Elsie Kessler
Bev Ketter
Mrs. John Korinko
Lois Kreiger
Mrs. John Lake
Linda Lang
Marilyn Lanz
Esther Lapiduss
Michael Lench
Mrs. Jack Lentz
Elima Leoni
Mary Lou Letterle
Lucy F. Lochhead
Mrs. Paul Losch
Shirley Losch
Mrs. Margaret V. Lyons
Jeannie Marino
Pearl Marrison
Pauline Master
Erla Maxwell
Cel McCabe
Mary Lou McCurdy
Ted McCurdy
Mrs. H. James McGill
Mrs. Kent McGlincy

Lilly S. McGregor
Mary Lou McLaughlin
Louise Meister
Mrs. Joseph A. Miller
Mrs. Walter H. Miller
Alison Moeller
Jane Molnar
Mrs. Sam Morris
Nila Myers
Mollie B. Nathenson
Gladys Ochsenhirt
Robbie Oppenheim
Mrs. Edward J. O'Rourke, Jr.
Claire Pandl
Diane Paul
Dee Perrotta
Myrtle Petty
Robin Pfeiffer
Leslie Pfiffner
Ann Pieprzny
Helen C. Pirillo
Jean Pleva
Helen Popovich
Mildred Miller Posvar
Douglas Praskach
Mari-Louise Rannow
Mrs. Raymond L. Rau
Roberta Ravasio
Regina Rectanus
Carolyn B. Reuter
Barly Rich
M. Richardson
Mr. Kenneth Roos
Sally Rose
Kate Rost
Mrs. Betty Rubinoff
Jean-Marie Ruebel
Judy Rugani
Marguerite Rush
Mrs. Samuel Ryave
Mona Saba
Doris Scott
Nancy Seagren
Pat Seiden
Anne Seeman
Sam Seeman
Francine Shapera
Gladys Shapera
Carol Shaugnessy
Eleanor B. Shaw
Sandra Shipkoski
Mrs. Seymour Sikov
Mary Jo Sinicrope
Lynn Smail
Frances L. Small
Anita Lynn Smith
Dolores W. Smith
Jean H. Smith
Mrs. Barry B. Sokolow
Mrs. David M. Spehar
Linda Spiker
Lually Stickle
Marge Stoudt
Mrs. Theodore Struk
Betsy Suatmi
Mrs. Francis Sullivan
Carolyn Swanson
Jane E. Swiech
Mrs. Maynard Swift
Madelain N. Tauberg
Betty Tenley
Judi Todd

Mrs. Raymond Tufts
Sophie Vargo
Mrs. Charles Veazey
Dorothy Vogelsinger
Aggie Wager
Flora A. Wager
Mrs. Alfred Waldbaum
Nancy Ward
Mrs. Richard Wardrop
Jeanne H. White
Carol Wieland
J. W. Wilmsfloet
Mrs. John Wilmsfloet
Lillian Wilson
Susan L. Wolf
Mrs. Raphael Wolpert
Kathy Yope
Rita J. Young
Anita Zebrovious
Mrs. H. J. Zubrow

If we have inadvertently omitted your name, please add it here.

____

TABLE OF CONTENTS

EXPOSITION

To insure your satisfaction in cooking with this book, please note the following:

1. Whenever salt is called for, a minimum amount is used.
2. All vegetables are cooked until just crisp-tender to insure the best flavor and to retain the maximum vitamin content.
3. Butter is used throughout, but margarine may be substituted, and the flour called for is all-purpose.
4. You will need more than 8 oz. sour cream or yogurt where 1 cup is called for; 8 oz. measures less than 1 cup.
5. Sour cream, yogurt and cottage cheese will remain fresher longer if stored upside-down in the refrigerator.
6. Wipe fresh mushrooms clean with a damp paper towel; they are miniature sponges that soak up water.
7. Remove the green center from garlic cloves or shallots to avoid a bitter taste.
8. When peeling the rind from citrus fruit, cut only the colored layer that contains the flavor-giving oils
9. Only partially defrost frozen berries when adding to batters; they will not bleed in cooking.
10. When making bread, you will find it easier to knead the dough if you rub a little oil on your hands.
11. 1 Tbsp. fresh herbs equals 1 tsp. dried crumbled herbs; 1 tsp. dried herb leaves equals 1/4 tsp. ground herbs.
12. Rub all dried herbs between palms to release the greatest flavor and aroma.
13. White pepper is milder than black pepper; use twice as much if you substitute.
14. Freezing increases the flavors of black pepper, cloves and garlic; salt and onions become weaker.
15. Most foods freeze well. Do not, however, freeze the following: foods containing hard-boiled egg white, potatoes, rice or mayonnaise. Aspics, gelatin salads and gelatin desserts will not freeze. Rice may be frozen separately.
16. Place a paper towel between hot food and the covering; it will absorb extra moisture.
17. Parsley is used generously as a garnish throughout; keep fresh by washing, spinning dry, wrapping in paper towels and enclosing in a plastic bag.
18. Keep this cookbook clean while using by covering it with an upside-down glass pie plate.

In the beginning . . .

Beverages

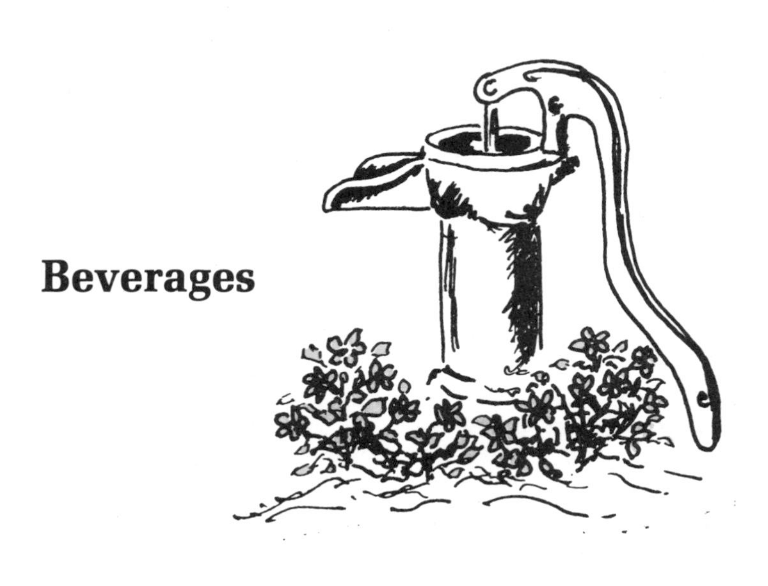

PINEAPPLE CUPS

Serves: 4

2 fresh pineapples
4 oz. Galliano
8 oz. dark rum
8 oz. pineapple juice
2 oz. lime juice
2 oz. sugar syrup
6 ice cubes
1 fifth champagne

Cut stems from pineapples, cut in half crosswise and carefully scoop out pineapple, leaving a 1/2″ intact shell. Shake next 5 ingredients together with ice, fill pineapple cups 1/2 full, then fill remaining part with champagne.

A terrific drink to serve in the summer out on the patio. Straws, either cocktail or regular ones cut in half, are a must.

SANGRITA

Serves: 12

3 qt. V-8 juice
1 Tbsp. dried basil
1 Tbsp. dried marjoram
1 Tbsp. dried thyme
1 qt. orange juice
1 tsp. celery salt
1/2 tsp. pepper
1/4 tsp. Tabasco sauce
Juice of 2 lemons
Parsley sprigs

Steep together overnight V-8 juice and herbs. To serve, strain V-8 juice. Add remaining ingredients, using parsley as garnish.

A surprising combination that is really good. Handsful of fresh herbs may be used.

WHISKEY SOUR PUNCH

Yield: 3 quarts

2 cups bourbon
2 6-oz. cans frozen lemonade, thawed
1 qt. apple juice, chilled
1 qt. ginger ale, chilled
Ice ring

Combine liquid ingredients and pour over ice ring in punch bowl. Garnish, if desired, with orange slices and stemmed maraschino cherries.

Add more bourbon if you prefer a more potent punch.

REVOLVING DOOR

Yield: 2 quarts

1 fifth bourbon
1 24-oz. bottle maple flavored syrup
2 cups lemon juice
Ice ring

Chill ingredients. Pour over ice ring in punch bowl and stir well.

And around and around we go!

RUM FRAPPÉ

Yield: 10 cups

1 6-oz. can frozen Hawaiian punch, thawed
1 6-oz. can frozen limeade, thawed
8 1/2-oz. cream of coconut
1 1/2 cups rum
3/4 cup water
Crushed ice

Combine all ingredients except crushed ice. Place half in blender and fill to within 1″ of top with crushed ice. Cover and blend well. Repeat.

Cool! Easy! Follow with Island-style food. Have a luau!

BRANDY ALEXANDER

Serves: 8

1 qt. French vanilla ice cream
4 oz. brandy
4 oz. Crème de Cacao
3 tsp. vanilla
3/4 cup milk

Fill blender jar with ice cream. Add remaining ingredients. Blend just to mix. Serve immediately with a dusting of nutmeg, if desired.

This is good enough to serve after dinner instead of dessert.

MULLED CIDER

Serves: 16

1 gallon fresh cider
3 apples
18 whole cloves
3 cinnamon sticks

Pour cider into large pan. Stud apples with cloves and add to cider with cinnamon sticks. Heat until piping hot. Serve in mugs.

For an added touch, place a cinnamon stick in each serving.

SPICED TEA

Yield: 2 1/2 cups

1 cup Tang
1/2 cup instant tea
1/2 cup lemonade mix
1 2/3 cups sugar
1 tsp. cinnamon
1/2 tsp. ground cloves

Mix ingredients together. Store in glass jar. To serve, use 2 tsp. stirred into either 1 cup boiling or ice water.

An easy-to-do instant mix that children especially enjoy. Also good as an afternoon pick-up for a tired adult.

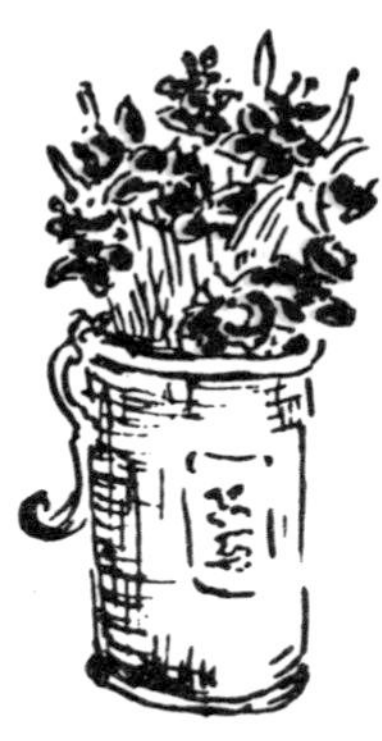

TEA PARTY PUNCH

Yield: 2 1/2 quarts

2 cups orange juice
3 Tbsp. lemon juice
1 cup sugar
1 cup grape juice
1 qt. tea
1 cup dark rum
1 cup ginger ale

Stir all ingredients together, except ginger ale. Chill. At serving time, pour over ice block in punch bowl and stir in chilled ginger ale.

Tastes really great with watercress sandwiches and petit fours.

APRICOT NECTAR PUNCH

Serves: 8-10

1 6-oz. can frozen pineapple-orange juice
1 1/2 cups water
3 cups apricot nectar
1 qt. bottle lemon-lime carbonated beverage

Combine all ingredients in large pitcher. Pour into tall glasses filled with ice.

An easy to prepare refreshing non-alcoholic beverage.

HOT MULLED WINE

Serves: 4-6

1 fifth burgundy
6 oz. sugar cubes
Grated rind of 1/2 lemon
Grated rind of 1/2 lime
2 whole cloves
1/2 cinnamon stick
1/8 tsp. mace
6 Tbsp. butter
4 Tbsp. brown sugar
1/2 cup brandy

In saucepan, pour burgundy over sugar cubes. Add next 5 ingredients. Stir together. Place over low heat until hot. Strain into goblets. Cream together butter and brown sugar. Spoon dollop into each goblet. Pour brandy equally over each serving.

This will warm the cockles of your heart. Perfect for after skiing and a grand holiday drink.

HOT SPICED CRANBERRY PUNCH

Yield: 3 3/4 quarts

4 6-oz. cans frozen lemonade
2 qt. cranberry juice cocktail
1/2 tsp. salt
1/2 tsp. cinnamon
1 tsp. allspice
1 qt. water

Combine all ingredients in large pan. Simmer uncovered 10-15 minutes. Do not boil. Serve hot.

The children will appreciate this after ice skating or sled riding.

MARGARITAS **Serves: 4**

1 wedge fresh lime
Coarse salt
1 6-oz. can frozen limeade, thawed
6 oz. tequila
6 oz. crushed ice

Rub outside edge of 4 wide rimmed glasses with cut lime. Dip in coarse salt. Set aside. Into blender, pour limeade, tequila and crushed ice. Blend 30-45 seconds. Pour into prepared glasses.

You will not find a better Margarita outside of Mexico.

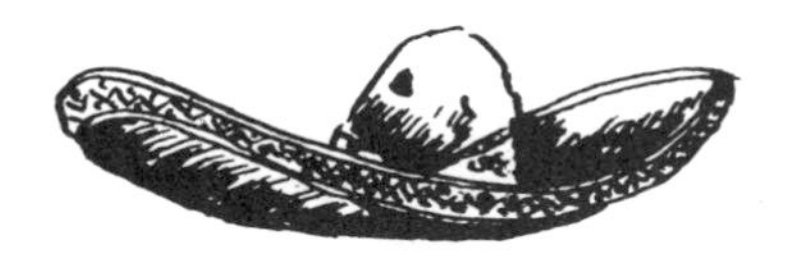

FROZEN STRAWBERRY DAIQUIRI **Yield: 3 cups**

1/2 10-oz. package frozen strawberries
1 6-oz. can frozen limeade, thawed
6 oz. light rum
6 oz. crushed ice

Partially defrost strawberries. Pour 1/2 package into blender with other ingredients and blend well.

On the sweet side, this drink tastes as good as it looks and can easily be doubled.

LEMON QUENCHER **Serves: 12-16**

2 6-oz. cans frozen pink lemonade, thawed
1 30-oz. can pineapple-pink grapefruit juice
1.5 liter rosé wine
1/3 cup brandy
2 cups ice cubes

Combine all ingredients and shake or stir together. May be topped with slices of fresh lemon and strawberries.

This is a most refreshing drink to place in a thermos and carry on a picnic.

ROSÉ SPARKLE

Serves: 24

4 10 1/2-oz. pkg. frozen strawberries, thawed
1 cup sugar
4 25 1/2-oz. bottles rosé wine
4 6-oz. cans frozen lemonade
Ice ring
2 qt. club soda

Combine strawberries, sugar and 1 bottle wine. Let stand 1 hour. Strain. To strained liquid add remaining wine and lemonade. Pour into punch bowl over ice ring. Add club soda just before serving.

This punch is delicious, and the marinated strawberries are a treat over ice cream.

VELVET PUNCH

Yield: 6 quarts

2 qt. cranberry juice cocktail
1 16-oz. can frozen orange juice, thawed
1 16-oz. can frozen pineapple juice, thawed
2 cups lemon juice
2 cups brandy
2 fifths champagne, chilled
Ice ring

Combine ingredients and serve over ice ring from punch bowl.

Two qt. ginger ale may be substituted for champagne and 2 cups grape juice for brandy.

PINK PANTHER PUNCH

Serves: 20

1 10 1/2-oz. jar maraschino cherries
1 qt. cranberry juice cocktail
1 46-oz. can pineapple-grapefruit juice
2 1-qt. bottles Cotts Half and Half
1 qt. raspberry sherbet

Pour cherries and juice into a ring mold. Fill with water and freeze. To serve, combine all ingredients and pour into punch bowl over ice ring.

A colorful summer drink that all ages will enjoy. And it is the perfect punch for a child's birthday party.

REALLY FROZEN DAIQUIRI **Yield: 2 1/2 quarts**

1 6-oz. can frozen lemonade
1 6-oz. can frozen limeade
1 fifth light rum
3 cups water
16 oz. 7-Up

Defrost lemonade and limeade. Combine with other ingredients and freeze. May be served as is or mixed in a blender.

Pour into a wide-mouth jar so that servings may be spooned out as needed.

GASPARILLA EGG NOG **Yield: 3 quarts**

6 eggs, separated
1 1/4 cups sugar
3/4 cup whiskey or bourbon
1/3 cup white rum
4 cups milk
2 cups whipping cream

A day ahead, beat egg yolks until creamy. Add 1/2 cup sugar. Beat until sugar dissolves. Add liquors. Stir well. Stir in milk. Refrigerate overnight. Just before serving beat egg whites until foamy. Add 1/2 cup sugar gradually, beating until stiff. Whip cream and stir in 1/4 cup sugar. Thoroughly fold egg whites into yolk mixture. Fold in whipped cream.

Serve from a large punch bowl with a sprinkle of nutmeg in each punch cup.

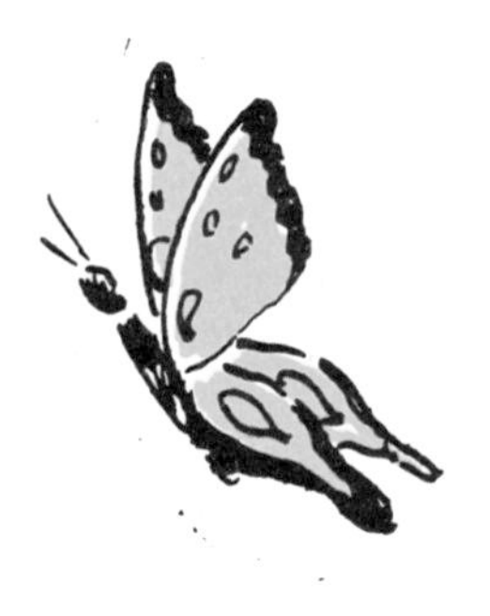

BRANDIED COFFEE VELVET **Serves: 6**

2 Tbsp. instant coffee
1/4 cup warm water
1/4 cup chocolate syrup
1/2 cup brandy
1 qt. vanilla ice cream
Whipped cream

Dissolve coffee in warm water. Add chocolate syrup, brandy and ice cream. Beat until smooth. Chill. Pour into frosted glasses. Garnish with whipped cream.

Smooth, rich and elegant!

PINEAPPLE COOLER **Serves: 6**

1 cup unsweetened pineapple juice
1 cup unsweetened pineapple chunks
4 Tbsp. plain yogurt
1 Tbsp. honey
1/8 tsp. nutmeg
1 cup ice cubes
Fresh mint sprigs

Place all but ice and mint in blender. Blend 30 seconds or until smooth. Continue blending as you drop in ice cubes. When ice is finely crushed, pour into chilled glasses. Top with mint.

A refreshing drink that will please any age. To double, just repeat.

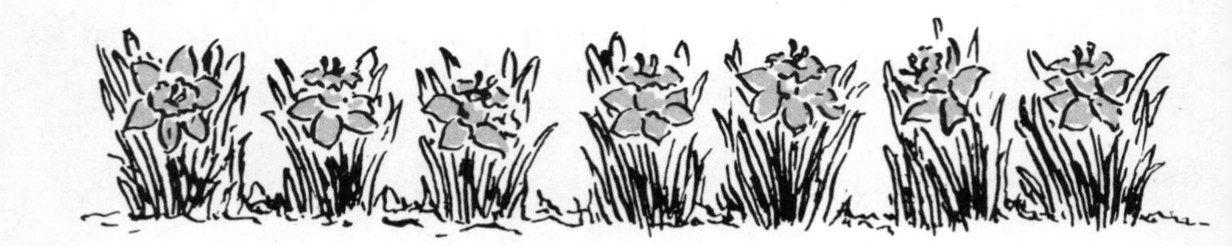

Appetizers

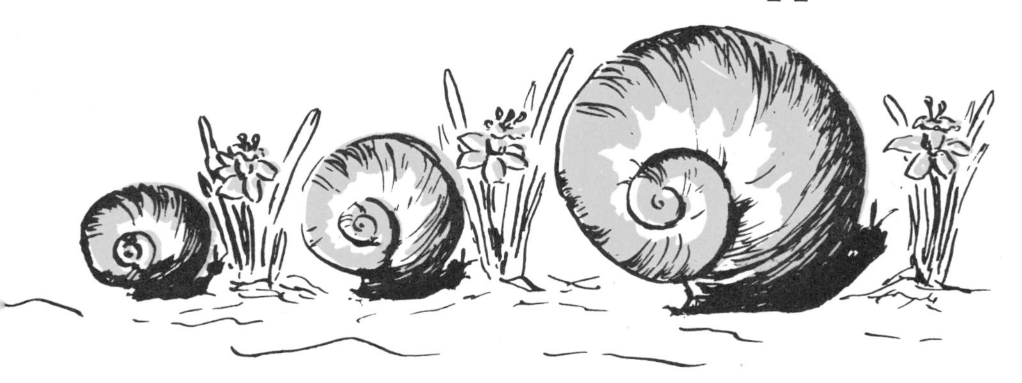

ESCALLOPED OYSTERS

Serves: 6-8

2 cups Ritz cracker crumbs
1 stick butter, melted
1/4 tsp. salt
1/8 tsp. pepper
1 pt. oysters
2 Tbsp. oyster liquor
2 Tbsp. cream
2 Tbsp. butter

Combine first 4 ingredients and spread 1/2 in 9″ pie plate. Cover with drained oysters. Combine liquor and milk and pour over oysters. Top with remaining crumbs. Dot with butter. Bake at 375° for 20-25 minutes.

Serve with forks on small dishes. To double, use 2 pints oysters and 1 1/2 times crumb mixture.

BLEU CHEESE MOUSSE

Serves: 12

4 egg yolks
2 Tbsp. water
1 envelope unflavored gelatin
2 Tbsp. water
1/2 lb. Bleu cheese, softened
1 cup whipping cream, whipped
4 egg whites, stiffly beaten
Parsley sprigs

Place egg yolks and 2 Tbsp. water in top of double boiler over hot, not boiling, water. Beat until mixture thickens and resembles cream sauce. Soften gelatin in 2 Tbsp. cold water, place over hot water and stir to dissolve. Add to egg yolks. Mash cheese or force through sieve. Add to yolk mixture. Beat until smooth. Cool. Fold in whipped cream and beaten egg whites. Pour into lightly oiled 6-cup mold. Chill until firm. Unmold and garnish with parsley.

Crisp toast rounds are a good cracker to serve with this delicate mousse.

MUSHROOM TARTS

Yield: 2 1/2 dozen

4 oz. cream cheese
4 Tbsp. unsalted butter
1 cup flour
1/2 tsp. salt
1/2 lb. fresh mushrooms, finely chopped
1/2 cup minced onion
4 Tbsp. butter
2 Tbsp. flour
2 Tbsp. cream
1 egg yolk
1/4 cup minced fresh parsley
1/4 cup grated Parmesan cheese
1/2 tsp. salt
1/2 tsp. white pepper

For pastry mix together well first 4 ingredients. Roll 1/4″ thick and cut in 2 3/4″ circles. Line 2 1/2″ muffin cups with pastry. For filling, sauté mushrooms and onion in butter until tender. Sprinkle with flour and stir in. Add remaining ingredients, stir well. Place filling in prepared muffin pans. Bake at 450° for 10 minutes. Reduce heat to 325° and bake 5 minutes more or until crust is golden.

There are two delicious bites to every tart. These can be made ahead and frozen.

CURRIED TUNA APPETIZERS

Yield: 40 pieces

Puffs:
1/2 cup water
4 Tbsp. butter
1/4 tsp. salt
1/2 cup flour
2 eggs

Filling:
1 6 1/2-oz. can tuna
1/2 cup mayonnaise
1/4 cup minced celery
2 hard-boiled eggs, chopped
1 Tbsp. curry powder
1/2 tsp. salt
Parsley sprigs

For Puffs: place water, butter and salt in 2-qt. saucepan over high heat until butter melts and mixture boils. Remove from heat. With wooden spoon, vigorously stir in flour until mixture forms ball and leaves side of pan. Beat in eggs until thoroughly blended. On greased cookie sheet, place heaping teaspoon dough 1″ apart to form 20 mounds. Bake at 375° for 20-25 minutes or until lightly browned. Cool on racks. To fill, cut each shell in half. Spoon 1 rounded teaspoon filling into each shell. Garnish with parsley. For Filling: stir undrained tuna with fork until finely flaked. Stir in next 5 ingredients and blend well. Cover and refrigerate.

Puffs may be made up to 1 month ahead and frozen. Bring to room temperature before cutting and filling.

LULU PASTE **Serves: 12**

2 eggs
4 Tbsp. sugar
2 Tbsp. butter
3 Tbsp. vinegar
11 oz. cream cheese, softened
1 4-oz. jar pimento, chopped
1 medium onion, chopped
1 green pepper, chopped

Beat together first 4 ingredients in top of double boiler. Cook, stirring, until thick. Add cream cheese and stir until melted. Remove from heat. Stir in remaining ingredients. Chill.

This is an old but still delicious recipe. Spread on crackers or use as dip for vegetables.

MUSHROOM-GARLIC ROUNDS **Yield: 2 dozen**

6 slices white or whole wheat bread
2 Tbsp. butter, melted
10 medium mushrooms, very finely chopped
1 Tbsp. butter
1/2 tsp. garlic salt
2 Tbsp. cut up pimento, drained

Cut each bread slice into 4 1 1/2″ circles. Brush 1 side of bread circles with 2 Tbsp. melted butter. Place butter side down on ungreased baking sheet. Bake at 400° until bottoms are light brown, about 5 minutes. Set aside. Cook and stir mushrooms in 1 Tbsp. butter over medium-high heat until mushroom pieces are brown, dry and separate, about 5 minutes. Stir in garlic salt. Spread about 1/2 tsp. mushroom mixture on unbuttered side of each bread circle. Cover and refrigerate up to 24 hours. Garnish each round with small piece of pimento. Bake at 350° for about 4 minutes.

One 8-oz. can mushroom stems and pieces, drained and finely chopped, can be substituted for fresh mushrooms.

SAUERKRAUT BALLS **Yield: 5 dozen**

1 lb. hot sausage
1 28-oz. can sauerkraut
1 cup Italian seasoned bread crumbs
2 eggs, lightly beaten
1 Tbsp. brown sugar

Crumble and sauté sausage over medium-high heat until done. Drain. Drain, squeeze dry, and snip sauerkraut. Mix all ingredients together and let stand 5 minutes. Roll into 3/4″ balls and place on cookie sheet. Bake at 350° for 3-5 minutes or until lightly browned.

These may be frozen before cooking. Increase cooking time to 10 minutes.

REUBEN ROLL-UPS

Serves: 8

1 8-oz. can crescent rolls
1 8-oz. can sauerkraut
1 Tbsp. Thousand Island dressing
8 1/2-oz. slices cooked corned beef or dried beef
2 slices Swiss cheese cut in 1/2″ strips

Unroll crescent dough and separate into 8 triangles. Drain sauerkraut thoroughly and snip or chop coarsely. Stir dressing into sauerkraut. To assemble, place one slice corned beef across wide end of dough triangle, spread with 2 Tbsp. sauerkraut, and top with 2 strips cheese. Roll up from wide end. Bake on ungreased sheet at 375° for 10-15 minutes until golden brown.

Neat to eat. When finger food only is being served, include this.

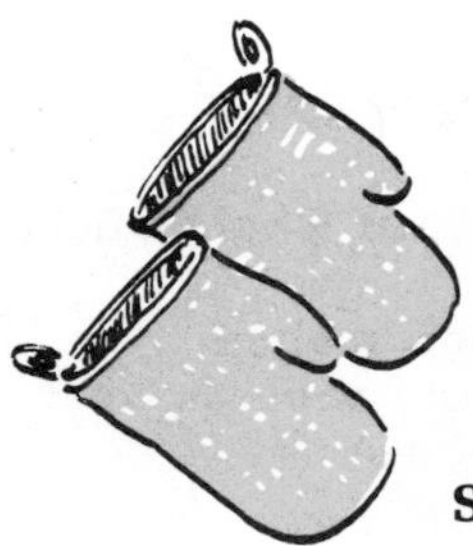

BAKED BRIE

Serves: 10-12

1 10-oz. pkg. frozen patty shells
3 4 1/2-oz. cans Brie
1 egg, beaten
1 Tbsp. water

Bring shells to room temperature. Roll each shell on lightly floured board into circle slightly larger than cheese. Place 3 pieces Brie on 3 circles. Combine egg and water. Brush edges of shells with egg mixture. Top with remaining circles, seal edges with fork and brush tops with egg mixture. Bake at 375° for 25-30 minutes. Let stand a few minutes before cutting into wedges.

These are delicious hot and equally good when cold.

CARAMELIZED BACON

Serves: 6

1/2 lb. regularly sliced bacon
1/2 cup firmly packed dark brown sugar

Cut bacon slices in half. Rub brown sugar into each piece. Place on rack in shallow pan. Bake at 250° for 50-60 minutes. May be made ahead. Do not refrigerate.

Guests will always ask how these were made and marvel at the ease.

OYSTER CHEESE ROLL

Serves: 6-8

1/2 clove garlic
1 8-oz. pkg. cream cheese, softened
1/4 tsp. salt
2 gratings fresh pepper
1 tsp. lemon juice
1 tsp. Worcestershire sauce
1 3 1/2-oz. can smoked oysters
1/4 cup chopped fresh parsley

Rub small bowl with garlic. Discard. In bowl beat together next 5 ingredients. Spread into 9″x7″ rectangle on cookie sheet. Drain oysters well, pat dry between paper towels and cut in small pieces. Sprinkle oysters over cream cheese. Press in lightly. Cover with wax paper and chill. From long side roll up firmly in jelly roll fashion. Sprinkle with parsley. Serve with crackers.

Easily doubled. Cheese mixture will almost cover cookie sheet.

SPINACH PIE

Serves: 8-12

3 eggs, beaten
1 cup sour cream
1/4 tsp. garlic powder
1/2 tsp. dill weed
1/2 tsp. salt
1/4 tsp. pepper
1/4 tsp. onion powder
1 10-oz. pkg. frozen chopped spinach, thawed and drained
8 oz. Cheddar cheese, grated
1 3-oz. can onion rings

Mix together all ingredients. Pour into buttered shallow 11″x7″ pan. Bake at 350° for 45 minutes or until golden brown. Cut into small squares.

Make ahead, refrigerate, cut and reheat. Or cut in larger squares and serve as a side dish for dinner.

SEAFOOD CHEESE SPREAD

Serves: 16

1 lb. Old English sharp cheese, grated
2 sticks butter, softened
2 tsp. Worcestershire sauce
1/4 tsp. salt
2 Tbsp. onion juice
1 1/2 - 2 cups lobster, crab, or shrimp

Mix first five ingredients well. Fold in seafood. Spread on toasted bread round or party rye. Broil until bubbly.

This recipe is equally good on a hamburger or hot dog roll, amply spread, broiled and served as a luncheon item with fruit or salad.

BROCCOLI BEIGNETS

Serves: 12

1/2 bunch fresh broccoli
1 stick butter
1 cup water
1 tsp. salt
1/8 tsp. garlic powder
1 cup sifted flour
4 eggs
Oil for deep frying
1/2 cup grated Parmesan cheese

Prepare broccoli and cut into small pieces to make 2 cups. Cook until tender, mash and set aside. Heat together next 4 ingredients until water boils and butter melts. Stir in flour, remove from heat, stir until dough pulls away from pan. Beat in eggs 1 at a time. Stir in broccoli. Chill 2 hours or overnight. Deep fry at 375° in 3″ oil by dropping batter in from heaping teaspoon. Do not crowd. Fry until puffed and golden, 3-4 minutes, turning once. Drain. Sprinkle with cheese. Serve warm.

These may be prepared ahead. Reheat on a cookie sheet at 350° for 10 minutes.

BACON CRISPS

Serves: 6-8

8 slices bacon
1/2 cup flour
1 egg, beaten
1/2 cup seasoned bread crumbs

Separate bacon slices and cut in half crosswise. Flour both sides of each piece, dip in beaten egg, and sprinkle with bread crumbs. Place on cookie sheet. Bake at 400° for 7-10 minutes on each side, watching carefully to prevent burning. Remove and place on paper towels.

Bacon thickly sliced will need the full cooking time.

CRISP BACON CRACKERS

Serves: 8

4 Tbsp. Parmesan cheese
24 oblong crackers
12 bacon slices, cut in half

Place 1/2 tsp. Parmesan cheese evenly on each cracker. Wrap lengthwise in 1/2 bacon slice, tucking in ends. Place on rack in shallow pan. Bake at 400° for 15-20 minutes or until bacon is cooked. Cool slightly before serving to allow the cracker to become crisp again.

These will disappear quickly and can be made in large amounts to serve a crowd.

CRABMEAT SPREAD

Yield: 2 cups

8-oz. fresh crabmeat or 6 1/2-oz. can crabmeat
1 tsp. grated onion
1 hard-boiled egg, chopped fine
1 Tbsp. lemon juice
1/2 cup mayonnaise
1/2 cup grated sharp Cheddar cheese
Parsley for garnish

Pick over crabmeat and remove shell, then carefully mix with remaining ingredients. Garnish with parsley and serve with assorted crackers.

This is rich, elegant and very easy.

MUSHROOM ARTICHOKE APPETIZER

Serves: 6-8

1 lb. small whole mushrooms
1 8-oz. can artichoke hearts, quartered
1 6-oz. can pitted black olives
1 large clove garlic, minced
1 small onion, grated
2 Tbsp. finely chopped fresh parsley
1/2 tsp. dried basil leaves
1/2 tsp. dried oregano
1/4 tsp. freshly ground pepper
2/3 cup light olive oil
6 Tbsp. red wine vinegar
8 cherry tomatoes

Wipe mushrooms clean with damp paper towel and trim stems. Drain artichokes and olives and place with mushrooms in large bowl. Shake together well next 8 ingredients and pour into bowl. Marinate several hours, stirring frequently. Before serving add cherry tomatoes.

Easy to make. Serve on small trays with hors d'oeuvres forks.

SHRIMP AND CHUTNEY DIP

Serves: 6-8

1 8-oz. pkg. cream cheese, softened
1 Tbsp. curry powder
1/4 tsp. garlic powder
1/4 cup Major Grey chutney, cut up
1 cup chopped cooked shrimp
1/2 cup sour cream
1/4 tsp. salt

Beat together first 4 ingredients. Fold in shrimp, sour cream and salt. Do not mash shrimp.

Serve as a spread with plain rice crackers or as a dip for fresh vegetables. Include baby green onions and snow peas.

EASY BACON WATER CHESTNUTS

Serves: 15

1 lb. lean bacon, cut in thirds
3 8-oz. cans whole water chestnuts
1 cup sugar
1 cup catsup

Roll chestnuts in cut bacon strips and secure with pick. Place on rack in 9″x13″ baking pan. Bake at 325° for 1 hour. Remove picks and place in a shallow 9″x13″ dish. Combine sugar and catsup. Pour over bacon and water chestnuts. Bake at 325° for 1 more hour. Serve warm with fresh picks.

After baking the first hour, you may refrigerate and complete them nearer serving time.

ANCHOVY CHEESE SPREAD

Serves: 8-10

1 2-oz. can flat anchovies
1 8-oz. pkg. cream cheese, softened
1 stick unsalted butter, softened

Mash anchovies and put all ingredients in blender. Blend until well mixed. Serve with pumpernickel bread.

Easy, inexpensive and quite flavorful.

GOURMET SHRIMP SAUCE

Yield: 2 cups

2 green onions with tops
2 Tbsp. prepared horseradish
6 Tbsp. finely chopped fresh green or red peppers
2 Tbsp. finely chopped capers
1 cup mayonnaise
1/2 cup chili sauce
1/2 tsp. freshly ground pepper
1/2 tsp. crushed red pepper
1/2 tsp. salt
1 clove garlic, mashed
2 lb. shrimp, cleaned, cooked and chilled

Slice onions and tops into small pieces. Drain horseradish in strainer for 5 minutes to remove excess liquid. Mix onions, peppers, capers and garlic. Set aside. Mix mayonnaise and chili sauce thoroughly. Add red and black pepper and whip together with a whisk. Add all ingredients except shrimp and mix well. Taste for salt. Refrigerate at least 1 hour. Serve with shrimp.

This sauce is elegant served over crabmeat or bites of lobster.

GOUDA CHEESE ROLLS

Serves: 10-12

1 8-oz. can crescent rolls
1 7-oz. ball Gouda cheese

Divide package of crescent rolls in half. Unroll and pat each half together to form 2 squares. Cut cheese in half horizontally to form two thin circles. Place each cheese circle on a square. Fold up edges and wrap tightly. Place wrapped side down on ungreased cookie sheet. Bake at 375° for 10-12 minutes or until golden. Let stand a few minutes before cutting into wedges.

The wrap tightly part is important or cheese will melt out of crust.

CHEESE CIDER COCKTAIL SPREAD

Serves: 12

1 8-oz. pkg. cream cheese
1/2 cup apple cider
1/2 lb. Swiss cheese, shredded
1/2 lb. Cheddar cheese, shredded
1 stick butter, melted
Paprika
Parsley sprigs

Soften cream cheese, beat until smooth. Add next 4 ingredients and beat until fluffy. Pack into 3 buttered coffee cups, mounding tops. Chill overnight. To serve, turn cheese out of cups keeping mounded side up. Press and cut cheese into apple shapes. Press stems from real apples into each. Dust each all over with paprika. Place on serving tray. Garnish with parsley.

Use 3-cup mold for 1 large apple, if desired. Flavors improve if made 2-3 days ahead.

FROSTED LIVER PATÉ

Serves: 10-12

1 lb. liverwurst
1 clove garlic, minced
1/2 tsp. basil
3 Tbsp. minced onion
1 8-oz. pkg. cream cheese, softened
1/2 clove garlic, minced
1/3 tsp. Tabasco sauce
1 tsp. mayonnaise
1/4 cup chopped fresh parsley

Mix together liverwurst, 1 clove garlic, basil and onion. Form into ball and chill. Beat together remaining ingredients. Spread on outside of liverwurst ball to cover completely. Sprinkle with chopped parsley. Chill until serving time. Serve with crisp crackers.

Use 1/2 cup chopped nuts instead of parsley for a different texture.

CEVICHE

Serves: 12

2 lb. fillet of sole
1 cup lime juice
1 1-lb. can tomatoes
1 large onion, chopped
1/2 cup catsup
1/2 cup olive oil
2 tsp. salt
1/2 cup minced fresh parsley
1 tsp. oregano, crumbled
1 tsp. bottled red pepper seasoning

If using frozen fish, defrost and press out excess water. Cut boneless fish into little cubes, smaller than 1/2″ square. Place in deep glass bowl and pour lime juice over fish. There should be enough to cover fish. Cover bowl and chill overnight. Drain fish, rinse under cold water and place back in large bowl. Break up tomatoes and add with juice and remaining ingredients to fish. Stir lightly to mix. Chill.

At serving time, spoon into sherbet glasses.

MEXICAN BEAN DIP

Serves: 12

1 1-lb. can refried beans
1 3-oz. can chopped green chilies
1 onion, chopped
1 8-oz. jar mild taco sauce
3 cups grated Monterey Jack cheese
1 recipe Guacamole
1/2 cup sour cream
1 bag tortilla chips

Spread beans in 8″x11″ shallow baking dish. Sprinkle with green chilies and onion and cover with taco sauce. Top with grated cheese. Bake at 350° for 20 minutes. To serve, make a well in center of beans, fill with guacamole. Make a well in guacamole and fill with sour cream. Stand tortilla chips "fence fashion" around this mound. Serve with remaining chips.

Though it can be tricky, the best eating is a chip dipped in the beans and topped with guacamole and sour cream.

GUACAMOLE

Makes: 1 1/2 cups

2 ripe avocados
1/4 cup mayonnaise
3 Tbsp. lemon juice
1 tsp. chili powder
1/4 tsp. Tabasco sauce
1/4 tsp. salt

Mash avocados with fork and stir in remaining ingredients. Chill before serving to blend flavors.

Have napkins handy. The guacamole may be served as a dip itself.

PIZZA APPETIZERS

Yield: 9 dozen

1 lb. mild sweet Italian sausage
1 lb. hot Italian sausage
1 medium onion, grated
2 lb. Velveeta cheese
1 Tbsp. Italian seasoning
3 loaves cocktail rye bread

Fry sausage and onion until done. Drain off fat. Cut cheese in chunks and add with Italian seasoning to sausage. Stir constantly over low heat until cheese melts. Spread on bread slices and place on cookie sheet. Freeze. Put in plastic bags in freezer until ready to serve. Bake from frozen state at 400° for 10 minutes.

Great with beer. Serve to the fans watching televised football games.

CAULIFLOWER FRITTERS

Serves: 12

1 head cauliflower
2 eggs
1 cup milk
3/4 cup flour
1/4 tsp. salt
1/8 tsp. pepper
1/8 tsp. garlic powder

Steam cauliflower until just crisp-tender. Cool, cut into flowerets and discard core. In blender mix remaining ingredients and let stand 1/2 hour. Dip flowerets in batter, deep fry in oil over medium-high heat until golden. Remove, drain on paper towels and serve immediately. Cauliflower may be cooked and batter prepared a day ahead.

The dip using 1 cup mayonnaise and 2 Tbsp. honey is delicious with this.

HAM LOAF SPREAD

Serves: 12

1 8-oz. pkg. cream cheese, softened
2 Tbsp. mayonnaise
4 Tbsp. sweet relish
1 Tbsp. prepared mustard
1 Tbsp. grated onion
1/4 tsp. white vinegar
1 lb. ground smoked ham
Chopped fresh parsley

Mix together well first 6 ingredients. Stir in ground ham. Shape into ball and chill. To serve cover with chopped parsley.

Slices of party rye or pumpernickel bread are a good accompaniment, or use the spread to fill celery stalks.

SALMON MOUSSE

Serves: 12

2 envelopes unflavored gelatin
1/2 cup cold water
1 cup boiling water
3/4 cup mayonnaise
2 1-lb. cans salmon, drained
1 tsp. lemon juice
1 Tbsp. grated onion
1 Tbsp. Worcestershire sauce
1 tsp. salt
1/4 tsp. pepper
8 oz. sour cream
Fresh parsley sprigs

Cucumber Sauce:
1 cucumber, peeled, grated and drained
1 cup sour cream
1 tsp. dill weed
1 tsp. capers, drained
1 tsp. prepared mustard
1 Tbsp. lemon juice
1 tsp. grated onion
1/2 tsp. salt

Soak gelatin in cold water until dissolved. Add boiling water, stir and let cool until thickened. Beat mayonnaise into gelatin mixture until frothy. Break up salmon and remove any skin and bones. Add to gelatin mixture with next 5 ingredients. Fold in sour cream. Pour into lightly oiled mold and chill until firm. Unmold onto platter, garnish with sprigs of parsley and serve with cucumber sauce in separate bowl. For Sauce: combine all ingredients and chill. Makes 1 3/4 cups.

The sauce is good as a dressing for tomato aspic.

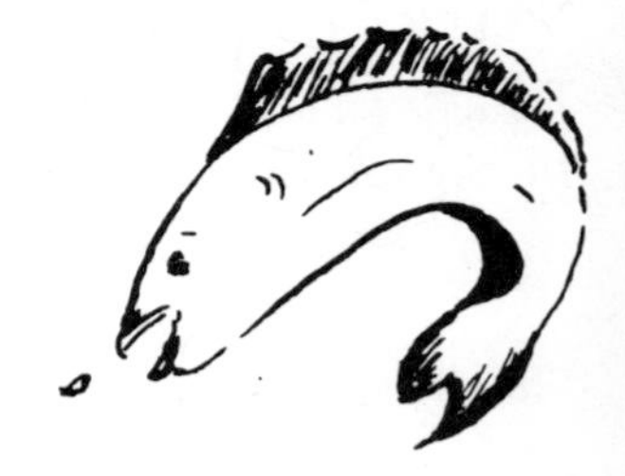

HOT SAUSAGE HORS D'OEUVRES

Yield: 8 dozen

1 lb. bulk sausage
1 lb. sharp Cheddar cheese, shredded
3 cups biscuit mix
3/4 cup water

Cook sausage 8-10 minutes. Drain and cool. In large bowl combine all ingredients with fork until just blended. Roll into 1″ balls. Place 2″ apart on baking pan. Bake at 400° for 10-12 minutes until golden brown. Serve hot.

These freeze well. Defrost and heat for only 5 minutes.

FRENCH APPETIZER TART

Serves: 10

Savory Butter Crust:
1 cup flour
1 tsp. grated lemon peel
1/2 cup cold butter
1 egg yolk

Filling:
6 oz. cream cheese, softened
4 Tbsp. sour cream
3/4 tsp. salt
1/4 tsp. white pepper
3 drops Tabasco sauce
2 Tbsp. chopped shallots or
1 Tbsp. grated onion
1 Tbsp. chopped fresh parsley
2-3 oz. sliced smoked salmon
3 hard-boiled eggs
2 green onions, sliced

For Crust: combine flour, lemon peel and butter with pastry blender or fingers until crumbly. Add egg yolk and mix until dough forms a ball. Pat dough on bottom and sides of 11" fluted pan with removable bottom. Bake at 425° for 8-10 minutes. For Filling: beat together cream cheese, sour cream, salt, pepper, Tabasco, shallots or onions and parsley. Spread over baked and cooled crust. Cut salmon in strips and place evenly around outer ring of tart. Finely chop egg yolks and whites separately. Make a ring of egg white just inside salmon. Arrange sliced onions in ring next to egg whites. Fill center with egg yolks. Cover and chill until serving time.

This will serve 6 as a beautiful luncheon dish. Consider chopped ripe olives, caviar, canned baby shrimp or crabmeat as topping variations.

CHICKEN WINGS PARMESAN

Serves: 12

2 lbs. chicken wings
1 cup grated Parmesan cheese
3 Tbsp. chopped fresh parsley
2 tsp. paprika
1 Tbsp. oregano
1 tsp. salt
1/2 tsp. pepper
1 stick butter, melted

Disjoint chicken wings and save tips for stock. Mix together next 6 ingredients. Dip chicken pieces in butter and roll in cheese mixture. Place on cookie sheet with rim. Bake uncovered at 300° for 1 1/4 hour.

Use small breast halves, legs and thighs for an entrée or picnic treat.

COGNAC BLEU CHEESE SPREAD

Serves: 6

1 stick butter
4 oz. Bleu cheese
1 3-oz. pkg. cream cheese
2 Tbsp. cognac

Bring first 3 ingredients to room temperature. Then blend all ingredients together. Chill overnight.

An original recipe recreated from memories of the past.

CALIFORNIA WINE AND CHEESE SPREAD

Serves: 10

1/2 lb. sharp Cheddar cheese
1 8-oz. pkg. cream cheese, softened
6 Tbsp. rosé wine
1/2 cup almonds, finely chopped
1 1/2 tsp. powdered ginger
1/8 tsp. salt
1/8 tsp. Cayenne pepper
4 fresh pears

Put cheese through ricer or shred on fine grater. Mix well with next 6 ingredients. Serve mounded on plate surrounded with wedges of pear.

Though pears are suggested and the flavor combination is just right, other fruits may be used.

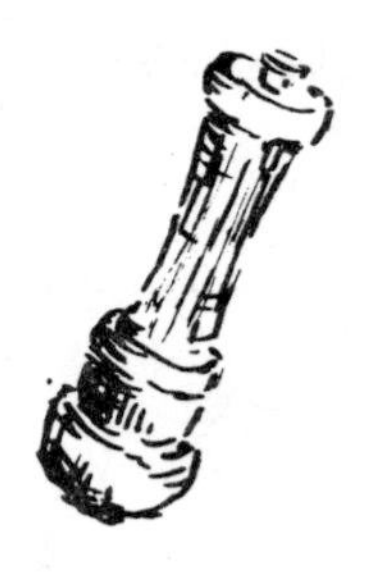

CHICKEN LIVER PATÉ I

Serves: 16-20

Sliced bacon
1/2 medium onion, cut in chunks
1 small clove garlic
1/4 tsp. ground ginger
1/3 cup diced bacon
1 1/2 tsp. salt
1/2 tsp. white pepper
1/2 tsp. ground allspice
1 lb. chicken livers, rinsed and patted dry
1 egg plus 1 egg white
3/4 cup cream
2 Tbsp. brandy
1/4 cup flour
4 medium bay leaves

Line 4″x8″ or 5″x9″ loaf pan with bacon strips. Set aside. With steel blade in processor bowl, place in next 7 ingredients. Process until very finely chopped. Add chicken livers and turn "on-off" a few times. Add next 4 ingredients and process until blended. Pour into prepared pan. Lay bay leaves on mixture. Cover with wax paper and double layer of foil and press tightly around lip of pan. Place loaf pan into larger pan and pour boiling water into outer pan. Bake at 325° for 1 3/4 hours. Cool on rack, remove bay leaves and turn out of pan onto serving plate and chill.

Serve with slices of small French bread, diced onion, sweet pickle and Poupon mustard. Do not freeze.

CHICKEN LIVER PATÉ II

Serves: 12-16

1 lb. chicken livers
1 stick butter
1/4 lb. mushrooms, chopped
1/4 cup chopped fresh parsley
1/4 cup chopped shallots or green onions
1/2 tsp. salt
1/2 tsp. dried thyme leaves
2 Tbsp. brandy
1/2 cup dry red wine
2 sticks butter

Cut chicken livers in half. Melt 1 stick butter, add livers and next 5 ingredients. Cook over medium heat until livers are firm but slightly pink in center. Warm brandy, set aflame, pour over livers and shake pan until flames die. Add wine and heat to simmer. Let mixture cool to room temperature. Put in blender or food processor, blend until smooth. Add 2 sticks butter, a chunk at a time. Blend until smooth. Mixture will resemble thick mayonnaise. Pour into foil lined rectangular quart pan. Chill covered overnight. Unmold and serve with crusty bread or toast.

This is best made 3 or 4 days ahead and will keep 1 week.

MUSHROOM CHEESE TOAST

Serves: 6-8

1 1/2 cups sharp cheese, grated
3/4 cup mayonnaise
1 cup chopped mushroom caps
1/2 cup chopped green onion with tops
Slices of party rye or white bread, toasted on one side

Combine first 4 ingredients. Spread on untoasted side of bread. Place on cookie sheet and broil until cheese melts and is golden.

Can be assembled ahead of time and refrigerated.

CHICKEN HORS D'OEUVRES

Serves: 12

3 whole chicken breasts
1/2 cup mayonnaise
1 tsp. dry mustard
1 tsp. grated onion
1/2 cup dry bread crumbs
2 Tbsp. sesame seeds
1 cup mayonnaise
2 Tbsp. honey

Poach chicken breasts until tender. When cool, skin, debone and cut in chunks. Mix together next 3 ingredients. Dip chicken pieces in mixture and roll in combined crumbs and sesame seeds. Place on cookie sheet. Bake at 425° for 10-12 minutes. Combine mayonnaise and honey. Use as dip for hot chicken served with toothpicks.

May be prepared ahead. Really delicious.

SWEET 'N SOUR MEATBALLS

Yield: 5 dozen

3/4 lb. ground round steak
1/4 lb. ground pork
3/4 cup rolled oats
1/2 cup milk
8 oz. finely chopped water chestnuts
1 tsp. Worcestershire sauce
1/2 tsp. onion salt
1/2 tsp. garlic salt
1/4 tsp. celery salt
Dash Tabasco sauce
1 bottle LaChoy Sweet'N Sour Sauce

Mix together well first 10 ingredients. Form small meatballs and place on cookie sheet. Bake at 400° for 10-12 minutes or until brown. Serve with LaChoy sauce.

You may make these ahead and freeze. Put in top of double boiler to thaw and heat.

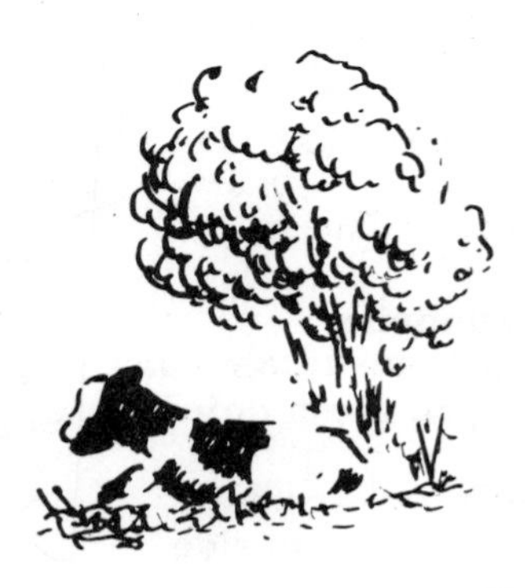

BEEF QUICHE

Yield: 8 dozen

Pastry for 9″ 2 crust pie
1 lb. ground beef
1 tsp. salt
12 oz. Swiss cheese, shredded
2/3 cup minced green onions, with tops
6 eggs, well beaten
2 1/2 cups light cream
3/4 tsp. salt
1/4 tsp. sugar
1/8 tsp. Cayenne pepper
Paprika

Prepare pastry and roll into a rectangle 17″x12″. Ease pastry into jelly roll pan 14 1/2″x10 1/2″x1″. Trim edges. In large skillet over medium heat brown ground beef. Drain well. Sprinkle with 1 tsp. salt. Layer cheese, onions and ground beef in pastry-lined pan. Mix eggs, cream, 3/4 tsp. salt, sugar and pepper. Pour slowly over ground beef. Bake at 425° for 15 minutes. Reduce oven temperature to 300° and bake 15-20 minutes or until knife inserted comes out clean. Sprinkle with paprika. Let stand 10 minutes before cutting.

This is another versatile recipe that can serve many as an appetizer or can be cut in larger pieces for an entrée.

ASPARAGUS CANAPÉS

Serves: 18

1 1-lb. loaf white sandwich bread
8 oz. cream cheese, softened
8 oz. Roquefort cheese
1 Tbsp. mayonnaise
1 egg, beaten
18 asparagus spears, canned or freshly cooked
1 stick butter, melted

Cut crusts from bread, roll flat. Combine next 4 ingredients and spread on bread. Roll 1 spear of asparagus in each bread slice, cut in thirds, dip in melted butter. Bake at 350° for 15 minutes or until golden.

These may be prepared up to the baking point a day ahead or frozen.

CHICKEN CURRY DIP

Serves: 6

1 4 3/4-oz. can chicken spread
1/2 cup sour cream
1 1/2 Tbsp. mayonnaise
1 tsp. curry powder
2 tsp. lemon juice
1/2 tsp. salt
Dash Cayenne pepper

Combine all ingredients and mix well. Serve in small bowl surrounded by crackers and crisp vegetables.

Quick to prepare and easily doubled.

SPINACH DIP

Serves: 16

2 10-oz. pkg. frozen chopped spinach, thawed and well drained
1/2 cup chopped green onion with tops
1 large onion, chopped
1/2 tsp. salt
1/2 tsp. pepper
3 4-oz. pkg. Original Ranch salad dressing mix with buttermilk
1 pt. sour cream
1 cup mayonnaise

Mix all ingredients together and chill. Serve with fresh raw vegetables.

Include fresh green beans or asparagus in season.

EGGPLANT HORS D'OEUVRES

Yield: 5 dozen

4 medium eggplants
2 cups Italian seasoned bread crumbs
1/2 cup chopped fresh parsley
1 cup grated Parmesan cheese
1/8 tsp. garlic powder
1 egg
1/4 tsp. salt
1/8 tsp. pepper
Oil for deep frying

Peel and dice eggplants. Cover with water and boil until soft when pierced with fork. Drain well. In large bowl, mash eggplant and add next 7 ingredients, mixing well. Form into 1″ balls. Deep fry in oil heated to 375° until golden brown. Drain on paper towels. Serve warm or cold.

May be frozen after frying but decrease garlic as freezing intensifies its flavor.

OLIVE BALLS

Yield: 32 pieces

16 mammoth stuffed green olives
1/4 cup flour
2 8-oz. pkg. cream cheese
Paprika
Fresh parsley, snipped

Drain olives well and pat dry with paper towels. Dust with flour. Cut each pkg. of cheese into 8 equal portions. Stick toothpick lengthwise through each olive as a guide for cutting later. Wrap each olive in one part of cream cheese, molding with hands into smooth ball, working carefully around protruding toothpick. Cover and refrigerate. When ready to serve, roll each ball in paprika or finely snipped parsley to completely coat outside. Cut each ball in half crosswise, removing toothpick. Arrange on serving platter, cut side up.

Perfect to pass with cocktails or as a garnish on a luncheon salad plate.

ARTICHOKE NIBBLES

Serves: 12

2 6-oz. jars marinated artichoke hearts
1 large onion, finely chopped
1 clove garlic, minced
4 eggs, beaten
1/4 cup dry bread crumbs
1/2 tsp. salt
1/8 tsp. pepper
1/8 tsp. oregano
1/8 tsp. Tabasco sauce
1/2 lb. sharp Cheddar cheese, grated
2 Tbsp. minced fresh parsley

Drain marinade from 1 jar of artichokes into skillet. Drain and discard marinade from second jar. Chop artichokes. Set aside. Sauté onion and garlic in marinade for 5 minutes. Remove from heat. Combine all ingredients. Pour into buttered 2-qt. shallow casserole Bake at 325° for about 30 minutes. Cool. Cut in 1″ squares.

Cut into larger squares and serve as a luncheon entrée.

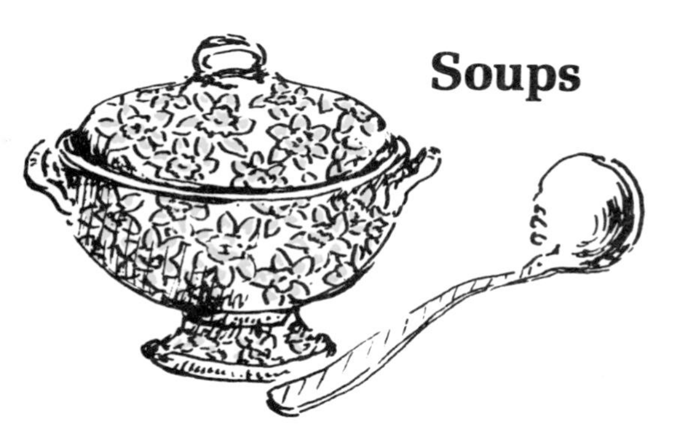

Soups

ITALIAN WEDDING SOUP

Yield: 6 quarts

1/2 lb. meat loaf mix
2 tsp. dried parsley
1/4 cup grated Parmesan cheese
1/4 tsp. salt
1/8 tsp. pepper
1 clove garlic, crushed
1/4 tsp. oregano
1/4 tsp. basil
2 slices bread
1/4 cup milk
1 stewing chicken
1 onion, quartered
1 carrot, thickly sliced
1 stalk celery with leaves, cut up
4 peppercorns
2 tsp. salt
6 qt. water
2 stalks celery, finely diced
2 carrots, grated
1 medium onion, finely diced
8 chicken bouillon cubes
1/2 head escarole, shredded

Combine first 10 ingredients. Form small 1/2″ balls. Drop into boiling salted water. simmer 5 minutes. Remove and refrigerate. Stew chicken with next 5 ingredients in 6-qt. water about 2 1/2 hours or until tender. Remove, skin, bone, cut up and refrigerate. Strain broth and return to pot. Add next 4 ingredients. Simmer 20 minutes. Parboil escarole in boiling salted water 10 minutes. Drain. Add to broth with 1 1/2 cups prepared chicken and meatballs. Simmer 10 minutes more.

This freezes well and can be doubled if you have a pot large enough. If desired add 2 cups cooked Acini di Pepe — tiny soup pasta.

TAVERN SOUP

Serves: 8

1/4 cup each chopped celery, carrot, green pepper and onion
3 13 3/4-oz. cans chicken broth
4 Tbsp. butter
3/4 tsp. salt
1/4 tsp. pepper
1/3 cup flour
3/4 lb. sharp Cheddar cheese, grated
1 12-oz. can beer, room temperature

Sauté vegetables in butter until tender. Add broth, salt and pepper. Cook, covered, 1 1/2 hours. Strain mixture, puree vegetables in blender and return to pan with broth. Dissolve flour in small amount of water and stir into broth. Over medium heat, add cheese 1/2 cup at a time, stirring until melted after each addition. Pour in beer and simmer for several minutes until heated through and thickened.

Quite good served to a crowd. Double the recipe and keep it warm in a crockpot.

GAZPACHO WITH SOUR CREAM

Serves: 4-6

1 cucumber, peeled, seeded and chopped
1 onion, chopped
1 clove garlic, crushed
5 green onions with tops, sliced
4 tomatoes, peeled, seeded and chopped
1 green and 1 red pepper, seeded and chopped
4 stalks celery, chopped
2 cups tomato juice
1/2 cup olive oil
1/4 cup wine vinegar
Juice of 2 limes
4 drops Tabasco sauce
1 tsp. salt
1/4 tsp. white pepper
Sour cream
6 slices bacon, fried crisp and crumbled
Croutons
4 Tbsp. chopped fresh parsley

Combine all vegetables in large bowl. Stir together next 7 ingredients. Pour over vegetables, stir, cover and chill 2-24 hours. Serve in bowls garnished with dollop of sour cream, bacon and parsley.

A food processor makes this delicious soup a joy to prepare.

SEAFOOD CHOWDER

Serves: 6

4 slices bacon, cut in 1/2″ pieces
1/2 cup finely chopped onion
1/2 cup finely chopped celery
2 Tbsp. fresh chopped parsley
1 cup diced potatoes
1 8-oz. can whole kernel corn, drained
1 cup clam juice
1/2 cup white wine
2 6 1/2-oz. cans minced clams, undrained
1/2 lb. scallops
5 Tbsp. butter
5 Tbsp. flour
2 cups milk
1 cup light cream
1 tsp. salt
1/2 tsp. white pepper

In large saucepan cook bacon until crisp, remove, set aside and drain off all but 2 Tbsp. fat. Add onion and celery and sauté until tender. Add next 7 ingredients, quartering scallops if large. Cover and simmer for 20 minutes. In another pan melt butter, add flour and cook, stirring for 5 minutes. Remove from heat, slowly stir in milk and cream. Return to heat, stirring until thickened and bubbling. Add to chowder with salt, pepper and bacon. Simmer but do not boil for 10 minutes more.

This is an excellent chowder and could be a complete meal served with crusty bread and butter.

BAY SCALLOP CHOWDER

Serves: 4

3 medium potatoes, diced
1 medium onion, chopped
1 small carrot, chopped
1 large stalk celery, chopped
2 cups chicken stock
1/2 tsp. salt
1/4 tsp. pepper
1/2 bay leaf
1/2 tsp. thyme leaves
1 1/2 Tbsp. butter
1/2 lb. fresh mushrooms, sliced
1 lb. fresh scallops
1/2 cup white wine
1 cup whipping cream
1 egg yolk, beaten

Place vegetables in large pot, cover with stock, bring to boil. Add seasonings, lower heat and simmer covered until vegetables are tender. Remove bay leaf. Puree vegetables and liquid. Return to pot and set aside. Melt butter and sauté mushrooms. Add scallops and wine and cook 1 minute only. Mix cream with egg yolk and stir in. Add to pureed stock and just heat through.

This can be doubled or tripled but it does not freeze well.

NEW YORK OYSTER STEW

Serves: 6

1/3 cup butter
1 Tbsp. Worcestershire sauce
1 tsp. salt
1/2 tsp. pepper
1 tsp. paprika
3 cups clam juice
1 pt. oysters
2 cups milk
1 cup cream

Heat together first 5 ingredients until butter melts. Add clam juice and oysters. Cook only until edges of oysters curl. Slowly stir in milk and cream. Serve when steaming hot.

This made-in-minutes stew is reminiscent of that served at the Grand Central Oyster Bar.

DUTCH CHICKEN CORN SOUP

Serves: 6-8

2 qt. chicken broth
2 cups diced cooked chicken
2 cups corn, fresh or frozen
1/3 cup chopped fresh parsley
5 hard-boiled eggs, chopped
1/2 tsp. salt
1/4 tsp. pepper

Heat broth. Add chicken and corn. Simmer 6-7 minutes. Stir in remaining ingredients. Heat through.

For heartier soup cook 1 cup noodles and add to broth before adding other ingredients.

CLAM CHOWDER

Serves: 6

1 2 3/4-oz. pkg. leek soup mix
2 cups water
1 10 3/4-oz. can New England clam chowder
2 7-oz. cans minced clams
1 cup Coffee Rich or cream

Slowly combine leek soup mix with water. Bring to boil, stirring constantly, then simmer uncovered 10 minutes, stirring occasionally. Stir in New England chowder. Drain juice from clams and add. Stir in Coffee Rich or cream and return to boil. Remove from heat, stir in clams and serve. May thin with extra Coffee Rich or cream if desired.

May be made ahead and refrigerated. Add clams after reheating.

CURRIED TURKEY CREAM SOUP

Yield: 4 quarts

1 turkey carcass
1/2 tsp. salt
1/4 tsp. pepper
Celery tops
1 onion, chopped
1 carrot, chopped
1 bay leaf
1 stick butter
1 large carrot, grated
2 stalks celery, chopped
1 onion, chopped
1/2 tsp. curry powder
1 1/2 cups flour
1 Tbsp. chicken flavored base
2 cups half and half
1 1/2 cups minced turkey
1/2 tsp. salt
1/2 tsp. white pepper
2 Tbsp. snipped fresh parsley

Cook turkey in enough water to cover with next 6 ingredients from 1 1/2 - 2 hours. Cut meat from bones. Set aside. Strain broth adding enough water to make 3 qt. Set aside. Melt butter in large pot over medium heat, stir in next 3 ingredients and cook 8 minutes stirring occasionally. Blend in curry, flour and chicken base. Slowly stir in reserved turkey broth. Simmer, stirring occasionally 1/2 hour. Heat half and half. Add to broth with 1 1/2 cups reserved turkey and remaining ingredients. Heat through but do not boil.

A very nice change from the soup one usually makes with the leftover holiday turkey.

POLISH SAUSAGE POTATO SOUP

Serves: 8

2 Tbsp. butter
1 lb. Polish sausage, sliced
1 cup chopped onion
2 cups chopped celery with leaves
4 cups shredded cabbage
2 cups sliced carrots
1 bay leaf
1/2 tsp. dried thyme
2 Tbsp. vinegar
1 1/2 tsp. salt
1 1/2 cups beef bouillon
5 cups water
3 cups cubed potatoes

Melt butter in large pan. Add next 3 ingredients. Cook until vegetables are tender. Add next 8 ingredients. Simmer, covered, 1 1/2 hours. Add potatoes and cook about 20 minutes more.

A wonderful winter supper for those who love Polish sausage a.k.a. kielbasi.

VEGETABLE CHOWDER

Serves: 6-8

4 Tbsp. butter
2 potatoes, cubed
3 carrots, sliced
1 onion, thinly sliced
1 10-oz. pkg. frozen lima beans
1 10-oz. pkg. frozen green beans
2 cups water
1 tsp. salt
1/8 tsp. pepper
1/4 tsp. celery seed
1/8 tsp. thyme
2 cups milk
1/2 lb. sharp cheese, grated

Melt butter in large saucepan. Stir in vegetables. Add water and seasonings, bring to boil, reduce heat and simmer 15 minutes. Add milk and cheese, stirring until cheese melts and chowder is heated through.

Serve this quick and easy chowder with hot buttered muffins and your meal is complete.

MUSHROOM SOUP

Yield: 4 quarts

1 lb. mushrooms, sliced
1 medium onion, chopped
4 qt. chicken stock
1/2 cup farfel
2 Tbsp. flour
1 stick butter, melted
6 Tbsp. white vinegar

Combine first 3 ingredients in stock pot. Simmer 2 hours. Add farfel. Cook another hour. Combine flour and butter. Add to broth with vinegar. Simmer 30 minutes more.

Farfel can be found in specialty stores. Soup will keep 2-3 days in refrigerator but do not freeze.

CRAB BISQUE

Serves: 6

2 10 3/4-oz. cans cream of asparagus soup
2 10 3/4-oz. cans cream of mushroom soup
2 soup cans milk
1 cup crab meat
1/2 soup can sherry
Chopped parsley

Pick over crab meat and remove shell. Pour soups into 3-qt. saucepan, add milk gradually and stir until smooth. Heat to boiling, add crabmeat and simmer 2 minutes. Add sherry and simmer 1 minute more. Garnish with parsley.

Delicious served for lunch with aspic salad and herbed bread.

BEAN AND BACON CHOWDER

Serves: 6

1 cup pea beans
8 slices bacon
3/4 cup chopped onions
1/4 cup chopped green onions with tops
1 clove garlic, crushed
1/4 cup diced celery
1 28-oz. can tomatoes
1/3 cup tomato paste
1 10 1/2-oz. can beef broth
1 tsp. salt
1/4 tsp. pepper
1/2 tsp. basil
1 Tbsp. sugar
1/2 cup hot water

Pick over pea beans and place in 3-qt. covered pan. Simmer in 2 cups water for 3-4 minutes, then let stand for 1 hours. Fry bacon until crisp, crumble and add to beans. In 3 Tbsp. bacon drippings, sauté onions, garlic and celery until golden. Add to beans. Add all other ingredients plus 1/2 cup hot water. Cover and simmer for 4-5 hours or until beans are cooked. Taste for seasoning. Add more beef broth, if necessary.

The flavor is enhanced if made a day ahead. This can serve as a meal.

CHILLED ZUCCHINI BISQUE

Serves: 6

2 10 1/2-oz. cans chicken broth
1 cup water
2 cups grated zucchini
1/4 cup chopped onion
4 Tbsp. rice
1/2 tsp. curry powder
1/2 tsp. ground ginger
1/2 tsp. dry mustard
1/2 tsp. salt
1/4 tsp. white pepper
1 1/2 cups half and half
1/2 cup yogurt

In large saucepan, simmer first 8 ingredients, covered, for 20 minutes. Place small amount at a time in blender and whirl until smooth. Add salt and pepper, chill for several hours or overnight. Just before serving, add half and half. Pour into chilled bowls and top with a spoonful of yogurt.

For those who grow and freeze their own zucchini, this can be made in the middle of winter.

YOUGHIOGHENY'S PRINCESS SOUP

Serves: 6

2 carrots, finely diced
2 small onions, finely diced
5 Tbsp. butter
4 Tbsp. flour
1 qt. chicken stock
1/8 tsp. mace
1 tsp. salt
1/8 tsp. pepper
2 cups milk, scalded
1/2 cup grated Parmesan cheese
1 Tbsp. chopped fresh parsley

Sauté vegetables in butter. Stir in flour. Slowly add chicken stock. Add seasonings. Simmer 15 minutes. Strain milk and add. Stir in cheese and parsley. Heat through but do not boil.

Warm bowls before serving hot soup. And chill bowls that will be used for cold soup.

LEMON SOUP

Yield: 1 quart

2 13 3/4-oz. cans chicken broth
1/4 cup uncooked rice
3 eggs
4 Tbsp. fresh lemon juice
1/2 tsp. salt
1/4 tsp. white pepper

Bring chicken broth to boil, stir in rice and simmer 25 minutes. Beat eggs. Stir in lemon juice. Add small amount of hot broth to eggs, stirring constantly. Slowly stir eggs into broth. Season with salt and pepper and serve promptly.

An easy to make, lovely, and light soup with the taste of springtime.

ASPARAGUS SOUP

Serves: 4-6

1 10-oz. pkg. frozen asparagus spears
1 10 3/4-oz. can cream of asparagus soup
1 cup milk
1/4 tsp. Tabasco sauce
1/4 tsp. salt
1/2 tsp. celery salt
1/2 pt. sour cream
1 Tbsp. chopped onion
Chopped chives

Cook asparagus according to directions, cut off tips and reserve. Cut spears in pieces and place in blender with remaining 7 ingredients. Blend until mixed. Heat and serve in mugs topped with chives and reserved asparagus tips.

May be made well ahead and refrigerated.

HERBED POTATO SOUP

Serves: 6

3 leeks, white part only, chopped
1/3 cup chopped shallots
1 medium onion, chopped
2 large stalks celery, chopped
3 Tbsp. butter
4 large potatoes, peeled and cubed
2 large Swiss Chicken Cubes
2-3 cups water
2 Tbsp. dry chervil
1/2 tsp. salt
1/4 tsp. white pepper
1 1/2 cups light cream
2 Tbsp. slivered carrot
2 Tbsp. slivered celery
1 tsp. chicken flavor base
1/2 cup boiling water

In large saucepan cook first 4 ingredients in butter until golden. Add potatoes, chicken cubes and water to cover. Cook until potatoes are well done. Puree entire mixture. Add salt, pepper and cream, stir well, heat but do not boil. Cook slivered carrots and celery with base in boiling water 2-3 minutes and use as garnish.

Thickness of this soup may vary. Thin with cream. Or thicken with 1-2 tsp. arrowroot dissolved in water.

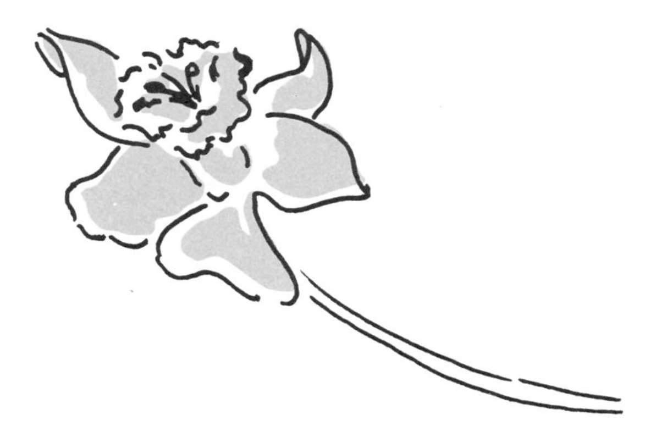

CHEESE SOUP

Serves: 6

1 10 3/4-oz. can cream of celery soup
1/2 cup white wine
1 1/2 cups diced sharp cheese
1/4 tsp. nutmeg
1/8 tsp. pepper
1/8 tsp. garlic powder
1 cup half and half

Combine ingredients over low heat until cheese melts and soup is piping hot. Do not boil.

Easily made and doubled, this soup keeps well in the refrigerator for 1 week.

CHICKEN AND VEGETABLE SUPPER SOUP

Serves: 4-6

3 1/2 cups chicken broth
1/4 cup uncooked rice
1 1/2 medium carrots, sliced
1 medium zucchini, sliced
1 1/2 stalks celery, sliced
3 Tbsp. butter
3 Tbsp. flour
1 cup milk
2 cups cut up cooked chicken
1 tsp. salt
1/2 tsp. pepper
1/4 cup sliced green onions with tops

Simmer broth and rice 10 minutes. Add vegetables. Simmer 10 minutes more. In another pan melt butter, add flour and cook, stirring until bubbling. Remove from heat. Slowly stir in milk and 1 cup broth from soup pot. Stir into vegetables and broth. Add remaining ingredients, heat through stirring often.

Serve this with a salad and hard rolls for a complete meal.

MUSHROOM CLAM VELOUTÉ

Serves: 6-8

1 stick butter
1/2 cup flour
1 8-oz. can minced clams with liquid
1 qt. clam broth
1 1/2 lb. mushrooms, coarsely chopped
1 1/2 cups water
2 cups whipping cream
1/2 tsp. salt
1/4 tsp. pepper
1/8 tsp. nutmeg

Melt butter in heavy pan. Add flour and cook, stirring until mixture turns hazel brown. Remove from heat. Slowly stir in next 4 ingredients. Return to heat and simmer 10 minutes. Add remaining ingredients. Heat through, but do not boil.

An excellent soup that would be a grand beginning for an important dinner.

Enter The Entrée

Beef and Veal

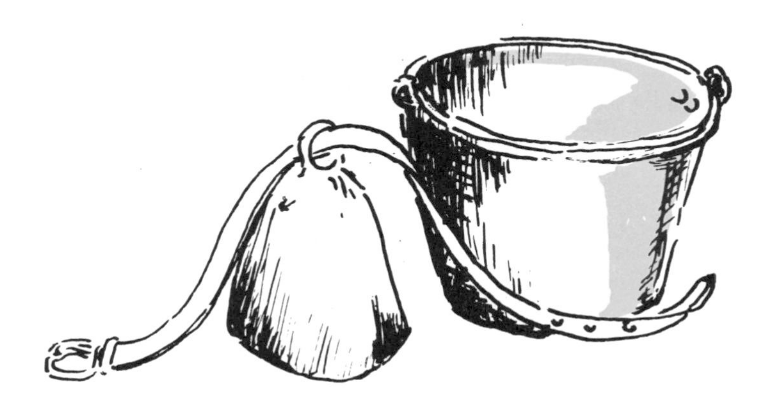

HERBED BEEF STEW **Serves: 16**

4 lb. beef chuck, cut in 1″ cubes
1/4 cup butter
1 lb. mushrooms, sliced
6 onions, sliced
2 cloves garlic, crushed
1 Tbsp. salt
1 tsp. dried dill weed
3/4 tsp. basil
1/4 tsp. pepper
1/2 tsp. thyme
1/2 tsp. savory
2 bay leaves
1 10 1/2-oz. can consommé
2 1-lb. cans tomatoes
1 lb. small white onions
1 bunch carrots, cut in 1″ chunks

Poppy Seed Noodles:
3 6-oz. pkg. bow knot noodles
5 oz. slivered almonds
2 sticks butter
1/4 cup poppy seeds
1 tsp. salt

Brown meat in butter and remove. Add mushrooms and onions. Sauté 5 minutes. Add garlic and cook 3 minutes. Add next 9 ingredients. Return meat to pan, cover and simmer 1 1/2 hours. Add onions and carrots. Simmer 45 minutes more. Remove bay leaves. To thicken gravy, stir in flour combined with water. Cook 5 minutes more. Serve with poppy seed noodles. For Noodles: cook noodles as package directs. Drain. Sauté almonds in butter 3-5 minutes. Add poppy seeds and salt. Pour over noodles.

This wonderfully flavored stew may be prepared ahead. Good company fare.

VEAL-PRINCE ORLOFF

Serves: 8

Roast:
3-3 1/2 lb. veal roast
2 Tbsp. salad oil
3 Tbsp. butter
1/2 cup sliced carrots
1/2 cup sliced onions
1/2 tsp. salt
1/2 tsp. thyme
1 bay leaf
4 slices bacon

Stuffing:
3 qt. water
1/2 tsp. salt
1/3 cup uncooked white rice
6 Tbsp. butter
4 cups thinly sliced yellow onion
3/4 tsp. salt

Duxelles:
1 cup finely diced mushrooms
1 1/2 Tbsp. butter
1/4 tsp. salt
1/4 tsp. white pepper

Sauce:
6 Tbsp. butter
6 Tbsp. flour
2 cups liquid from veal and milk
1/2 tsp. salt
1/4 tsp. white pepper
1/4 tsp. nutmeg
1/4 cup whipping cream
1 cup grated Swiss cheese
3 Tbsp. butter, melted

Have butcher bone and tie sirloin or rump roast of veal. Brown all sides in oil over medium-high heat. Melt butter in roasting pan. Sauté carrots and onions until crisp-tender. Place veal over vegetables. Sprinkle with salt. Add thyme and bay leaf. Lay bacon slices over veal. Cover veal with foil like a blanket. Place lid on pan. Bake at 325° for 1 hour. Remove lid, place meat thermometer into center of veal, through foil, and continue baking until thermometer registers 175°. Cool and refrigerate. Reserve pan juice. For Stuffing: bring water to boil, add 1/2 tsp. salt and rice. Boil 5 minutes. Drain. Melt 6 Tbsp. butter in 2-qt. casserole. Add onions and stir to coat. Add rice and 3/4 tsp. salt. Mix well. Bake covered at 350° for 1 hour or until tender and golden. Cool. Refrigerate. For Duxelles: in skillet stir mushrooms and butter together over medium-high heat. Sauté, stirring occasionally, until all liquid evaporates and mushroom pieces separate. Cool. Add salt and pepper. Set aside. For Sauce: in saucepan stir together butter and flour for 2 minutes over medium heat. Combine liquid from veal with enough milk to make 2 cups. Remove butter mixture from heat. Slowly add liquid, stirring constantly. Return to heat and cook until bubbling. Add salt, pepper and nutmeg. Add 2/3 cup of sauce and 3 Tbsp. cream to stuffing mixture. Purée in blender or processor. Stir in duxelles. Place remaining sauce in small bowl. Pour over 1 Tbsp. cream to cover top. Refrigerate stuffing and sauce. To Assemble: evenly slice veal slightly less than 1/4″ thick. Butter 3-qt. shallow casserole. Place 1 slice veal at end. Spread with spoonful of stuffing. Overlap with next slice of veal, spread with stuffing. Continue until all slices are used. Spread any remaining stuffing over and around veal. Heat sauce. Add 1/2 cup cheese. Stir to melt. Spoon over veal. Sprinkle with remaining cheese and butter. Bake at 375° for 30-35 minutes until heated through and golden.

Taken step by step, this classic dish is not difficult. Prepare all ingredients a day ahead. Assemble roast in the morning. Refrigerate until near baking time. Increase baking time to 45-50 minutes. Then relax and collect your compliments.

VEAL RING

Serves: 8-10

2 eggs
3/4 cup milk
1 1/2 cups coarse cracker crumbs
1 tsp. salt
1/4 tsp. pepper
1 1/2 Tbsp. Worcestershire sauce
1/2 cup minced onion
1/3 cup minced green pepper
2 1/2 lb. ground veal
3/4 lb. ground lean pork

Raisin-Coconut Pilaf:
4 cups cooked long grain rice
1 cup golden raisins
1/2 cup coconut chips or shredded, toasted coconut
2 Tbsp. slivered orange rind
2 Tbsp. minced fresh parsley

Curry Sauce:
1/2 cup minced onion
3 Tbsp. butter
1/4 cup flour
1/4 tsp. salt
1/4 tsp. pepper
1/4 tsp. nutmeg
2 tsp. curry powder
1 13 3/4-oz. can chicken broth

Beat together eggs and milk. Stir in next 6 ingredients. Add veal and pork. Blend thoroughly. Pack into greased 8-cup ring mold. Place mold in larger pan to catch drips. Bake at 325° for about 1 1/2 hours. Let stand 5 minutes. Unmold on serving platter. Fill center with raisin-coconut pilaf. Serve with curry sauce. For Pilaf: stir raisins into hot rice to plump them. Add coconut chips. Fill center of veal ring. Top rice with orange rind and parsley. For Sauce: sauté onion in butter until golden. Blend in flour and seasonings. Remove from heat. Slowly add broth. Return to heat and cook, stirring until thickened and smooth. Simmer about 1/2 hour, stirring occasionally.

Attractive as is but even more so surrounded by parsley and kabobs of fresh fruit.

MARINATED EYE OF THE ROUND

Serves: 8-10

1 3 1/2-lb. eye of the round
1/2 cup salad oil
1/4 cup lemon juice
1 Tbsp. paprika
2 Tbsp. Worcestershire sauce
Dash of Tabasco
2 Tbsp. vinegar
2 tsp. salt
2 tsp. sugar
2 cloves garlic, crushed
Lemon-pepper marinade

Carefully trim away all fat and fiber from meat. Save fat. If one end is narrow, tuck under and secure with picks. Combine next 9 ingredients and shake together. Place meat and prepared marinade in plastic bag. Twist closed. Place in shallow pan. Refrigerate 24 hours, turning often. Bring to room temperature. Place meat on rack in shallow pan. Place tip of meat thermometer into center of meat. Sprinkle generously with lemon-pepper marinade. Cover with reserved fat. Bake at 200° for 3 hours or until meat thermometer registers 140°. To serve let stand 10-15 minutes before carving into thin slices.

This is excellent chilled and sliced thinly. Use this recipe whenever cold roast beef is called for.

CHUCK BARBECUES

Serves: 8

2 lb. boneless chuck roast
1 Tbsp. shortening
1 cup water
3 Tbsp. butter
1 medium onion, chopped
1 cup diced celery
1 cup water
1 cup catsup
1/2 tsp. dry mustard
1 Tbsp. Worcestershire sauce
2 Tbsp. pickle relish
4 tsp. onion juice
2 Tbsp. brown sugar
2 Tbsp. vinegar
1/2 tsp. garlic salt

In Dutch oven brown chuck roast in shortening. Add water, cover and simmer 2 hours or until very tender. Melt butter and lightly brown onion and celery. Combine remaining ingredients, add to onion mixture and bring to simmer. Shred chuck roast, cutting away any fat and simmer in sauce 1 hour. Serve on buns.

The flavors blend when made ahead. Serve topped with coleslaw or coleslaw on the side.

BEER BURGERS

Serves: 12

4 lb. ground chuck
2 Tbsp. bacon fat
6 medium onions, thinly sliced
3 12-oz. cans beer
1 Tbsp. seasoned salt
1 tsp. pepper
1/8 tsp. garlic powder
2 tsp. Worcestershire sauce
1 10 1/2-oz. can beef broth
12 semi-hard rolls

Form ground chuck into 12 patties, brown in skillet in bacon fat and arrange in large pan. Lightly brown onions in same skillet and combine with remaining ingredients. Pour over patties and simmer 1 hour covered and 1 hour uncovered. Serve on rolls with sauce.

For barbecue flavor, brown the patties on an outdoor grill. These are surprisingly good!

DILLED ROAST OF VEAL

Serves: 6-8

1 1/2 cups sour cream
1 envelope dry onion soup mix
1/4 cup fresh snipped dill or 2 Tbsp. dry dill weed
1/4 tsp. freshly ground pepper
1 3-4 lb. veal shoulder roast
Parsley sprigs

In small roasting pan combine first 4 ingredients. Add veal, cover and bake at 325° for 2 1/2 hours. Uncover and cook 30 minutes more or until meat is brown and tender. To serve, slice across grain, pour sauce over and garnish with parsley.

A delicious sauce forms, so consider serving this over a cooked pasta.

CANDLELIGHT CUTLETS

Serves: 2

2 veal cutlets
1 thin slice cooked ham
1/4″ round slice Gouda cheese
1/4 tsp. sage
2 Tbsp. flour
4 Tbsp. butter
1/4 cup dry sherry

Pound cutlets on both sides until very thin. Place ham and cheese on 1 cutlet. Sprinkle with sage. Top with second cutlet. Secure edges with skewers or toothpicks. Dredge with flour. In large skillet, over medium heat, brown cutlet in butter, about 8 minutes per side. Remove and keep warm. Add sherry to pan over high heat. Cook and stir a few seconds. Remove skewers, divide cutlet in half and pour sauce over.

The name brings to mind a romantic setting . . . wine and roses and soft music.

SUKIYAKI

Serves: 8-10

1 1/2 lb. beef fillet
2 Tbsp. salad oil
2 stalks celery, sliced in 1″ pieces
1/2 lb. broccoli, cut in bite-size pieces
1 cup sliced fresh mushrooms
1/2 head cauliflower, cut in small flowerets
1 8-oz. can bamboo shoots, drained and thinly sliced
1/2 lb. spinach, torn into large pieces
1 bunch green onions, cut in 2″ pieces
1 1/2 cups beef broth
1/2 cup soy sauce
3 Tbsp. sugar
Hot cooked rice

Cut beef into very thin strips across grain. Arrange meat and vegetables on platter in separate piles. Combine beef broth, soy sauce and sugar. Heat oil in large skillet or wok. Add 1/3 beef. Stir-fry 1 minute. Add 1/3 celery, broccoli, mushrooms and cauliflower. Stir-fry 2 minutes. Add 1/3 bamboo shoots, spinach, onions and broth mixture. Toss gently together, cover and steam 3-4 minutes or until vegetables are just crisp-tender. Remove from pan. Repeat twice with remaining ingredients. Serve with hot cooked rice.

Have a cook-at-the-table dinner using an electric skillet or wok. Pass servings as each batch is done.

ROLATINI OF BEEF

Serves: 6-8

1 1/2 lb. round steak
3/4 lb. ground veal
1/2 lb. bulk sausage
3/4 cup bread crumbs
4 eggs
4 Tbsp. grated Parmesan cheese
1/2 tsp. salt
1/4 tsp. pepper
1 large onion, chopped
1 large clove garlic, minced
2 Tbsp. salad oil
1 29-oz. can tomato puree
1/2 tsp. salt
1/4 tsp. pepper
1 tsp. crushed basil
1 Tbsp. snipped fresh parsley
1-2 cups water
Grated Parmesan cheese

Pound meat very thin. Combine next 7 ingredients. Spread on steak. Roll up jelly-roll fashion. Tie with string in several places. In Dutch oven sauté onion and garlic in oil for 5 minutes on medium-low heat. Add meat roll and brown. Add next 5 ingredients and 1 cup water. Add remaining cup water as needed during cooking. Simmer covered 1 1/2 hours stirring occasionally. Remove meat from sauce. Cut string. Let stand 10 minutes. Slice and arrange on serving plate. Pour sauce over slices and sprinkle with grated Parmesan cheese.

Save some sauce to serve over pasta and top with more grated cheese.

OSSO BUCO ROMA

Serves: 6

4 lb. veal shin bones, cut in 1″-1 1/2″ pieces
1/3 cup olive oil
3/4 cup flour
1 tsp. salt
1/2 tsp. pepper
1 Tbsp. dried parsley
1/4 tsp. garlic powder
1 cup white wine
1 cup chicken broth
1 cup peeled, seeded and chopped tomatoes

Gremolata:
Rind of 1/2 lemon, grated
2 Tbsp. finely chopped fresh parsley
1 cup finely chopped celery leaves
1 clove garlic, minced

Brush veal pieces with olive oil. Combine next 5 ingredients. Roll veal in flour mixture. Reserve extra flour. Brown veal slowly in remaining olive oil for about 15 minutes. Add wine, broth and tomatoes. Cover and bake at 350° for 1 1/2 hours or until meat pulls away from bones. Remove meat. Keep warm. Thicken broth with about 1 Tbsp. reserved flour mixed with 2 Tbsp. water. Pour sauce over veal and sprinkle with gremolata.
For Gremolata: combine all ingredients and stir well.

Serve buttered noodles or rice with this rich and flavorful stew.

VEAL WITH RIPE OLIVES

Serves: 4-6

2 lb. lean cubed veal
1/4 cup flour
1/2 tsp. salt
1/4 tsp. pepper
1/4 cup salad oil
1 small onion, sliced
1 clove garlic, minced
2/3 tsp. dried rosemary
1/2 cup dry white wine
1 Tbsp. tomato paste
1 cup chicken stock
12 pitted ripe olives, sliced
2 Tbsp. chopped fresh parsley

Dredge veal with flour, salt and pepper. Heat oil in Dutch oven. Brown veal. Add onion and garlic. Cook 3 minutes. Stir in next 4 ingredients. Bake covered at 300° for 2 hours. Stir in olives. Bake 30 minutes more. Garnish with parsley to serve.

A good recipe to serve buffet style for no knives are needed.

CHUCK WAGON STEAK

Serves: 8-10

2-3 lb. chuck roast, cut 2″ thick
2 tsp. unseasoned meat tenderizer
1 cup wine vinegar
3 Tbsp. lemon juice
1/2 cup salad oil
2 tsp. instant minced onions
2 tsp. thyme
1 tsp. marjoram
1 bay leaf, crushed

Sprinkle meat evenly on both sides with meat tenderizer. Pierce deeply with fork. Mix remaining ingredients in glass dish. Marinate meat covered in refrigerator at least 3 hours or up to 3 days. Turn occasionally. Broil 4″-6″ from heat for 10 minutes. Turn and brush with marinade. Broil 15-20 minutes. If 3 lb., turn, brush again with marinade. Broil about 10 minutes more or until done as desired. Slice diagonally across grain in thin slices.

This is also excellent done on an outdoor grill.

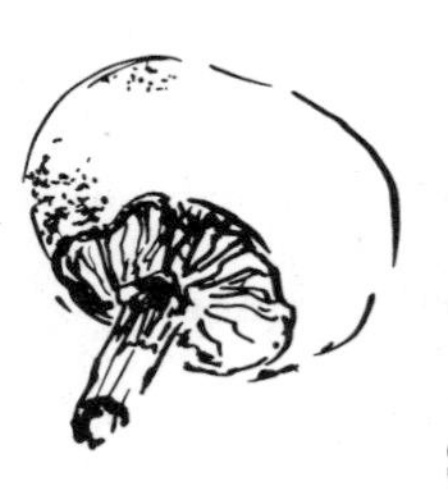

BEEF AND MUSHROOMS VINAIGRETTE

Serves: 4-6

1 lb. mushrooms
3 Tbsp. olive oil
Juice of 1 lemon
2 tsp. chicken stock base
1 1/2 lb. beef, rump or eye of round, baked medium-rare and chilled
4 Tbsp. olive oil
1/4 cup dry red wine
3 Tbsp. red wine vinegar
1/4 tsp. each chervil, thyme, basil and marjoram
2 Tbsp. chopped fresh parsley
1/2 tsp. salt
1/4 tsp. pepper
4 artichoke hearts, cooked and cut in wedges
6 cherry tomatoes

Slice mushrooms and sauté 5 minutes in next 3 ingredients. Cool and set aside. Cut beef into strips 1/4″ thick and 1″ wide. Mix together oil, wine, vinegar, seasonings, parsley and juices from mushrooms. Arrange beef strips in shallow serving dish. Spoon mushrooms down center and pour dressing over. Cover and refrigerate at least 3 hours, basting several times. At serving time, garnish with artichoke wedges and tomatoes.

Should the beef be well-done, cut 1/8″ thick to assure tenderness.

EASY TAMALE PIE

Serves: 6-8

1 lb. ground beef
1/2 Tbsp. olive oil
1/2 Tbsp. butter
2 medium onions, chopped
1 clove garlic, minced
1/2 cup diced celery
2 8-oz. cans tomato sauce
1/4 cup water
1 Tbsp. chili powder
1 Tbsp. flour
2 Tbsp. water
1 cup sliced ripe olives
1/2 tsp. salt
1/4 tsp. freshly ground pepper
2 cups grated Cheddar cheese
2 cups corn chips, lightly crushed

Brown beef in oil and butter. Pour off drippings. Stir in next 6 ingredients and simmer, covered, for 20 minutes. Make paste of flour and water, add and cook, stirring until mixture comes to boil. Add olives, salt and pepper. Layer 1/3 meat mixture, 1/3 cheese and 1/3 chips in 2-qt. casserole. Repeat. Bake at 350° for 25-30 minutes.

Introduce your friends and family to South-of-the-Border style cooking with this uncomplicated recipe.

VEAL STEW ITALIEN

Serves: 4-6

1 small onion, chopped
3 Tbsp. butter
2 Tbsp. salad oil
2 lb. boneless veal shanks or shoulder, cubed
1 cup canned Italian tomatoes, coarsely chopped
1/2 cup dry white wine
1/2 tsp. sage
2 Tbsp. chopped fresh parsley
1 tsp. salt
1/2 tsp. freshly ground pepper
1 10-oz. pkg. frozen peas, thawed

In large skillet, sauté onion in butter and oil. Set aside. In same skillet brown veal well. Return onions, add next 6 ingredients, bring to boil, lower heat and simmer covered about 1 1/2 hours. Add peas and cook 10 minutes more.

Sprinkle hot cooked rice with Parmesan cheese and top with stew.

MEXICAN STEW

Serves: 6-8

2 lb. cubed beef chuck or cubed pork butt
2 Tbsp. salad oil
3 small zucchini, sliced
3 medium green peppers, sliced in rings
1 large onion, sliced in rings
1 lb. fresh mushrooms, sliced
1 28-oz. can tomatoes with juice, chopped fine
3 cloves garlic, minced
1/2 tsp. crushed red pepper
1/2 tsp. each oregano, basil and cumin
1 tsp. salt
1/2 tsp. pepper
Hot cooked rice
3-4 tortillas

Brown meat in oil in Dutch oven. Add next 10 ingredients and simmer 2 1/2-3 hours or until meat is very tender. Serve over cooked rice with wedges of warm tortillas.

Use 1 lb. each of beef and pork cubes for a contrast in flavor and texture.

STEAK MONTROSE

Serves: 6

6 fillets, 1 1/4″ thick
2 Tbsp. olive oil
1/2 tsp. garlic salt
Freshly ground pepper
2 sheets frozen puff pastry, thawed
6 Tbsp. bottled steak sauce
1 egg yolk
1 Tbsp. water

Trim fat from steaks, brush with olive oil, sprinkle with garlic salt and gratings of fresh pepper. Heat heavy skillet on high until quite hot, sear steaks 30 seconds on each side, remove and cool. Cut each pastry sheet in thirds. Roll each out to 9″×6″. Brush each steak with bottled sauce, wrap in pastry, brush seams with combined yolk and water and press firmly to seal. Place seam side down on ungreased baking sheet with sides. Brush tops with remaining yolk mixture. Preheat oven to 500°. Place pan in center of oven, reduce heat to 450° and bake for 15 minutes or until pastry is puffed and golden. Serve with quick Bordelaise sauce found in "Sauces and Et Ceteras."

Strip steaks or Delmonico steaks cut in half may be used in place of fillets.

HEAVENLY STEAK

Serves: 6-8

2 lb. round steak, cut in 1/8″ strips
1/2 cup flour
2 Tbsp. salad oil
3 medium onions, sliced and separated into rings
1 beef bouillon cube
1 cup water
1 4 1/2-oz. can mushrooms with liquid
1 clove garlic, minced
1 10 3/4-oz. can cream of mushroom soup
1 tsp. salt
1/2 tsp. pepper
1/2 cup sour cream

Dredge meat strips in flour. Brown quickly in oil. Add onions and cook until golden. Add next 7 ingredients, stir well and simmer covered for 1 1/2 hours. Stir occasionally and add a little water if needed. Remove from heat, stir in sour cream and heat through.

Toss hot cooked noodles with butter, chopped fresh parsley or chives and chopped toasted nuts. Serve topped with this rich, saucey steak.

LIVER SCALLOPINI

Serves: 4

2 Tbsp. butter
1 medium onion, chopped
1 stalk celery, diced
1 medium carrot, shredded
1 Tbsp. flour
1/4 lb. mushrooms, sliced
1 Tbsp. tomato paste
1/2 cup dry red wine
1/2 cup beef broth
1/2 tsp. salt
1/4 tsp. pepper
2 Tbsp. butter
1 1/4 lb. calves liver
1/2 cup chopped fresh parsley
Hot cooked rice or pasta

Melt 2 Tbsp. butter, add onion, celery and carrot. Sauté until crisp-tender. Stir in flour, add next 6 ingredients and simmer uncovered for 10 minutes, stirring occasionally. Melt 2 Tbsp. butter in frying pan, add liver cut into bite-size pieces and brown quickly over medium-high heat. Pieces should remain pink in center. Stir into sauce, sprinkle with parsley, and serve over rice or pasta.

Those who like liver will enjoy this change from the bacon and onion bit.

BEEF MALAGA

Serves: 10-12

4 lb. round steak
4 Tbsp. salad oil
2 large onions, chopped
1 clove garlic, minced
1 10 3/4-oz. can cream of mushroom soup
1/2 lb. mushrooms, sliced
3/4 cup sherry
1/4 tsp. dried marjoram leaves
1/4 tsp. dried thyme leaves
1/2 tsp. dried basil leaves
1 cup sour cream
1/2 lb. Cheddar cheese, shredded
2 canned peach halves, mashed
Hot cooked rice or noodles
1/2 cup chopped fresh parsley

Trim fat from meat and cut in 3/4" cubes. Heat 1 Tbsp. oil in Dutch oven and brown 1 lb. meat. Remove meat and pour off any drippings and repeat until all meat is browned. Return meat to pan. Stir in next 8 ingredients, cover and simmer 2 hours. Add next 3 ingredients, stirring until cheese melts and mixture simmers. Serve over rice or noodles. Garnish with chopped fresh parsley.

Prepare ahead to blend flavors. Stir butter-browned chopped nuts into rice or noodles.

BEEF PARMIGIANO

Serves: 6

2 lb. round steak
1 egg
1 Tbsp. water
1/3 cup grated Parmesan cheese
1/3 cup dry bread crumbs
1/3 cup salad oil
1 onion, chopped
1 6-oz. can tomato paste
2 cups hot water
1 tsp. salt
1/4 tsp. pepper
1/2 tsp. sugar
1/2 tsp. marjoram
1/2 lb. Mozzarella cheese, sliced

Cut steak in serving-size pieces. Beat together egg and water. Stir together Parmesan and crumbs. Dip steak in egg, then coat with crumbs. Shake off excess. Brown in oil in skillet over medium heat. Remove and arrange in single layer in baking pan. Add chopped onion to skillet. Sauté until golden. Add next 6 ingredients. Stir and cook 5 minutes. Pour 3/4 sauce over steak. Cover with Mozzarella. Pour remaining sauce over cheese. Bake covered at 350° for 1 1/4 hours. Uncover for 15 minutes more.

Can be completely assembled up to a day before and baked just before serving.

VEAL SCALLOPS

Serves: 4

1 lb. veal scallops
1/4 cup Parmesan cheese
1/4 cup flour
1 Tbsp. butter
1 Tbsp. olive oil
1/4 tsp. basil
2 cloves garlic, crushed
1/4 cup white wine
1/4 cup water
Parsley sprigs

Sprinkle scallops with Parmesan and pound until very thin. Dust lightly with flour. Sauté in butter and oil about 2 minutes per side. Remove from skillet and keep warm. Sauté basil and garlic about 1 minute. Add wine and water. Boil hard 1-2 minutes to deglaze pan. Pour over veal and serve. Garnish with parsley.

This proves there is elegance in simplicity.

BAVARIAN POT ROAST

Serves: 10-12

2 Tbsp. salad oil
4 lb. boneless chuck roast
1 cup apple juice
1 8-oz. can tomato sauce
1 medium onion, sliced
3/4 tsp. ground allspice
1/4 tsp. pepper
3/4 cup water
1 tsp. salt

Heat oil over medium-high heat in Dutch oven. Brown chuck roast well on all sides. Stir in remaining ingredients, bring to boil, cover and simmer 2 1/2-3 hours or until fork tender.

For the last hour of cooking you may add quartered potatoes, carrots, etc. — vegetables of your choice.

SAVORY BEEF

Serves: 6-8

2 lb. round steak, cut in serving pieces
2 Tbsp. salad oil
2 medium onions, sliced
1 clove garlic, minced
1/2 lb. fresh mushrooms, sliced
1 green pepper, chopped
3/4 cup chili sauce
1/2 cup dry red wine
1 Tbsp. Worcestershire sauce
1 cup ripe olives
1/2 tsp. salt
1/4 tsp. pepper
1/4 cup chopped fresh parsley

Brown meat quickly in oil. Place in shallow 2-qt. baking dish. In steak drippings, sauté next 4 ingredients. Place on top of steak. Add remaining ingredients to pan, stirring well. Bring to simmer and pour over steak. Bake covered at 350° for 1 hour.

Double the recipe and freeze the extra for a needed last minute meal.

VEAL A LA SWISS

Serves: 4

1/4 cup chopped onion
1 clove garlic, minced
1 Tbsp. olive oil
1 8-oz. can tomato sauce
1/2 tsp. basil leaves
1/4 tsp. oregano
1/4 tsp. salt
1/8 tsp. pepper
1 lb. veal cutlet or round steak
1/4 cup flour
3 Tbsp. salad oil
1 ripe avocado, peeled, seeded and sliced
4 oz. Swiss cheese, grated

Sauté onion and garlic in olive oil until transparent. Add next 5 ingredients. Simmer 5 minutes. Set aside. Cut veal in 4 pieces, pound very thin, dust with flour. Sauté quickly in oil over medium-high heat on both sides, 3-4 minutes altogether. Place in shallow baking dish. Spoon over reserved sauce. Arrange avocado over top, reserving 4 slices. Sprinkle with cheese. Place under broiler until cheese melts. Garnish with 4 avocado slices.

This dish, often served in restaurants, is quite easy to prepare at home.

STUFFED VEAL CUTLETS

Serves: 6

1 1/2 lb. veal cutlets in 6 slices
Juice of 1 lemon
6 thin slices liverwurst
6 slices Mozzarella cheese
6 thin slices prosciutto
1/4 cup flour
1 egg, well beaten
1/2 cup fine dry bread crumbs
3 Tbsp. olive oil
3 Tbsp. butter
1/2 cup dry white wine

Pound cutlets flat. Sprinkle with lemon juice. Place slices of liverwurst, cheese and prosciutto on each. Roll up and secure with toothpicks or skewers. Dip in flour, then egg, then bread crumbs. Brown in oil and butter. Place in shallow buttered baking dish. Pour wine over. Bake covered at 350° for 45 minutes, basting occasionally with pan juice. Remove picks and serve.

This may be prepared, up to baking point, a day ahead and refrigerated.

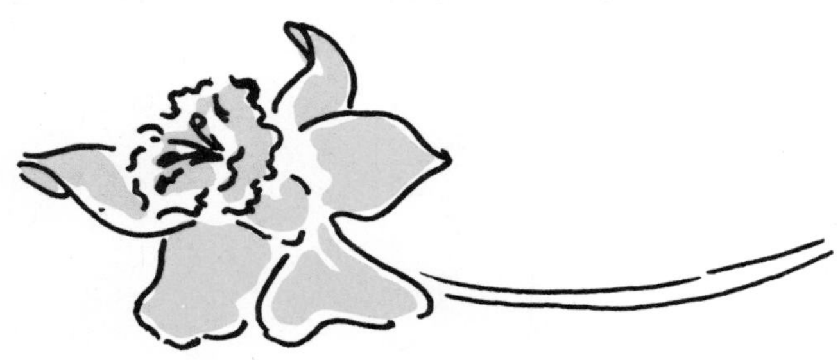

PARTY PATTIES

Serves: 6

1/2 cup mayonnaise
1/2 cup sour cream
1/2 cup finely chopped onion
2 Tbsp. chopped fresh parsley
2 lb. ground beef
1/2 tsp. salt
1/4 tsp. pepper
1 cup shredded sharp Cheddar cheese
6 rye bread slices, toasted and buttered
Lettuce leaves
2 large tomatoes, sliced

Combine first 4 ingredients, mix well, set aside. Shape meat into 6 oval patties. Broil on both sides to desired doneness. Season with salt and pepper. Top patties with sauce and cheese. Broil until cheese melts. Layer toast, lettuce, tomato and patties. Serve hot.

For an added touch skewer 1 ripe and 1 green olive on pick and place on each patty.

MEAT LOAF WITH PROSCIUTTO AND CHEESE

Serves: 6

1 1/2-lb. lean ground beef or meat loaf mixture
3/4 cup dry bread crumbs
1 egg, beaten
3/4 tsp. salt
1/2 tsp. pepper
1/4 cup grated Parmesan cheese
1 clove garlic, crushed
1/4 cup catsup
1/4 cup water
1/4 lb. prosciutto
1/4 lb. Mozzarella cheese, shredded
1/3 cup finely diced celery
1/3 cup finely diced onion

Combine first 9 ingredients. Roll out on wax paper to about 9″ × 12″ rectangle. Cover to within 1″ of edges with prosciutto, then cheese, celery and onion. Using wax paper to lift, roll up lengthwise. Pinch ends and seams to seal. Remove wax paper and place seam-side down in 9″ × 5″ loaf pan. Bake at 350° for 1 hour.

Thin sliced baked ham can be substituted for prosciutto, and you may use any white cheese of your choice.

STUFFED BEEF TENDERLOIN

Serves: 6-8

3 lb. beef tenderloin, trimmed
4 Tbsp. butter
1 medium onion, chopped
1/2 cup diced celery
1/4 lb. fresh mushrooms, sliced
2 cups soft bread crumbs
1/2 tsp. salt
1/8 tsp. pepper
1/2 tsp. basil
4 Tbsp. chopped fresh parsley
6 strips bacon

Make lengthwise cut 3/4 way through meat. Melt 2 Tbsp. butter and sauté onion and celery 2 minutes. Sauté mushrooms separately in remaining butter until all juice is released. Drain. Combine onions, celery and mushrooms with next 5 ingredients. Lightly stuff meat. Secure opening with skewers or toothpicks. Lay bacon strips across top. Place on rack in shallow pan. Bake at 375° for 45-60 minutes.

This is best served medium-rare and a meat thermometer is a must.

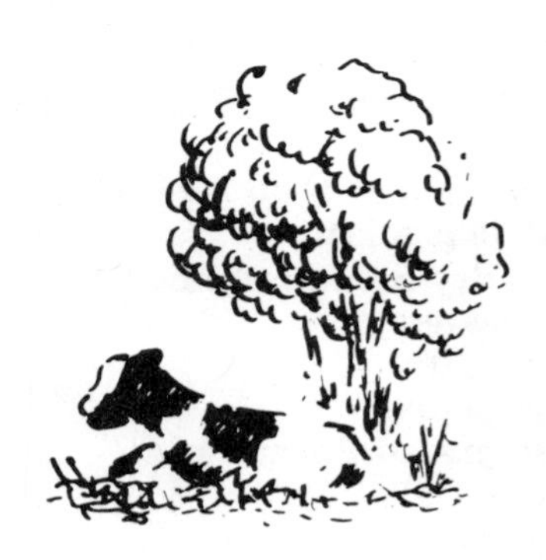

CHIPPED CORNED BEEF CASSEROLE

Serves: 8-10

1 10 3/4-oz. can cream of mushroom soup
1 10 3/4-oz. can cream of celery soup
1 cup milk
4 oz. Cheddar cheese, shredded
2 hard-boiled eggs, sliced
3 Tbsp. chopped onion
1 1/4 cups uncooked macaroni
4 oz. chipped corned beef, cut in bite-size pieces
1/4 cup chopped green pepper

Combine all ingredients and spoon into buttered casserole. Refrigerate 5-6 hours or overnight. Bake uncovered at 350° for 1 hour.

Every busy cook needs a dozen easy recipes like this one.

BEEF BRISKET

Serves: 8

3 lb. fresh beef brisket
4 Tbsp. flour
1 tsp. garlic salt
1/2 tsp. pepper
1 tsp. paprika
2 tsp. dried parsley flakes
1/2 cup wine vinegar
1/2 cup Worcestershire sauce
2 cups water
4 carrots, sliced
4 onions, sliced

A day ahead, moisten brisket with water. Mix together next 5 ingredients. Rub into both sides of brisket. Brown on both sides under broiler. Place in Dutch oven. Pour liquids over. Place sliced carrots and onions around and on top of roast. Cover and bake at 350° for 4 hours. Chill meat. Chill pan juices with carrots and onions. Next day slice meat and place on ovenproof platter. Remove grease from pan juice mixture, heat, and puree in blender to make gravy. Pour over sliced meat and reheat at 350° for 15-20 minutes. Serve extra gravy separately.

Easy, flavorful and good with noodles or mashed potatoes.

REUBEN CASSEROLE

Serves: 10-12

1 27-oz. can sauerkraut, well drained
3 tomatoes, sliced
1 1/2 cups Thousand Island dressing
4 Tbsp. butter
1 lb. corned beef, sliced thin
1 lb. baby Swiss cheese, sliced
1 8-oz. can Hungry Jack biscuits
1/2 tsp. caraway seed

Spread sauerkraut in bottom of 9″ × 13″ casserole. Top with tomato slices. Spread dressing over evenly and dot with butter. Cover with corned beef slices, then cheese. Bake uncovered at 425° for 30 minutes. Open biscuits and separate each into 3 layers. Arrange slightly overlapping on casserole. Sprinkle over caraway seeds. Bake 10-15 minutes more.

A hearty winter casserole that would be delicious served with a large bowl of mashed potatoes and a fresh green vegetable.

COLD JAMOCA BEEF

Serves: 10-12

1 cup catsup or chili sauce
1/2 cup water
1/3 cup vinegar
1/4 cup salad oil
2 Tbsp. instant coffee
1 tsp. salt
1/2 tsp. pepper
1 tsp. chili powder
1 tsp. celery seed
1 clove garlic, crushed
3-4 drops Tabasco sauce
1 3-4 lb. eye of the round roast

Combine first 11 ingredients. Place meat, trimmed of all fat and fiber, in plastic bag. Pour marinade over meat, close bag, place in shallow dish and refrigerate several hours or overnight, turning often. Reserve marinade. Barbecue roast over medium coals for 45-60 minutes or until rare. Or bake at 200° for 3-4 hours. Chill. To serve, cut in thin slices and brush each slice with reserved marinade.

A meat thermometer can be used as satisfactorily on a barbecue grill as in the oven.

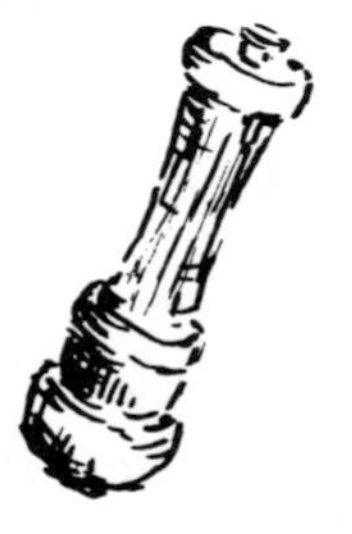

MOCK TOURNEDOS

Serves: 6

1 1/2 lb. beef flank steak
1/2 cup salad oil
1/4 cup lemon juice
1 Tbsp. grated onion
1 tsp. coarsely ground pepper
6 slices bacon, partially cooked
1 recipe Béarnaise sauce

Cut steak into strips 3/4″ wide. Combine next 4 ingredients, pour over strips, stir and marinate overnight, stirring occasionally. Lay out strips so that there are 6 equal portions. You may need to cut and piece. Roll up each portion pinwheel fashion to form "fillet." Wrap each with bacon slice and secure edges with toothpicks. Broil 3″-4″ from heat 6 minutes. Turn and broil 4-6 minutes for medium-rare. Serve with Bearnaise Sauce found under "Sauces and Et Ceteras."

This is an economical way to serve delicious steak to company.

BAKED FLANK STEAK

Serves: 4-6

1 1/2-2 lb. flank steak, scored
2 large tomatoes, quartered
1 large green pepper, sliced in rings
1 large onion, sliced in rings
1/3 lb. fresh mushrooms, sliced
2 Tbsp. butter
3 Tbsp. chili sauce
3 Tbsp. catsup
1 Tbsp. Worcestershire sauce
1/2 tsp. salt
1/2 tsp. pepper

Place steak in shallow baking pan. Arrange vegetables over steak. Dot steak with butter. Combine last 5 ingredients and pour over steak. Bake at 350° for 45 minutes or until tender. Slice steak thinly on diagonal across grain. Arrange on serving platter surrounded by vegetables. Pour sauce from pan over all.

This is a colorful, eye-catching entrée that gives off a mouth-watering aroma while baking.

LEMON BARBECUED MEAT LOAVES

Serves: 6

1 1/2 lb. ground chuck
4 slices day old bread, diced
1/4 cup lemon juice
1/4 cup minced onion
1 egg, beaten
2 tsp. seasoned salt
1/2 cup catsup
1/3 cup brown sugar, packed
1 tsp. dry mustard
1/4 tsp. allspice
1/4 tsp. ground cloves
6 thin lemon slices

Combine first 6 ingredients, mix well, shape into 6 individual meat loaves and place in 9″ × 13″ pan. Bake at 350° for 30 minutes. Combine next 5 ingredients. Pour over loaves. Top each with lemon slice. Bake 30 minutes more, basting occasionally. To serve, spoon sauce over each loaf.

Double the recipe for it freezes well and can be kept on hand for a surprise guest.

EASY BRISKET OF BEEF **Serves: 6-8**

1 cup catsup
1 cup ginger ale
1 envelope dry onion soup mix
1 3-lb. beef brisket, well trimmed
1/2 cup red wine
Hot rice or noodles

Combine first 3 ingredients in Dutch oven or heavy frying pan. Add brisket and turn to coat all sides with sauce. Bring just to boil over medium heat. Add wine, reduce heat to simmer and cook covered 2 hours or until tender. Add water or more wine, if necessary. To serve, cut meat thinly on diagonal across grain. Return to sauce to heat through. Serve over rice or noodles.

A well trimmed chuck roast, browned first, may be used with equally good results.

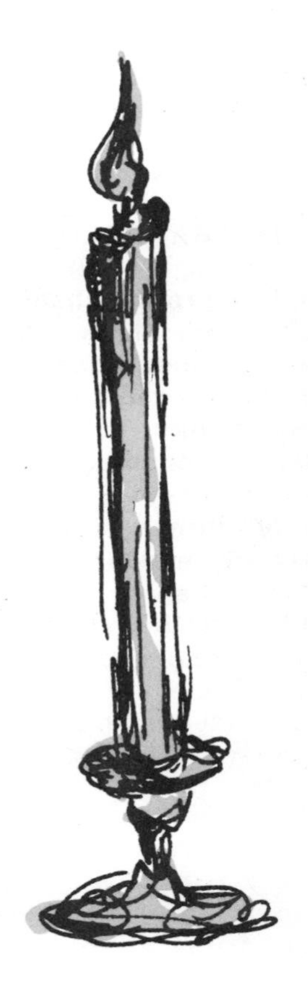

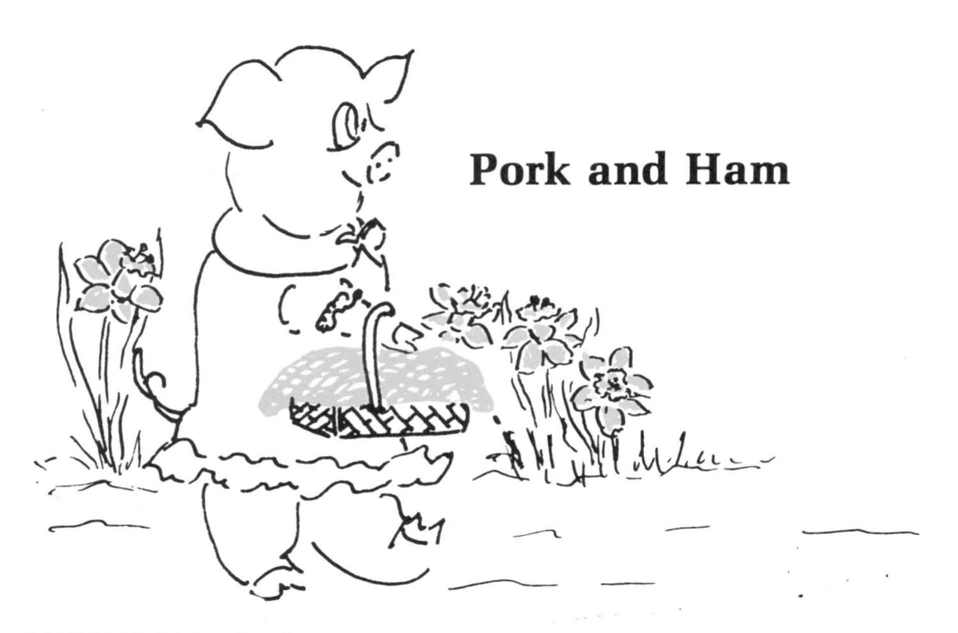

Pork and Ham

MARINATED PORK ROAST

Serves: 12

1/2 cup dry sherry
1/2 cup soy sauce
2 cloves garlic, minced
2 Tbsp. dry mustard
1 tsp. thyme leaves
1 tsp. ground ginger
1 4-5 lb. pork loin, boned, rolled and tied
1 10-oz. jar apricot preserves
1 Tbsp. soy sauce
2 Tbsp. dry sherry

Combine first 6 ingredients in shallow bowl. Add roast and marinate covered in refrigerator 4 hours turning occasionally. Remove roast, place on rack in roasting pan. Insert meat thermometer. Roast at 325° until temperature reaches 170°, about 2 1/2 - 3 hours. Combine last 3 ingredients in small pan over low heat until preserves melt. Serve with sliced roast.

Because of the number it serves, this is a fairly economical entrée.

ROAST GLAZED LOIN OF PORK

Serves: 8-10

1 5-6 lb. pork loin
2/3 cup currant jelly
3 Tbsp. port
2 tsp. vinegar
1 tsp. dry mustard

Place pork loin on rack in roasting pan. Place in 325° oven and roast about 3 hours or 35 minutes per pound. Combine remaining ingredients. Bring to boil, then simmer 10 minutes stirring occasionally. Baste roast several times during last 1/2 hour. Let roast stand 15 minutes before carving.

The addition of port to this simple glaze gives it a special flavor.

HUNGARIAN BRAISED PORK ROAST

Serves: 8-12

4 Tbsp. shortening
3-4 lb. boneless loin of pork
1 cup finely chopped onion
1 cup diced carrots
1 1/2 tsp. sweet Hungarian paprika
1 cup chicken or beef stock
2-3 Tbsp. flour
1 cup sour cream
1 1/2 Tbsp. chopped fresh parsley
1 tsp. chopped capers
1 Tbsp. caraway seeds
1 cup tart applesauce
1/2 tsp. salt
1/4 tsp. pepper

In Dutch oven heat shortening over medium-high heat. Add roast and brown on all sides. Remove and set aside. Pour off all but thin film of fat. Sauté onions over medium heat until golden. Add • carrots. Cook 3 minutes more. Add paprika, stir quickly to coat vegetables and immediately stir in stock. Scrape pan and bring to boil. Place roast in pan. Bake covered at 350° 1/2 hour per pound, 1 1/2 - 2 hours. Baste roast occasionally with pan juices. Keep roast warm. Pour liquid and vegetables into sieve over saucepan. Skim fat from liquid. Press as much vegetable through sieve as possible, then discard. Stir flour into sour cream. Add to saucepan. Bring to simmer stirring constantly. Add remaining ingredients and heat again. Carve roast and dress slices with some sauce. Pass remaining sauce in gravy boat.

Red cabbage, cooked separately, would be the right vegetable to accompany this roast.

PORK AND PAPRIKA

Serves: 10-12

3 strips bacon, chopped
1 Tbsp. butter
3 large onions, coarsely chopped
4 Tbsp. Hungarian paprika
3 lb. lean pork, cubed
2 cups beef broth
3 lb. sauerkraut, rinsed and drained
3 Tbsp. tomato paste
1 tsp. caraway seeds
1 tsp. salt
1/2 tsp. freshly ground pepper
Sour cream

Blanch bacon by bringing 2 cups water to boil, add bacon and boil 3 minutes. Drain and dry between paper towels. Place bacon and butter in heavy 4-qt. pan, brown bacon over medium heat, remove, set aside. Add onions and cook over medium-high heat until golden. Reduce heat to low, stir in paprika, add pork and combine well. Add broth, cover and simmer 1 hour. Stir in sauerkraut, bacon, tomato paste and caraway seeds. Cover and cook 30 minutes more, adding more broth if necessary. Add salt and pepper. Serve and pass sour cream separately.

May be prepared 3-4 days before serving. In fact, this will enhance flavors. Perfect for New Year's Day buffet.

STUFFED SAUSAGE PATTIES

Serves: 6

1 1/2 lb. bulk pork sausage
1 cup herb seasoned stuffing mix
1/4 cup boiling water
2 Tbsp. butter, melted
1 cup pared and finely chopped tart apple
1/2 cup finely chopped celery
1/4 cup minced onion
1/4 cup minced fresh parsley
2 Tbsp. chili sauce
1/4 tsp. dry mustard
1/4 tsp. pepper
6 spiced apple rings
6 parsley sprigs

Shape sausage into 12 1/4" thick patties. Toss stuffing mix with water and butter. Stir in next 7 ingredients. Place 6 patties in shallow baking pan. Top each with stuffing. Place remaining patties over and press edges together. Put toothpick down through center of each. Bake at 375° for about 45 minutes. Remove picks and top each with apple ring and parsley sprig.

Serve these for an easy dinner, good for a brunch or hearty breakfast.

SAUSAGE-APPLE RING

Serves: 8

2 lb. lean bulk sausage
1 1/2 cups cracker crumbs
2 eggs, slightly beaten
1/2 cup milk
1/4 cup minced onion
1 cup finely chopped, peeled tart apple

Break up sausage and mix well with remaining ingredients. Pack into greased 6-cup ring mold and turn out or shape into ring and place in shallow baking pan. Bake at 350° for 1 hour. Drain off fat. Cut in wedges to serve.

Fill center with scrambled eggs, garnish with fruit and serve to 12 people for brunch.

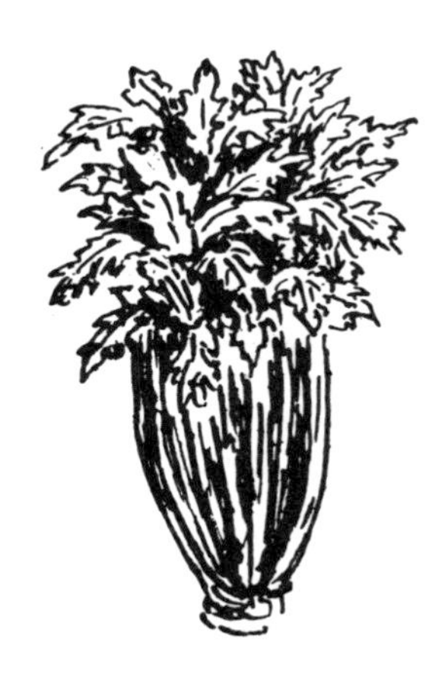

PORK AND SAUERKRAUT ROLL

Serves: 4-6

1 lb. ground pork
1/2 cup fine dry bread crumbs
1 egg, beaten
1 tsp. salt
1/4 tsp. pepper
1/2 tsp. Worcestershire sauce
1 16-oz. can sauerkraut, drained and snipped
1/2 cup chopped onion
5 slices bacon

Mix together first 6 ingredients. On wax paper pat out to 10″x7″ rectangle. Roll up jelly-roll fashion and place in shallow baking dish. Arrange sauerkraut and onion evenly over. Cover with bacon slices. Bake at 350° for 40-45 minutes.

Be energy efficient and bake yams or potatoes with meat.

JAMBALAYA

Serves: 6-8

8 small pork sausages
1/2 cup chopped onion
1/2 cup chopped green pepper
1 clove garlic, crushed
1 cup diced cooked chicken
1 cup diced cooked ham
1 28-oz. can tomatoes
2 cups chicken broth
1 cup long grain rice
1/4 tsp. thyme
1/2 tsp. salt
1 tsp. Worcestershire sauce
16 cooked shrimp

In heavy skillet, cook sausages until brown. Remove and cut in thirds. Leave 2 Tbsp. fat in pan. Sauté onion, pepper and garlic until crisp-tender. Add next 3 ingredients. Cook over medium heat 7-10 minutes or until liquid partially evaporates. In large saucepan combine next 5 ingredients. Bring to boil, cover and cook 15 minutes. Stir rice, shrimp and sausage into tomato mixture. Heat through.

The flavors blend wonderfully if this is made ahead. The sausage is a marvelous addition.

BLEU CHEESE PORK CHOPS

Serves: 6

6 large pork chops for stuffing
3 Tbsp. butter
1 tsp. minced onion
1/4 cup chopped mushrooms
3 oz. Bleu cheese
3/4 cup fine dry bread crumbs

Trim excess fat from chops. Melt butter. Sauté onions and mushrooms for 5 minutes. Stir in cheese and crumbs. Stuff chops. Secure opening with toothpicks. Over medium-high heat lightly brown chops, turn heat to low and cook covered 1 hour or until tender.

These are delicious barbecued on a covered grill.

CARIBBEAN PORK CHOPS

Serves: 6

6 thick pork chops, well trimmed
3 Tbsp. salad oil
1 large onion, chopped
1 clove garlic, minced
1/4 cup peanut butter
1 1/2 Tbsp. brown sugar
1 tsp. salt
1/2 tsp. curry powder
2 tsp. soy sauce
1/4 tsp. pepper
1 cup warm water
1/2 cup orange juice
1 small orange, sliced
1 small green pepper, seeded and cut in rings

Brown chops well in oil. Drain off all fat. Sprinkle onion and garlic over and around chops. Combine next 7 ingredients and mix well. Stir in juice. Pour over chops. Place orange slices and pepper rings on chops. Simmer covered for about 50 minutes or until chops are tender. Stir sauce and baste chops occasionally while cooking. Add small amount of water if needed.

Garnish with sections of fresh orange and pineapple chunks, if desired.

HAM LOAF

Serves: 12

2 lb. ground smoked ham
1 lb. ground pork
10 graham crackers, crushed
1 cup milk
1 egg
1 Tbsp. brown sugar
2 Tbsp. vinegar
1/4 tsp. pepper
1/3 cup brown sugar
1 tsp. dry mustard
1/4 cup vinegar
Pineapple rings
Maraschino cherry halves

Mustard Sauce:
2 egg yolks, slightly beaten
1/4 cup vinegar
1/4 cup sugar
2 Tbsp. dry mustard
1 5 1/2-oz. can evaporated milk
1/4 tsp. salt

Combine first 8 ingredients. Shape into loaf. Pour 1/4 cup water into pan around loaf. Bake at 350° for 45 minutes. Combine next 3 ingredients and pour over. Decorate with pineapple rings and cherries. Bake 15 minutes more. For Mustard Sauce: combine all ingredients. Cook, stirring over low heat for 5 minutes. Sauce will thicken when cool.

Everyone has a favorite ham loaf recipe, but this one is well worth trying.

PORK CHOPS AND APPLES IN MUSTARD SAUCE

Serves: 4

2 lb. apples
4 pork loin chops, 3/4" thick
1/4 tsp. salt
1 Tbsp. butter
1/4 cup dry white wine
1 cup whipping cream
1/3 cup Dijon mustard
1/4 tsp. salt
1/4 tsp. white pepper

Peel, core and slice apples thinly. Spread in buttered 8"x11" baking dish. Bake at 400° for 15 minutes. Trim fat from chops, salt and brown in butter over medium-high heat 7-8 minutes per side. Arrange chops over apples. Deglaze pan with wine, reducing by half. Pour over pork chops. Mix remaining ingredients, pour over chops and shake dish so sauce goes through to apples. Bake at 400° for about 15 minutes.

The taste combination is superb and this can be presented proudly to company.

BAKED HAM IN CIDER WITH CIDER SAUCE

Serves: 20

10-12 lb. fully cooked ham, bone in
3/4 cup sliced onion
1 bay leaf, crumbled
4 cups apple cider
1 cup brown sugar, packed
1 Tbsp. lemon juice
Whole cloves

Cider Sauce:
4 cups cider
2 lb. McIntosh apples
1/2 cup sugar
1 cup golden raisins
1/4 tsp. cinnamon

Place ham in shallow roasting pan without rack. Arrange 1/2 cup onion slices over ham. Sprinkle with bay leaf. Pour 2 cups cider into pan. Cover pan tightly with foil. Bake at 325° for 2 1/2 hours. While ham bakes, combine 2 cups cider, brown sugar, lemon juice and 1/4 cup sliced onion. Boil uncovered 5 minutes. Strain. Pour all liquid from roasting pan. With sharp knife make diagonal cuts in ham, 1/4" deep and 1" apart. Place clove in center of each cut. Pour cider mixture over ham. Bake uncovered 45 minutes more, basting every 15 minutes. Let stand 20 minutes before carving. Serve cider sauce separately. For Cider Sauce: bring 4 cups cider to boil. Boil gently over medium heat for 20 minutes or until cider is reduced to 1 cup. Pare and quarter apples and add with sugar. Simmer gently until apples are soft, about 20 minutes. Add raisins and cinnamon last 5 minutes. Makes 3 1/2 cups sauce.

An excellent recipe. And sauce would be good with roast pork or ham loaf.

APRICOT PORK CHOPS

Serves: 6

1/2 cup boiling water
18 dried apricot halves
6 pork chops, 3/4″-1″ thick
1 tsp. salt
1/4 tsp. pepper
1/2 tsp. thyme, crushed
1/4 cup maple syrup

Pour boiling water over apricots, cool to room temperature, drain and save liquid. Trim fat from chops. Heat fat in skillet, render 1 Tbsp., remove fat and brown chops on both sides. Pour off excess fat. Combine remaining ingredients with apricot liquid. Pour over chops. Top each with 3 apricot halves. Cover and cook over low heat about 1 hour. Cook uncovered last few minutes, spooning sauce over chops.

Prepare these ahead, place in baking dish and cover. Then bake at 350° for 1 hour, remove cover last 10 minutes and baste.

HAM 'N NOODLES DANDY

Serves: 6-8

1/2 lb. green noodles
1 clove garlic, crushed
1/2 cup chopped onion
2 Tbsp. butter
1/2 lb. ham, cubed
1 8-oz. carton large curd cottage cheese
1 10 1/2-oz. can cream of mushroom soup
1/2 cup milk
1/4 cup grated Parmesan cheese

Cook noodles according to package directions, using minimum cooking time. Drain. Sauté garlic and onion in butter. Add ham. Brown lightly. Remove from heat. Stir in cheese, soup and milk. Combine with noodles. Pour into buttered 2-qt. casserole. Sprinkle over Parmesan cheese. Bake at 350° for 40-45 minutes.

Another good way to use leftover ham. May be prepared ahead. Serve with salad and garlic toast.

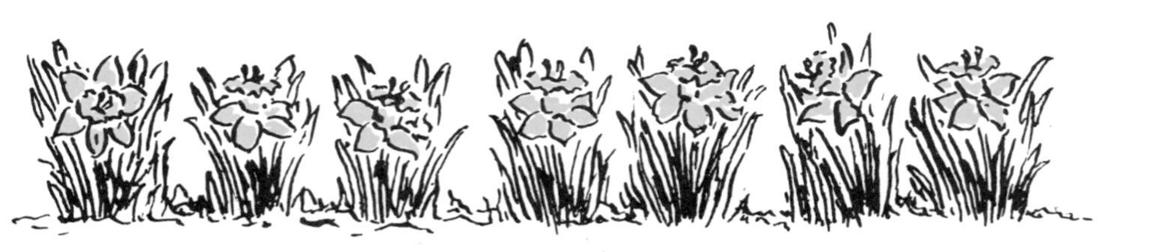

HAM LOGS WITH RAISIN SAUCE

Serves: 4

1 lb. ground ham
1/2 lb. freshly ground pork
3/4 cup millk
1/2 cup quick rolled oats
1/2 tsp. salt
1 egg, beaten
2 Tbsp. horseradish
1/2 tsp. pepper
1 Tbsp. cornstarch
3/4 cup cold water
2 Tbsp. lemon juice
2 Tbsp. vinegar
1/2 cup brown sugar, packed
1/4 cup raisins

Combine first 8 ingredients. Mix well. Shape into 8 logs. Place in 2-qt. shallow baking dish. Blend together cornstarch and water, add remaining ingredients and cook, stirring until mixture bubbles. Pour over ham logs. Bake at 350° for 40-45 minutes, basting several times with sauce.

An easy entrée for an informal dinner and could also be served at brunch.

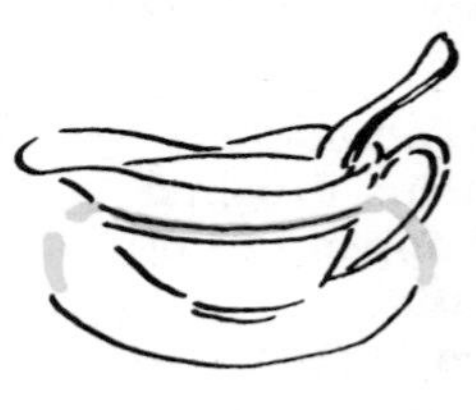

HAM-STUFFED PORK CHOPS

Serves: 6

6 pork chops for stuffing
1/2 tsp. salt
1/4 tsp. ground sage
1/4 tsp. dried thyme leaves
3 cups fresh bread crumbs
1 cup chopped cooked ham
1/8 tsp. pepper
1/4 tsp. nutmeg
1 egg, beaten
1 10 1/2-oz. can beef broth
2 Tbsp. salad oil
1/4 cup water

Rub pork chops with salt and herbs. Combine next 5 ingredients and stir in 1/2 cup beef broth. Stuff pork chops. Rub with salad oil. Brown well on both sides in heavy skillet. Place in baking pan. Pour over remaining beef broth and water. Bake covered at 350° for 1 hour.

Stir a little horseradish into sour cream with a dash of salt and white pepper for a sauce to serve separately.

GLAZED HAM LOAF

Serves: 8-10

2 lb. ground smoked ham
1 lb. ground fresh pork
2 cups soft bread crumbs
3/4 cup milk
2 eggs, slightly beaten
1 Tbsp. prepared mustard
1/2 tsp. salt
1 cup brown sugar, packed
1/2 cup vinegar
1/4 cup water
1/4 tsp. cinnamon
1/4 tsp. ground cloves

Combine first 7 ingredients. Shape into 2 loaves and place in 9″x13″ pan. Bake at 350° for 1 hour. Combine remaining ingredients and boil 3 minutes. Pour off all fat from ham loaves. Spoon sauce over meat. Bake 30 minutes more, basting occasionally to glaze loaves. Let stand 10 minutes before slicing.

There are dozens of recipes for ham loaf, but this basic one is one of the best!

SPINACH STUFFED HAM

Serves: 20

8-10 lb. semi-boneless fully cooked ham
10 oz. fresh spinach
1 bunch parsley
8 green onions with tops
3/4 cup dry red wine
1/2 cup honey

With sharp knife, make X-shaped cuts 3″ deep and 1″ apart all across top of ham. Trim stems and coarse ribs from spinach. Trim stems from parsley. Rinse and dry all greens well, chop coarsely and mix together. With fingers press and pack greens mixture into cuts. Place ham, stuffed side up on rack in shallow pan. Pour 1/4 cup wine over ham. Bake at 300° for 2 hours. After 1 hour, pour another 1/4 cup wine over ham. Combine last 1/4 cup wine with honey and baste ham frequently last 1/2 hour. Let stand 20 minutes before carving.

If you carve well, do so at the table, for this ham is most attractive before it is cut.

CHINESE SPARERIBS

Serves: 4

3 lb. spareribs
3 cloves garlic, crushed
1 tsp. seasoned salt
1/2 tsp. salt
1/2 cup honey
1/4 cup soy sauce
1/4 cup catsup
1/2 tsp. prepared mustard
2 chicken bouillon cubes
1 cup boiling water

Cut spareribs into serving size pieces. Mix next 7 ingredients. Dissolve bouillon cubes in water, add to sauce. Pour over ribs and marinate overnight, turning occasionally. Remove ribs from marinade, place on rack in roasting pan and bake at 325° for 1 hour 15 minutes, basting frequently with marinade. Turn ribs for even browning.

These adapt easily to an appetizer that serves 8. Just cut into pieces that can be held in the fingers.

RIBS AND RED CABBAGE

Serves 6-8

4 lb. country style pork spareribs in serving size pieces
1/2 tsp. salt
1/4 tsp. pepper
1 medium red cabbage, coarsely shredded
1/4 cup flour
3 Tbsp. firmly packed brown sugar
1 tsp. salt
1/4 tsp. pepper
1/2 cup chopped onion
1/2 cup vinegar
1/2 cup raisins
1/3 cup water
2 tsp. caraway seeds
1 apple, peeled, cored and diced

Sprinkle spareribs lightly with salt and pepper, place on rack in roasting pan and bake at 350° for 1 hour and 15 minutes. Remove ribs and rack from pan. Pour off drippings. Into pan stir together all remaining ingredients, place ribs on top, cover and bake 1 hour more or until ribs and cabbage are tender. Remove cover and stir cabbage mixture once or twice while baking.

Combine red and green cabbage, if you like or add a shredded carrot or two.

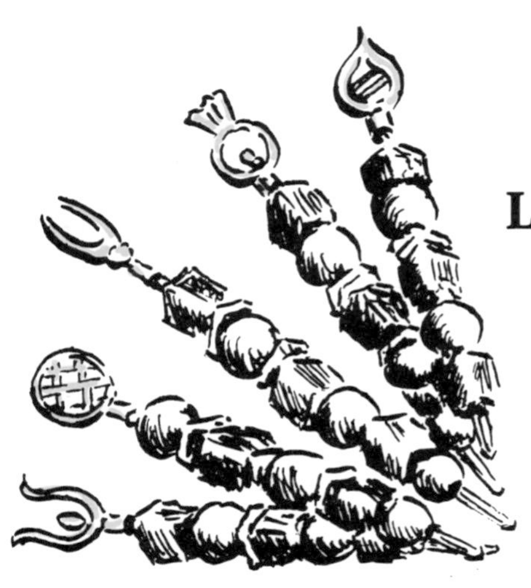

Lamb

LAMB PILAF CASSEROLE

Serves: 8-10

4 Tbsp. butter
3 lb. boned lamb cut in 1″ cubes
1 large onion, thinly sliced
1/2 tsp. cinnamon
1/2 tsp. freshly ground pepper
1 1/2 cups uncooked rice
1 cup white raisins
1 tsp. salt
1 10 1/2-oz. can consommé
1 1/4 cups water
1/4 cup lemon juice
3 oz. almonds, sliced and toasted
4 Tbsp. chopped fresh parsley

In large skillet over high heat melt 2 Tbsp. butter and quickly brown 1/2 cubes lamb. Remove to paper towels, wipe pan clean and repeat, saving fat. Lower heat to medium. Sauté onion with cinnamon and pepper 3-5 minutes. Sprinkle 1/2 rice in buttered 2 1/2-qt. casserole. Layer 1/2 meat, onions and raisins. Repeat. Combine salt, consommé and water. Carefully pour over. Bake covered at 400° for 50 minutes. Remove cover. Sprinkle lemon juice and almonds over meat. Bake 10 minutes more. Sprinkle with parsley to serve.

Assemble early in the day. Pour consommé over meat just before baking.

MINTED LAMB

Serves: 8

5 lb. leg of lamb
3 cups cider vinegar
1/4 cup dried mint leaves
1 Tbsp. salt
1 tsp. whole cloves
1/4 tsp. pepper

Marinate lamb in remaining ingredients 12-24 hours, turning occasionally. Bake on rack in roasting pan at 300° for 30-35 minutes per pound or until meat thermometer registers 175°.

If you have fresh mint, by all means use it, but double the quantity and crush it thoroughly.

BROILED OR BARBECUED BONED LAMB **Serves: 8-10**

1 7-lb. leg of lamb
1 1/2 cups French dressing
1 clove garlic, crushed
1 1/2 cups chopped onion
2 tsp. barbecue spice
1 tsp. salt
1 tsp. freshly ground pepper
1/2 tsp. oregano
1 bay leaf, crushed

Have butcher trim, bone and cut leg to lie flat. Place in plastic bag. Combine remaining ingredients, pour over lamb and secure bag. Place in pan and refrigerate 2-3 days, turning often. Barbecue on grill for about 45 minutes, brushing with marinade and turning once with tongs. Or broil in oven 4″ from heat for 10 minutes, turn with tongs, baste and broil 10 minutes. Turn oven to 450° and bake for 25-35 minutes. Center should be pink. Carve against grain in 1/4″ thick slices.

Even those who dislike lamb will like this. Serve with Béarnaise sauce, in "Sauces and Et Ceteras."

LAMB KABOBS AND PEACHES **Serves: 4**

1 1-lb can pitted purple plums
2 Tbsp. lemon juice
1 Tbsp. soy sauce
1 tsp. Worcestershire sauce
1/2 clove garlic, minced
1/4 tsp. dried basil, crushed
1 lb. lean lamb, cut in 1″ cubes
1/2 tsp. salt
1/4 tsp. pepper
4 canned peach halves
2 tsp. butter
Hot cooked rice

Drain plums, saving 1/2 cup plum juice. Puree plums by pressing through sieve. Combine juice, plums and next 5 ingredients. Add lamb cubes, stir together and marinate, covered, several hours at room temperature or in refrigerator overnight. Stir often. Preheat broiler. Place lamb cubes on skewers and season with salt and pepper. Broil 4″ from heat for 8-10 minutes, turning and basting with marinade. Dot each peach half with 1/2 tsp. butter and place on broiler rack. Broil 3-5 minutes more until heated through and lamb is done. Place kabobs on rice, heat and pass remaining marinade.

A cousin to shish kabobs, this is somewhat sweet.

LAMB SHANKS MEDITERRANEAN

Serves: 4

4 lamb shanks, trimmed
2 Tbsp. lemon juice
1/2 tsp. salt
1/2 tsp. pepper
2 Tbsp. olive oil
1 clove garlic, minced
1 large onion, quartered
1/2 tsp. oregano
1/2 cup hot bouillon
1/2 cup dry white wine
1 10-oz. pkg. frozen artichoke hearts, defrosted
2 Tbsp. minced parsley
Rind of 1 lemon, grated
1 Tbsp. cornstarch
1/4 cup water

Rub shanks with 1 Tbsp. lemon juice, salt and pepper. In Dutch oven brown in oil on all sides. Sprinkle with 1 Tbsp. lemon juice, garlic, onion and oregano. Bake covered at 300° for about 2 1/2 hours. Add next 5 ingredients, raise heat to 350° and bake covered 20-30 minutes more. Remove meat and artichoke hearts to warm platter. Blend cornstarch and water and thicken pan juices. Serve sauce separately.

If you wish, you may add dried apricots to the pan with the artichokes. Colorful!

LAMB STUFFED EGGPLANT

Serves: 6

12 small, oval Italian eggplants
1/2 cup olive oil
1/2 cup salad oil
1 large onion, chopped
2 cloves garlic, minced
1 lb. ground lamb
1/3 cup pine nuts
1/4 tsp. ginger
1/4 tsp. pepper
1/2 tsp. allspice
1/4 tsp. cinnamon
1/4 tsp. cumin
1 tsp. salt
1 1-lb. can tomatoes

Partially peel eggplants in stripes, leaving on stem. Combine oils, reserving 2 Tbsp., and lightly fry eggplants. Arrange side by side in rectangular baking dish. Make a pocketlike slit in each. Sauté onion and garlic in reserved oil until golden, add lamb and nuts and brown lightly. Stir in spices. Fill pockets evenly with mixture. Cut up tomatoes in can and pour over. Bake at 375° for about 15 minutes.

If served in combination with another meat dish, this authentic Middle-Eastern recipe serves 12.

LAMB AND WHITE BEAN CASSEROLE

Serves: 4-6

2 Tbsp. butter
1 large onion, sliced
1 clove garlic, minced
1/2 tsp. salt
1/2 tsp. dried basil
1/4 tsp. dried rosemary
1 1-lb. can tomatoes
1 Tbsp. chopped fresh parsley
2 cups cooked lamb, cubed
2 20-oz. cans navy beans
1 bay leaf
1 cup lamb or rich beef gravy

Melt butter. Sauté onion and garlic 3 minutes. Add salt, basil and rosemary. Break up and add undrained tomatoes. Simmer uncovered 20 minutes. Stir sauce, parsley, lamb and beans into 2-qt. casserole. Top with bay leaf. Bake uncovered at 350° for about 30 minutes. Remove bay leaf. Heat gravy and stir in before serving.

A good way to turn a little bit of leftover lamb into a big meal.

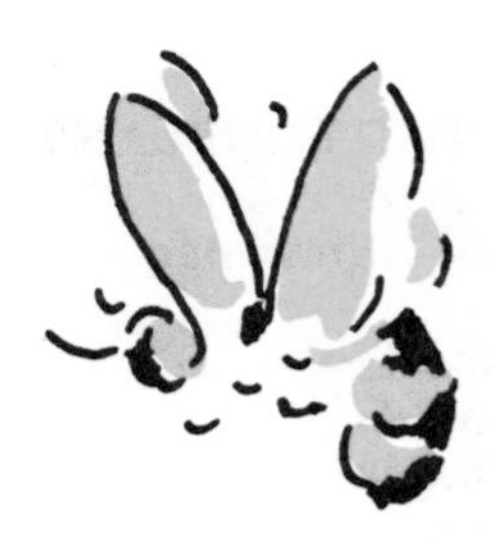

LAMB AND BEEF CURRY BALLS

Serves: 6-8

1 lb. ground lamb
1 lb. ground meat loaf mixture
1/2 cup uncooked rice
1/2 cup tomato juice
1 medium onion, chopped
1 tsp. garlic salt
1/2 tsp. curry powder
1 large onion, sliced
1 large green pepper, cut in large squares
1 10 3/4-oz. can tomato soup
1/2 cup water
1 Tbsp. sugar
1 tsp. curry powder

Break up ground meats and mix well with next 5 ingredients. Shape into 12-16 balls. Place in single layer in shallow baking dish. Top with onion and green pepper. Combine remaining ingredients and pour over. Cover tightly and bake at 400° for 1/2 hour. Reduce heat to 325° and bake 2 hours more.

Use this meat mixture to stuff green peppers. Pour sauce over but omit sliced onion and green pepper squares.

ROAST LEG OF LAMB

Serves: 8-10

1 6-lb. leg of lamb
1 tsp. dried thyme
1 1/2 tsp. dried rosemary
1 tsp. salt
1 tsp. pepper
1 cup chopped green onions with tops
2 cups chicken stock
8 medium potatoes, peeled
2 Tbsp. water
2 Tbsp. flour
1 lb. spinach, steamed and drained
1 cup sour cream

Trim leg of lamb and rub in seasonings. Place on rack in roasting pan. Cover with green onions. Bake at 400° for 20 minutes. Reduce heat to 325° and bake about 2 1/2 hours. Baste every 1/2 hour with chicken stock. Arrange potatoes around roast for last 1 hour of cooking. Remove meat and potatoes to large platter and keep warm. Add any remaining chicken stock to roasting pan. Bring to boil. Stir flour and water together. Add slowly and stir until thickened. Simmer 5 minutes. Arrange spinach topped with sour cream on platter with meat and potatoes. Slice roast and pass gravy.

A lamb shoulder roast may be substituted. Increase cooking time by an hour.

LAMB CHOPS WITH ORANGE

Serves: 6

6 1/2″ thick loin lamb chops
2 Tbsp. salad oil
1/2 cup orange juice
1/4 cup soy sauce
1 1/2 tsp. ground ginger
1/4 tsp. garlic salt
1/4 tsp. pepper
1/2 tsp. sugar
2 oranges, peeled and sectioned

Trim fat from chops, brown lightly in oil, and drain on paper towels. Place chops in shallow baking dish. Combine orange juice, soy sauce and seasonings. Pour over chops. Cover and refrigerate 4 hours, turning once. Bake chops covered in marinade at 350° for 45 minutes. Place orange sections on chops, baste with pan juices, and bake uncovered 10 minutes more.

These actually may be marinated many hours or overnight.

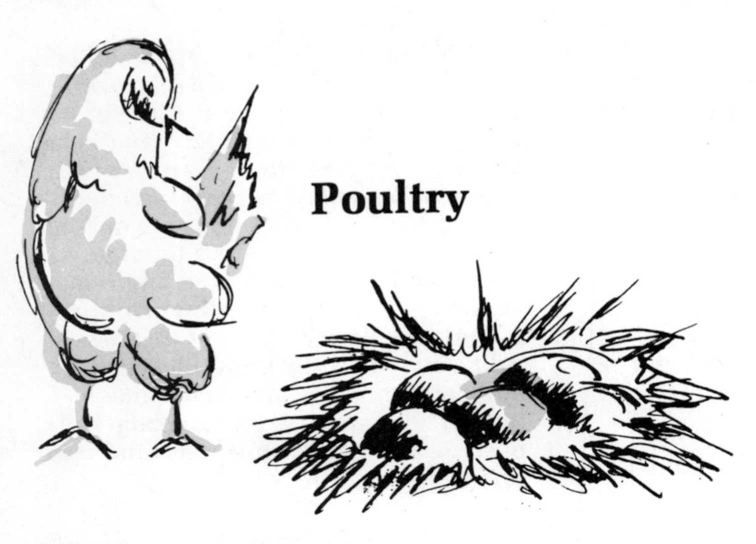

Poultry

CHICKEN BROCCOLI CRÊPES

Serves: 8

Crêpes:
1 cup flour
1 1/2 cup milk
2 eggs
1 Tbsp. salad oil
1/2 tsp. salt

Sauce:
6 Tbsp. butter
6 Tbsp. flour
1 tsp. salt
3 cups milk
1 5 1/2-oz. jar sharp cheese spread
1/4 cup dry white wine

Filling:
1 cup sauce
1 10-oz. pkg. chopped broccoli, cooked and drained
2 1/2 cups chopped cooked chicken
1 2 1/2-oz. jar mushroom pieces, drained

For Crêpes: beat ingredients with rotary beater until well blended. Refrigerate 1 hour. Pour 2 Tbsp. batter into buttered 6″ crêpe pan and cook over medium-high heat for about 1 1/2 minutes, turning once. Repeat. Cool and stack. For Sauce: melt butter in saucepan. Stir in flour. Slowly add salt and milk. Cook, stirring until thickened and smooth. Add cheese and stir until melted. Add wine, stirring until smooth. Set aside to cool. For Filling: combine all ingredients. Spread 1/4 cup filling on each crêpe. Roll up and place seam side down in baking dish. Top each crêpe with more sauce. Bake at 325° for 30 minutes or until heated through.

A good make-ahead dish for a ladies' luncheon or an effortless and elegant company dinner.

ALMOND TOPPED CHICKEN PIE

Serves: 6

1 Tbsp. cornstarch
1/2 tsp. salt
1 tsp. Worcestershire sauce
1 8-oz. carton sour cream
2 cups cooked chicken, diced
1 cup grated American cheese
2 Tbsp. pimento
2 Tbsp. chopped green pepper
3-4 drops Tabasco sauce
2 Tbsp. minced onion
1 9″ pie shell, unbaked
1/2 cup slivered almonds
2 tsp. butter

Stir first 3 ingredients into sour cream. Add next 6 ingredients. Spoon into pie shell. Bake at 400° for 25 minutes. Toast almonds in butter. Sprinkle over pie. Bake 5-10 minutes more or until set.

Another versatile dish that can be a luncheon or dinner entrée or can be served as an appetizer.

COUNTRY STYLE CHICKEN KIEV

Serves: 4

1/2 cup bread crumbs
2 Tbsp. grated Parmesan cheese
1 tsp. basil
1 tsp. oregano
1/2 tsp. garlic salt
1/4 tsp. salt
2 whole chicken breasts, split
2/3 cup butter, melted
1/4 cup white wine or apple juice
1/4 cup chopped green onion
1/4 cup chopped fresh parsley

Combine first 6 ingredients. Dip chicken pieces in butter. Set remaining butter aside. Roll in crumbs. Place skin side up in 1 1/2-qt. shallow casserole. Bake at 375° for 50-60 minutes. To leftover butter add remaining ingredients. Pour over baked chicken. Bake 2-3 minutes more.

Though not boned and rolled as is a true Kiev, these chicken breasts taste surprisingly like the original.

CASHEW CHICKEN

Serves: 4-6

3 whole chicken breasts
1 4-oz. pkg. cashew nuts
1 1/2 Tbsp. salad oil
1/2 lb. snow peas, ends removed
1 1/2 lb. fresh mushrooms, sliced
1 tsp. salt
1 1/2 tsp. sugar
1 cup chicken broth
2 Tbsp. cornstarch
1/4 cup soy sauce
4 whole green onions, cut in 1 1/2″ lengths, ends of each slashed to form brush
Hot cooked rice

Skin and bone chicken. Cut in bite-size chunks. Sauté cashews in 1 Tbsp. oil 1 minute until toasted. Remove from skillet. Add remaining oil. Add chicken and cook quickly until opaque. Add next 5 ingredients. Cover and cook 2 minutes. Mix cornstarch and soy sauce. Add to pan and cook until thickened, stirring gently. Stir in onions. Immediately serve over rice and sprinkle with nuts.

This is meant to be cooked in a wok, though a large skillet will work well.

CHICKEN BAKED WITH CURRY SAUCE

Serves: 8

8 large chicken breast halves
6 Tbsp. flour
1/2 tsp. salt
1 tsp. ginger
6 Tbsp. butter
1 medium onion, chopped
6 slices bacon, diced
1 Tbsp. curry powder
2 Tbsp. flour
1 Tbsp. sugar
1 10 1/2-oz. can beef broth
1/4 cup coconut
2 Tbsp. applesauce
2 Tbsp. catsup
2 Tbsp. lemon juice

Shake chicken breasts in 6 Tbsp. flour, salt and ginger. Melt butter in shallow 3-qt. baking dish. Roll chicken pieces in butter and turn skin side up. Bake chicken uncovered at 375° for 20 minutes. Combine remaining ingredients, bring to boil stirring constantly, then simmer 15 minutes, stirring often. Baste chicken with 1/2 curry sauce. Bake 20 minutes. Pour over remaining sauce. Bake 20 minutes more.

For a quick dinner, cut leftover cooked chicken into chunks, make sauce, add chicken and heat through. Serve over rice.

BHUNA CHICKEN

Serves: 4-6

2 Tbsp. butter
1 medium onion, chopped
3 cloves garlic, finely chopped
1 tsp. powdered ginger
1 tsp. tumeric
2 tsp. salt
1 1/2 tsp. garamsala
1 tsp. chili powder
1 28-oz. can whole or crushed tomatoes
2 Tbsp. yogurt
4 whole chicken breasts, boned and cut in 1″ pieces
1 tsp. lemon juice
1 Tbsp. grated coconut
3 Tbsp. chopped fresh parsley
Cooked rice

Garamsala:
3 Tbsp. ground black pepper
1 Tbsp. cumin powder
1 tsp. ground cinnamon
2 tsp. cardamom
3 Tbsp. coriander
1 tsp. ground cloves
1 1/2 tsp. mace
1/2 tsp. nutmeg

Melt butter in large heavy skillet over medium heat. Add onion and cook 2 minutes, stirring. Add garlic and ginger. Sauté 1 more minute. Add next 4 ingredients. Sauté 1 more minute. Mixture will be very dry. Add tomatoes and yogurt. If whole tomatoes are used, cut coarsely. Mix well. Stir in chicken pieces. Cover with tight fitting lid. Cook until chicken is tender, about 35 minutes. Stir in lemon juice, parsley and coconut. Cook 5 more minutes. Serve over rice. For Garamsala: mix together all ingredients. Store in glass jar with tight lid.

Garamsala, used in place of curry powder for seasoning Eastern meat dishes, will keep many months, though you may choose to cut recipe in half.

CHICKEN-TORTILLA CASSEROLE

Serves: 6

4 whole chicken breasts
12 corn tortillas
1 10 3/4-oz. can cream of mushroom soup
1 10 3/4-oz. can cream of chicken soup
1 cup milk
1 medium onion, chopped
1 7-oz. can green chile salsa
1/2 lb. Cheddar cheese, shredded

Skin, bone, and cut chicken breasts in quarters. Cut tortillas in 1″ strips. Combine next 5 ingredients. Cover bottom of buttered 2-qt. casserole with 1/3 tortillas, 1/3 chicken breasts, 1/3 soup mixture. Repeat twice. Top with cheese. Let stand 24 hrs. in refrigerator. Bake at 325° for 1 1/2 hrs.

Margaritas served before dinner would make this good casserole taste even better.

ELEGANT STUFFED CHICKEN QUARTERS

Serves: 4

3 Tbsp. butter
2 medium zucchini, shredded
3 slices white bread
1 egg, beaten
1/2 cup shredded Swiss cheese
1/2 tsp. pepper
1 2 1/2-3 lb. chicken, quartered
2 Tbsp. honey
1/4 tsp. salt

Melt butter, add zucchini and cook, stirring 2 minutes. Tear bread in small pieces. Stir into zucchini with next 3 ingredients. Carefully loosen skin on chicken quarters by pushing fingers between skin and meat to form pockets. Insert 1/4 stuffing in each. Place in 9″ × 13″ pan and bake at 400° for 50 minutes or until tender. To serve brush with honey and salt.

Minced onion, sautéed with the zucchini, would be good addition as would a bit of oregano.

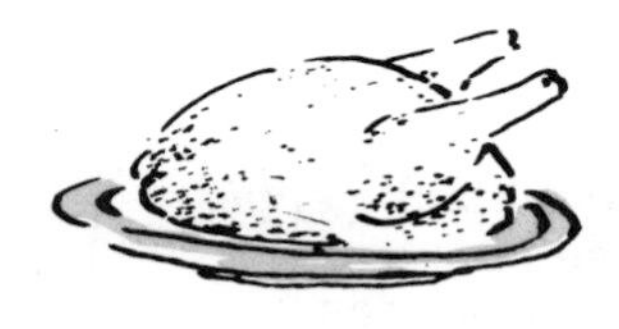

CHICKEN PARMESAN

Serves: 4-6

2 lb. chicken pieces
1 egg
1 tsp. water
1 cup bread crumbs
1/2 cup grated Parmesan cheese
1/4 cup salad oil
2 15-oz. cans tomato sauce
1/2 cup chopped onion
1/2 tsp. garlic powder
1/2 tsp. basil
1/2 tsp. oregano
1/2 tsp. salt
1/2 tsp. sugar
6 oz. Mozzarella cheese, shredded
3 Tbsp. grated Parmesan cheese

Remove skin from chicken. Combine egg and water. Stir together crumbs and cheese. Dip chicken in egg, then roll in crumbs. Brown in oil in heavy skillet. Pour off excess oil and stir in next 7 ingredients. Bake covered at 350° for 1 hour. Sprinkle with cheese. Return to oven uncovered for 10 minutes.

Serve with either pasta or hot mashed potatoes and a good green salad.

CHICKEN MONTEREY

Serves: 8

4 large whole chicken breasts
1/2 tsp. salt
1/4 tsp. white pepper
1/4 cup flour
1 stick butter
1/2 cup chopped onion
1 clove garlic, minced
8 large mushrooms, chopped
2 Tbsp. flour
1/2 tsp. celery salt
1/2 tsp. white pepper
1 cup chicken stock
1/2 cup white wine
1 1/2 cups grated Monterey Jack cheese

Skin, bone, cut in half and pound chicken breasts thin between 2 sheets of wax paper. Sprinkle with salt and pepper. Dust with flour. Melt 4 Tbsp. butter in skillet. Quickly sauté breasts until golden, no more than 2-3 minutes per side. Place on platter and keep warm. Melt remaining butter in same skillet and sauté onion, mushrooms and garlic 3 minutes. Stir in flour. Remove from heat, stir in seasonings, stock and wine. Cook, stirring until bubbling and thick. Add 1/2 cup cheese, stirring to melt. Arrange chicken breasts in buttered 3-qt. shallow casserole. Pour over cheese sauce. Top with remaining cheese. Bake at 350° for 10-15 minutes.

There is no end to delicious ways to serve chicken breasts.

CHICKEN BREAST ALFREDO

Serves: 4-6

3 whole chicken breasts
1/2 cup flour
3 eggs, beaten
3 Tbsp. water
1 cup Romano cheese, grated
1/4 cup snipped fresh parsley
1/2 tsp. salt
1 cup fine bread crumbs
3 Tbsp. butter
2 Tbsp. salad oil
1 cup whipping cream
1/4 cup water
4 Tbsp. butter
1/2 cup grated Romano cheese
1/4 cup chopped fresh parsley
6 slices Mozzarella cheese

Split and bone chicken breasts. Coat with flour. Mix together next 5 ingredients. Dip chicken in egg mixture, then in crumbs. Sauté chicken in butter and oil until golden, no more than 3-4 minutes per side. Place in buttered 2-qt. shallow casserole. Stir cream, water and butter together over medium heat until butter melts. Add cheese. Cook, stirring 5 minutes. Stir in parsley. Pour over chicken. Top each breast with Mozzarella slice. Bake at 425° for 8-10 minutes.

Prepare ahead and refrigerate. Increase baking time 5-10 minutes. Grand served with wild rice.

INTRIGUING CHICKEN

Serves: 8

2 3-lb. chickens, cut up
1/2 cup strong coffee
1/2 cup brandy
1/2 cup salad oil
1/4 cup honey
2 Tbsp. lemon juice
1 tsp. grated lemon rind
3/4 cup prepared mincemeat
1 Tbsp. cornstarch
2 Tbsp. water

Place chicken in shallow 3-qt. glass baking dish. Combine next 6 ingredients, pour over chicken and marinate over night. Pour off marinade and reserve. Bake chicken uncovered at 375° for 45 minutes, basting frequently with marinade. Save 3/4 cup, place in saucepan, add mincemeat, cornstarch dissolved in water and cook until thickened. Place chicken on platter. Spoon over mincemeat sauce.

Guests will never guess the marinade ingredients in this surprisingly good recipe.

CHICKEN STRATA

Serves: 9-10

8 slices bread
4 cups cooked cut up chicken
1/2 cup finely diced green pepper
1 cup diced celery
1/2 cup Hellmann's mayonnaise
1/2 tsp. chicken stock base
4 eggs
3 cups milk
1/2 tsp. salt
1/4 tsp. pepper
1 cup grated sharp Cheddar cheese
1/2 tsp. paprika
1 10 3/4-oz. can cream of mushroom soup
1/4 cup sour cream

Cut crusts from bread and cube. Place 1/2 bread in buttered 2-qt. shallow casserole. Combine next 5 ingredients. Spoon over bread. Top with remaining bread. Blend together next 4 ingredients and pour over. Cover and refrigerate overnight. Bake uncovered at 350° for 15 minutes. Sprinkle with cheese, paprika and 1/2 can soup. Bake 1 hour more. Heat remaining soup and sour cream together. To serve, cut strata in in squares topped with heated soup sauce.

This calls for large sprigs of fresh parsley and even some pimento for garnish.

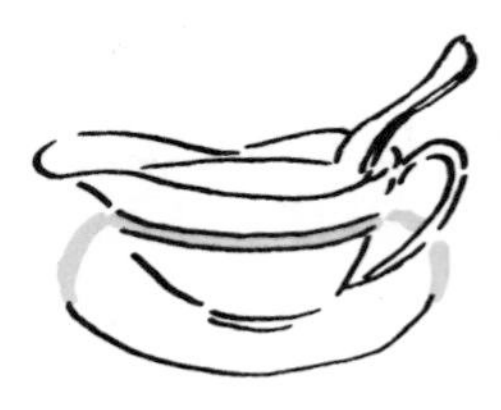

BAKED CHICKEN WITH BARBECUE SAUCE

Serves: 4

2 lb. chicken thighs and drumsticks
1/3 cup flour
1/4 tsp. salt
1/8 tsp. pepper
2 Tbsp. salad oil
1 10 3/4-oz. can tomato soup
1/4 cup chili sauce
1 large onion, chopped
1/4 cup brown sugar packed
1/3 cup sweet pickle relish
1 1/2 tsp. Worcestershire sauce
1/4 tsp. salt
1/8 tsp. pepper

Rinse and pat chicken dry. Shake together with flour, salt and pepper. In heavy skillet, heat oil over medium-high heat, add chicken and brown on all sides. Place in single layer in baking dish. Combine remaining ingredients and pour over chicken. Bake covered at 350° for 1/2 hour. Uncover and bake 1/2 hour more.

The barbecue sauce is marvelous served over mashed potatoes. The recipe doubles easily and also freezes well.

HOT-SAUCED CHICKEN

Serves: 4

1 Tbsp. vinegar
1 tsp. chili powder
1 tsp. salt
3/4 tsp dry mustard
1 Tbsp. sugar
1 Tbsp. Worcestershire sauce
1/8 tsp. cayenne pepper
1/2 tsp. Tabasco sauce
1 tsp. pepper
1 cup water
1 onion, chopped
2 1/2 lb. chicken, cut up
1 stick butter

Combine first 11 ingredients in saucepan. Simmer for 15 minutes. Fry chicken pieces in butter until golden. Pour sauce over chicken. Cover and bake at 350° for 1 hour. Uncover and bake 1/2 hour more.

This could well be called Chili Chicken. For 8 servings, use 2 chickens and 1/2 again as much sauce.

CHICKEN BREAST SUPREME

Serves: 6

6 whole chicken breasts
1 pt. sour cream
1/4 cup lemon juice
4 tsp. Worcestershire sauce
4 tsp. celery salt
1/2 tsp. garlic powder
2 tsp. paprika
1 1/2 cups Italian-seasoned bread crumbs
1 1/2 sticks butter, melted

Bone, skin and cut chicken breasts in half. Combine next 6 ingredients. Pour over chicken and marinate overnight. Remove breasts from marinade. Roll in bread crumbs. Place in buttered 9″x13″ pan. Pour 1/2 melted butter over chicken. Bake covered at 350° for 25 minutes. Pour on remaining butter. Bake uncovered 20 minutes more.

An easy but excellent way to prepare the ever-popular breast of chicken.

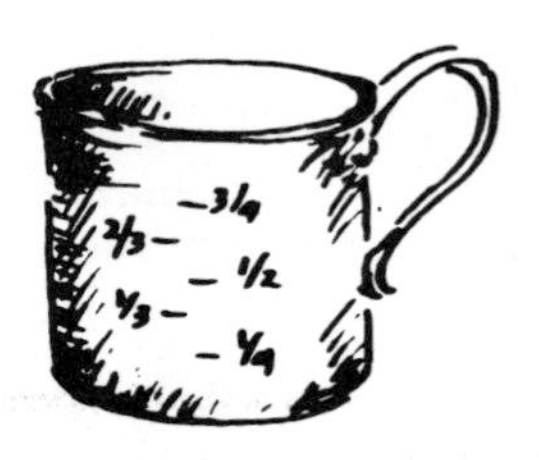

CHEESE BAKED CHICKEN BREASTS

Serves: 8

4 large whole chicken breasts
8 1-oz. slices Swiss cheese
1 10 3/4-oz. can cream of chicken soup
1/4 cup dry white wine
2 cups seasoned stuffing mix
1/3 cup butter, melted
Paprika

Split chicken breasts, remove skin and bone them if desired. Rinse, pat dry and arrange chicken in 2-qt. shallow casserole. Place slice of cheese on each. Stir soup and wine together and pour over. Coarsely crush stuffing mix, sprinkle over, and evenly drizzle on butter. Sprinkle top generously with paprika. Bake uncovered at 350° for 45-55 minutes.

To ensure a rich cheese sauce, double the amount of soup and wine. Serve with rice.

WINE-GLAZED CHICKEN AND VEGETABLES

Serves: 4

1 3-lb. chicken, quartered
1/2 tsp. salt
1/4 tsp. pepper
1/4 cup salad oil
2 Tbsp. flour
1 tsp. sugar
1/4 tsp. dried thyme leaves
1/4 tsp. dried rosemary
2 Tbsp. lemon juice
1/2 cup chicken broth
1/2 cup dry red wine
1 lb. baby carrots, parboiled
12 small onions, peeled and parboiled
1/2 lb. fresh small mushrooms
2 Tbsp. chopped fresh parsley

Sprinkle chicken with salt and pepper. Lightly brown chicken in oil in heavy skillet over medium heat. Remove chicken. Mix together flour, sugar and herbs. Stir into pan drippings. Add juice and broth stirring until mixture boils. Add wine, vegetables and chicken. Reduce heat, cover and simmer 30 minutes. Remove cover and continue cooking at medium heat until most liquid is evaporated and a rich glaze coats chicken and vegetables. Garnish with parsley.

Red wine and chicken do go together. Try this dish and see.

CHICKEN LINDOS

Serves: 6

1/4 cup salad oil
1 clove garlic, minced
1 3-lb. chicken, cut up
6 slices bacon, cut in half
1/2 pt. sour cream
1 10 3/4-oz. can cream of chicken soup
1 Tbsp. lemon juice
1 tsp. dried thyme leaves
1/4 lb. fresh mushrooms, sliced
1/2 cup sliced green onions, with tops
1/2 cup sliced black olives
1/4 tsp. celery salt
1/4 tsp. salt
1/8 tsp. white pepper

Heat oil in heavy skillet over medium heat. Lightly brown garlic. Add chicken and brown on all sides. Place chicken in shallow 2-qt. casserole. Cover with bacon pieces. Bake uncovered at 425° for 25 minutes. Pour off fat. Combine remaining ingredients, spoon over chicken, covering each piece entirely. Lower heat to 375° and bake 25 minutes more.

Our rice ring has chili peppers and would accompany this perfectly.

CHICKEN LIVER CASSEROLE

Serves: 4

1 10-oz. pkg. frozen peas and carrots
1 lb. chicken livers
6 Tbsp. flour
1 stick + 2 Tbsp. butter
1 cup milk
1/4 tsp. poultry seasoning
1 chicken bouillon cube

Cook carrots and peas as package directs. Drain and place in shallow 1-qt. casserole. Dredge chicken livers in 4 Tbsp. flour. In skillet sauté quickly in 1 stick butter until browned on all sides. Arrange over vegetables. Add remaining 2 Tbsp. butter to skillet, stir in flour. Slowly add remaining ingredients and cook, stirring constantly until mixture bubbles. Pour into casserole. Bake at 350° for 15 minutes.

This is an ideal recipe to serve at a brunch.

CRAZY CHICKEN

Serves: 8-10

6 whole chicken breasts
1 8-oz. bottle Russian dressing
1 envelope Lipton's dry onion soup mix
1 1-lb. can whole cranberry sauce

Skin, bone and split chicken breasts. Roll into compact shapes and place in 8″ × 11″ baking dish. Mix together remaining ingredients. Cover with foil. Refrigerate 12 hours or overnight. Bake uncovered at 325° for 1 1/2 hrs.

Having weekend guests? Prepare this ahead and pop in oven when needed along with casserole of rice.

CHICKEN LIVERS IN WINE

Serves: 6

6 slices bacon
4 Tbsp. butter
4 green onions with tops, chopped
1/4 cup chopped green pepper
1 lb. chicken livers
4 Tbsp. flour
1 cup dry white wine
2 Tbsp. chopped fresh parsley
1/8 tsp. ground thyme
1/4 tsp. salt
1/8 tsp. freshly ground pepper
Toast points

Cook bacon until crisp, drain, crumble and set aside. Melt butter in same pan and sauté green onions and pepper until crisp-tender. Rinse and dry livers. Coat with flour. Add to vegetables and cook over medium heat stirring often for 5 minutes. Add wine and seasonings and simmer for 5 minutes or until livers are done. Serve over toast points and sprinkle with bacon.

Substitute all or part of the wine with chicken broth, if you wish.

CRAB STUFFED CHICKEN BREASTS

Serves: 6

3 large whole chicken breasts
1/2 tsp. salt
1/4 tsp. pepper
1/2 cup chopped onion
1/2 cup chopped celery
3 Tbsp. butter
3 Tbsp. dry white wine
1 7 1/2-oz. can crabmeat, drained and flaked
1/2 cup herb seasoned stuffing mix
2 Tbsp. flour
1/2 tsp. paprika
2 Tbsp. butter, melted

Sauce:
1 pkg. Hollandaise sauce mix
3/4 cup milk
2 Tbsp. dry white wine
1/2 cup shredded Swiss cheese

Skin, bone and cut chicken breasts in half. Pound between wax paper to flatten. Sprinkle with salt and pepper. Sauté onion and celery in butter to soften. Add wine, crab and stuffing mix. Toss together. Divide between breasts. Carefully roll up, tucking in ends and secure with picks. Combine flour and paprika. Coat chicken. Place in buttered shallow casserole. Drizzle with butter. Bake uncovered at 375° for 45-50 minutes. Baste occasionally. For Sauce: combine mix and milk. Cook, stirring until thick. Add wine. Stir in cheese until melted. Arrange breasts on platter. Cover generously with sauce.

This may be prepared ahead. Coat with flour just before baking.

CHICKEN CANNELLONI

Serves: 8

4 whole chicken breasts
1/2 tsp. salt
1/2 tsp. pepper
2 tsp. Italian seasonings
8 slices Mozzarella cheese
1/4 cup flour
1/4 cup salad oil
1 cup chopped green onions with tops
1/2 lb. mushrooms, sliced
4 medium tomatoes
1 cup chicken stock
1 cup vermouth

Skin, bone, cut in half and pound chicken breasts between sheets of wax paper until thin. Sprinkle with seasonings. Place slice of Mozzarella cheese on each and roll up. Secure with toothpicks. Dredge in flour and sauté in oil until golden on all sides. Remove from pan and set aside. Into same pan sauté onions and mushrooms. Squeeze juice from tomatoes, chop and add. Stir in chicken stock and wine. Bring to a simmer, add chicken breasts and cook covered 1/2 hour. Sauce may be thickened with flour, if desired.

A serving idea would be to dress pasta with sauce, place on warm platter and arrange chicken to top. Garnish with parsley sprigs.

CORNISH HENS MANDARIN

Serves: 8

4 Cornish hens
4 Tbsp. butter
1 11-oz. can mandarin oranges
1 6-oz. jar orange marmalade
1/4 cup Grand Marnier
1 tsp. salt
1/2 tsp. pepper

Have butcher cut frozen hens in half. Remove giblets and place frozen hens cut side down in shallow baking dish. Butter generously. Bake at 350° for 1 hour. Drain oranges, reserve sections, combine juice and marmalade and simmer 10 minutes or until slightly thickened. Remove from heat and stir in sections and liqueur. Salt, pepper and pour sauce over hens. Bake 15-30 minutes more or until hens are brown and glazed. Serve sauce separately.

Serve with wild rice, fresh asparagus and hot homemade rolls. These hens are truly elegant.

HERBED TURKEY

Serves: 12

1 12-lb. turkey
4 Tbsp. butter
1/4 cup minced onion
1/4 cup chopped fresh parsley
1 Tbsp. dried dill
1/2 cup minced celery and leaves
2 small bay leaves, crumbled
1 clove garlic, crushed
1 1/2 tsp. salt
1 tsp. dried thyme
1/2 tsp. white pepper
2 sticks butter, melted
1 tsp. tumeric
1/2 tsp. salt
1/2 tsp. white pepper
1/4 cup chopped fresh parsley
2 Tbsp. snipped fresh dill or 1 Tbsp. dried dill weed

If turkey is frozen, thaw. Rinse and pat dry. Combine next 10 ingredients. Rub inside cavities with mixture. Fasten neck and back openings with skewers. Stir 2 Tbsp. melted butter and tumeric together. Carefully brush entire surface of turkey. Fasten wings and legs. Place on rack in roasting pan. Bake at 325° for about 3 1/2 hours, basting twice with melted butter. When done, brush with remaining butter, season with salt and pepper. Sprinkle with parsley and dill. Return to oven for 5 minutes. Let stand 20 minutes before carving.

The butter and herbs inside the turkey make for the most moist and tender meat. Bake stuffing separately and baste with juice from turkey.

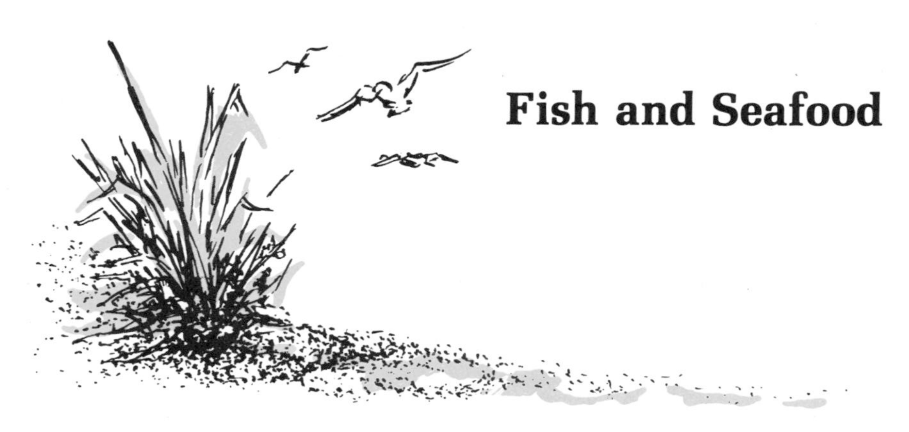

Fish and Seafood

SEAFOOD LASAGNA

Serves: 10-12

9 lasagna noodles
3/4 cup chopped onion
2 Tbsp. butter
1 8-oz. pkg. cream cheese, softened
1 1/2 cups cream style cottage cheese
1 egg, beaten
2 tsp. dried basil, crushed
1/2 tsp. salt
1/4 tsp. pepper
2 10 3/4-oz. cans cream of mushroom soup
1/2 cup milk
1/2 cup dry white wine
1 lb. shelled cooked shrimp, halved
1 7 1/2-oz. can crabmeat, drained, flaked and cleaned
1/4 cup grated Parmesan cheese
3/4 cup grated American cheese

Cook and drain noodles according to package directions. Sauté onion in butter until crisp-tender. Blend in cream cheese. Stir in next 5 ingredients. Arrange 3 noodles in bottom of buttered 9″x13″ baking dish. Spread with 1/3 cheese mixture. Combine soup, milk and wine. Fold in shrimp and crab. Spread 1/3 over cheese layer. Repeat twice. Sprinkle top with Parmesan. Bake uncovered at 350° for 45 minutes. Top with American cheese. Bake 2-3 minutes more. Let stand 15 minutes before serving.

An elegant casserole that may be prepared ahead of time and refrigerated.

SHRIMP IN FRESH TOMATO SAUCE

Serves: 6-8

1/2 cup chopped onion
2 cloves garlic, minced
1/3 cup olive oil
6 cups peeled, seeded and chopped fresh tomatoes
1 1/2 tsp. honey
1 tsp. dried tarragon
3/4 tsp. dried basil
1/2 tsp. dried oregano
1 lb. cooked shrimp
1/8 tsp. Cayenne pepper
1/2 tsp. salt
8 cups cooked linguine
Parmesan cheese

Sauté onion and garlic in oil until crisp-tender. Add next 5 ingredients. Cook covered on low heat for 15 minutes. Stir in shrimp, Cayenne and salt. Heat through. Serve over hot linguine and sprinkle with Parmesan.

Use tiny shrimp, if you can find them, or 2 cans drained minced clams.

STUFFED SOLE WITH SAUCE NEWBURG

Serves: 8

1 1/4 cups finely minced celery
1 1/4 cups finely minced onion
1 medium green pepper, finely minced
1 1/2 sticks butter
1/2 tsp. salt
1/4 tsp. freshly ground pepper
3 tsp. paprika
12 medium shrimp, shelled, deveined and finely chopped
1 1/2 cups fresh bread crumbs
16 small sole or flounder fillets, about 2 lb.

Sauce Newburg:
4 Tbsp. butter
1 Tbsp. flour
1/4 tsp. paprika
2 cups whipping cream
1/2 tsp. salt
1/4 tsp. white pepper
3 egg yolks, beaten
1/4 cup dry sherry

Sauté celery, onion and green pepper in 1 stock butter until just crisp-tender. Stir in salt, pepper and 1 tsp. paprika. Add shrimp and cook, stirring about 1/2 minute. Remove from heat, add bread crumbs and cool. Place 8 fillets on flat surface. Spread filling equally on each and cover with remaining fillets. Place 1 layer in large buttered baking dish. Melt 4 Tbsp. remaining butter and pour over fish. Sprinkle remaining 2 tsp. paprika through sieve over fish. Bake at 450° for 15 minutes or until fish flakes easily. Serve with Sauce Newburg: For Sauce Newburg: melt butter, whisk in flour and paprika and cook, stirring for 1 minute. Remove from heat, add cream, stirring constantly. Return to heat, cook and stir until mixture bubbles. Add salt and pepper. Whisk small amount of hot mixture into yolks, quickly blend yolks into hot mixture. Add sherry and heat through but do not boil.

Flounder may be used instead of sole. Cover skin side with stuffing, top with fillet, skin side down.

FLORIDA FILLETS

Serves: 8

2 lb. skinless snapper
1/2 cup unsweetened frozen orange juice, thawed
1 Tbsp. salad oil
1/4 cup soy sauce
1/4 cup cider vinegar
1/2 tsp. salt
1/4 cup fresh parsley, chopped
Orange slices

Place fish skinned side up in buttered 10″x15″ baking dish. Combine next 5 ingredients and brush fish with sauce. Broil about 4″ from heat for 5 minutes. Turn and brush again. Broil 5-6 minutes more. To serve, sprinkle with parsley and garnish with orange slices.

Though snapper is the best, try broiling other fish fillets with this sauce.

CLAM CASSEROLE

Serves: 6

1 8-oz. pkg. green noodles
1/2 lb. fresh mushrooms, sliced
2 Tbsp. chopped onion
2 Tbsp. butter
2 10 3/4-oz. cans cream of mushroom soup
2 7-oz. cans minced clams, drained
1 pt. sour cream
2 tsp. Worcestershire sauce
2 tsp. curry powder
1 tsp. chopped fresh parsley
1/2 cup white wine
1/8 tsp. oregano
1/4 tsp. salt
3 oz. sharp Cheddar cheese, shredded

Cook noodles as package directs. Drain and set aside. Sauté mushrooms and onions in butter until tender. Stir in next 9 ingredients. Place 1/2 noodles in buttered 2-qt. casserole. Spoon clam mixture over noodles. Top with remaining noodles. Bake at 350° for 45 minutes. Sprinkle cheese over and bake 15 minutes more.

One more can of clams could be used. This is a good addition to a buffet menu.

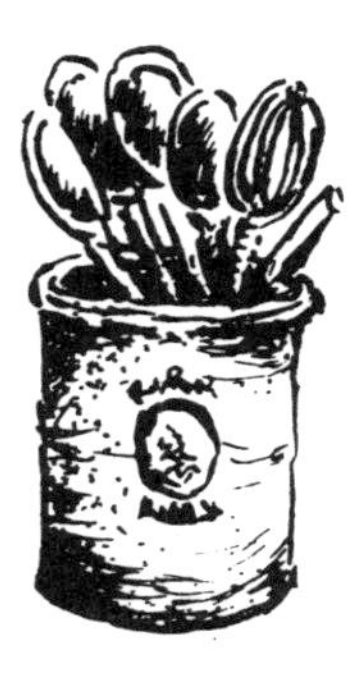

SHRIMP SCAMPI

Serves: 2

1 lb. shrimp
6 Tbsp. butter
2 Tbsp. chopped onion
1 1/2 Tbsp. chopped garlic
1/2 tsp. salt
Freshly ground pepper
1 Tbsp. lemon juice
2 Tbsp. chopped fresh parsley

Shell and clean shrimp, leaving on tails. In heavy skillet, melt butter. Sauté shrimp, onion and garlic 4-6 minutes. Remove shrimp to serving plate. Stir salt, 2 gratings of pepper and lemon juice in skillet. Heat. Pour over shrimp. Sprinkle with parsley.

The classic way to prepare shrimp. Serve with homemade pasta for an extra treat.

BAKED SCALLOPS WITH CHIVES AND PIMENTO

Serves: 8

1 lb. sea scallops
1/2 tsp. salt
1/4 tsp. white pepper
6 Tbsp. unsalted butter
5 large shallots, minced
1 5-oz. jar pimentos
2 Tbsp. lemon juice
1/2 tsp. salt
1/4 tsp. Hungarian paprika
Freshly ground pepper
1/3 cup minced fresh parsley
2 Tbsp. minced fresh chives

Wash and pat scallops dry. Cut into quarters. Sprinkle with salt and pepper. Divide among 8 shells or ramekins. Place on baking sheet. Melt butter. Sauté shallots 5 minutes. Drain, pat dry and puree pimento. Stir into shallots with lemon juice, salt, paprika and 3 gratings of pepper. Stir together parsley and chives, reserve 2 Tbsp. and add remainder to shallots. Pour over scallops. Cover with foil. Bake at 425° for about 10 minutes. Do not overcook or scallops will be tough. Immediately remove foil and serve topped with reserved parsley and chives.

These may be prepared several hours ahead and refrigerated. Serve as a first course.

MOCK LOBSTER

Serves: 4

1 lb. monk fish
4 cups water
2 tsp. vinegar
1 tsp. salt
4 tsp. Old Bay Seasoning

Rinse fish and cut in bite-size pieces. Bring remaining ingredients to boil, drop in fish, return to boil. Cover, lower heat and simmer 6-8 minutes. Drain. Serve hot with melted butter or cold with cocktail sauce.

You may even fool Mother Nature. Use in lobster newburg or thermidor or wherever lobster is called for.

MANDARIN SHRIMP

Serves: 4

1 stick butter
1 clove garlic, minced
1/4 cup chopped onion
1/4 cup chopped celery
2 lb. shrimp, shelled and cleaned
1/4 cup dry white wine
1/2 cup chili sauce
1/4 cup chopped fresh parsley
2 Tbsp. minced shallot
1/2 tsp. salt
1/4 tsp. pepper
1/8 tsp. Cayenne pepper
Hot cooked rice

Melt butter and cook garlic gently for 3 minutes and remove. Stir in celery and onion. Sauté until crisp-tender. Add shrimp, wine and chili sauce. Cook until shrimp loses its transparency, about 3-5 minutes. Stir in parsley, shallot and seasonings. Serve immediately over rice.

A tossed salad and hot garlic toast would complete this easy recipe.

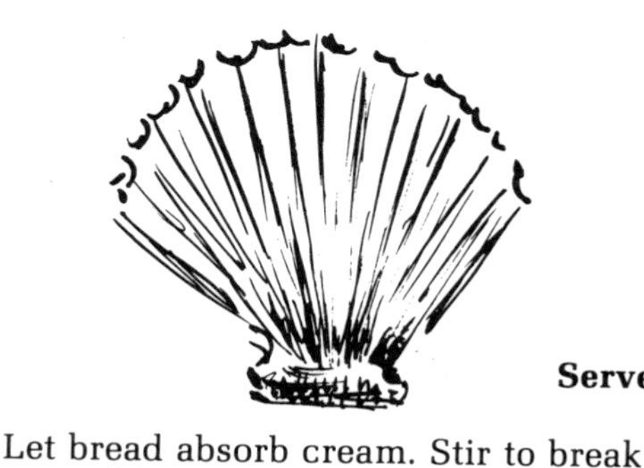

EASY DEVILED CRAB

Serves: 4

4 slices fresh bread
3/4 cup light cream
1 7-oz. can crabmeat, drained or frozen 8-oz. pkg., thawed
1 tsp. dry mustard
1/2 tsp. salt
1 tsp. fines herbs
2 Tbsp. diced celery
2 Tbsp. diced green pepper
1 Tbsp. minced onion
2 dashes Worcestershire sauce
1/2 cup fresh bread crumbs
1 Tbsp. butter, melted

Let bread absorb cream. Stir to break up. Fold in next 8 ingredients. Place in 4 buttered ramekins or shells. Top with bread crumbs mixed with butter. Bake at 350° for 12-15 minutes.

This may be baked in one buttered dish. Increase baking time to 20 minutes.

OYSTER PIE

Serves: 6-8

3/4 cup crushed soda crackers
1 pt. oysters
Heavy cream
3 Tbsp. butter
2 Tbsp. flour
2 egg yolks
1/2 cup heavy cream
2 Tbsp. dry sherry
3-4 drops Tabasco sauce

Toast cracker crumbs at 350° for 10 minutes. Drain oysters and add cream to liquor to measure 1 1/2 cups. Scald liquid. Melt 2 Tbsp. butter, add flour and cook, stirring for 3 minutes. Remove from heat, slowly whisk in scalded liquid, return to heat, stirring until mixture simmers. Simmer over moderate heat 10 minutes. Stir egg yolks into 1/2 cup heavy cream. Reduce heat to low and slowly stir in with sherry and Tabasco. Barely simmer 3 minutes more. Add oysters and remove from heat. Sprinkle 12″ gratin dish with 1/2 crumbs. Spread oyster mixture over. Top with remaining crumbs and dot with 1 Tbsp. butter. Bake at 350° for about 20 minutes.

This very rich dish may be served at a luncheon or as part of an elegant evening supper.

OYSTER SOUFFLÉ

Serves: 4-6

3 Tbsp. butter
3 Tbsp. flour
3/4 cup oyster liquor
1/2 cup light cream
1/2 tsp. salt
1/4 tsp. white pepper
4 eggs, separated
24 large oysters, cut in pieces
2 Tbsp. chives, chopped
1 Tbsp. lemon juice

Melt butter in saucepan. Add flour. Cook and stir 5 minutes. Remove from heat. Slowly stir in oyster liquor and cream. Return to heat. Cook, stirring until bubbling. Add salt and pepper. Beat egg yolks. Stir small amount of sauce into yolks. Slowly stir yolks into sauce. Heat through but do not boil. Remove from heat and add oysters, chives and lemon juice. Beat egg whites until stiff. Fold into sauce. Spoon into 1 1/2-qt. buttered soufflé dish. Bake at 350° for 40 minutes or until firm when lightly touched in the middle. Serve immediately.

This may be prepared ahead up to adding the egg whites. The pleasing result is worth the last minute work involved.

SCANDINAVIAN FISH BALLS

Serves: 4

1 lb. turbot or other fish fillet
1 egg
2 Tbsp. finely chopped green onion
1/2 cup cracker meal
1/4 cup light cream
1/2 tsp. salt
2 Tbsp. butter
2 Tbsp. flour
1/2 tsp. salt
1/4 tsp. dill weed
3/4 cup light cream
1 cup sour cream
1 Tbsp. chopped fresh parsley
Paprika

If frozen, thaw, dry well and cut fish in small chunks. Chop coarsely in blender or processor. Stir together with next 5 ingredients. Form into 16 balls. Melt butter, stir in flour, salt and dill weed. Cook, stirring 1/2 minute. Remove from heat, slowly stir in cream, return to heat, cook, stirring until mixture thickens and boils 1 minute. Remove from heat. Stir in sour cream. Pour 1/2 sauce into 2-qt. shallow baking dish. Arrange fish balls in dish. Cover with remaining sauce. Bake at 350° for about 25 minutes. To serve garnish with parsley and paprika.

For a lower calorie and equally delicious dish, substitute skim milk for cream and yogurt for sour cream.

SEAFOOD CASSEROLE

Serves: 6-8

1 lb. fresh canned crabmeat
1 lb. shrimp, cooked
6 Tbsp. butter
1/2 lb. fresh mushrooms, sliced
1 cup diced celery
1 cup diced onion
3/4 tsp. salt
1/4 tsp. pepper
1/4 tsp. paprika
6 Tbsp. flour
1 pt. light cream
3 Tbsp. sherry
2 tsp. Worcestershire sauce
3/4 cup bread crumbs
3 Tbsp. butter, melted
1/2 cup grated Parmesan cheese

Pick over seafood. Remove any shell. Melt 6 Tbsp. butter. Sauté mushrooms, celery and onion 4 minutes. Stir in next 4 ingredients. Remove from heat and slowly stir in liquids. Return to heat. Cook, stirring until sauce bubbles. Stir in seafood. Pour into buttered shallow 2-qt. casserole. Mix together remaining 3 ingredients and sprinkle over top. Bake at 350° for about 20 minutes.

Fresh canned crabmeat can be found in the refrigerated seafood section of the grocery store.

SHRIMP CURRY

Serves: 8

1 stick butter
6 Tbsp. flour
2 cups applesauce
1 envelope onion soup mix
2 cups water
2-3 tsp. curry powder
1/2 tsp. ginger
1/4 cup lemon juice
2 lb. fresh shrimp, shelled and deveined
Cooked rice

In large skillet, melt butter and blend in flour. Stir in next 6 ingredients. Cook, stirring until thickened. Add shrimp and simmer 3-5 minutes, just until shrimp are pink. Serve over rice.

Real curry lovers will use 3 tsp., but 2 tsp. gives a good bite. Serve with condiments.

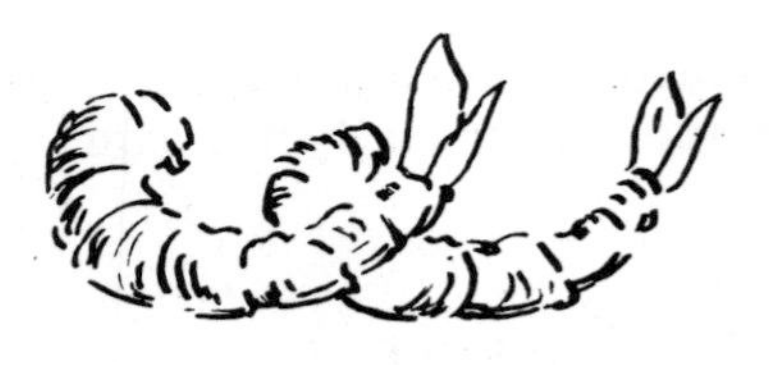

HOT SHRIMP CASSEROLE

Serves: 4

1/2 cup chopped onion
1 1/2 Tbsp. butter
1 3/4 cups canned tomatoes
1/2 cup chopped green pepper
1/3 cup crumbled Saltine crackers
1 tsp. salt
1/8 tsp. pepper
2 drops Tabasco sauce
1/8 tsp. nutmeg
1/8 tsp. thyme
1/8 tsp. mace
1 lb. raw shrimp, shelled and deveined
2 hard-boiled eggs
2 Tbsp. chopped fresh parsley

Sauté onion in butter 2 minutes. Stir in next 9 ingredients. Simmer 15 minutes, stirring occasonally. Add shrimp. Simmer 3 minutes. Chop eggs, reserving 1 yolk. Add eggs to shrimp. Pour into 1 1/2-qt. casserole. Bake at 350° for 15 minutes. To serve, garnish with sieved yolk and parsley.

Served over rice this is a splendid luncheon dish or a light dinner entrée.

PAELLA

Serves: 8

1 3-4 lb. chicken, cut up
1/4 cup olive oil
1/4 lb. pepperoni, sliced
2 tomatoes, peeled, seeded and sectioned
1/4 cup chopped onion
1/2 lb. raw shrimp, peeled
1 clove garlic, crushed
1 tsp. paprika
2 Tbsp. chopped fresh parsley
1 tsp. seasoned salt
1/16 tsp. saffron
1 tsp. salt
1/4 tsp. pepper
2 tsp. chicken stock base
1 1/2 cups rice
3 cups water
1 9-oz. pkg. frozen artichoke hearts
1 pimento, sliced
1 8-oz. can clams
1 10-oz. pkg. frozen peas

Brown chicken in oil. Remove. Brown pepperoni. Add tomatoes and onions. Sauté 2 minutes. Return chicken. Add remaining ingredients except peas. Cover and simmer 30 minutes. Add peas. Cook uncovered 5 minutes.

This is prepared more quickly than assembling the ingredients! Though fairly expensive to make, it is delicious and can be doubled or tripled.

PASTA SHELL SALMON

Serves: 6

6 oz. spaghetti, cooked and drained
3 Tbsp. butter
1/3 cup grated Parmesan cheese
2 eggs, beaten
1 15 1/2-oz. can salmon
1 10-oz. pkg. chopped spinach, cooked and drained
1 cup cottage cheese
1/2 cup chopped onion
1/4 cup chopped green pepper
1/2 tsp. garlic salt
1/2 cup grated Swiss cheese
6 triangular slices Swiss cheese

Combine spaghetti with 2 Tbsp. butter, Parmesan and eggs. Spread on bottom of 9″ pie plate. Drain and flake salmon. Add spinach and cottage cheese. Sauté onion and pepper in remaining 1 Tbsp. butter. Add to salmon with garlic salt and shredded Swiss cheese. Spread over spaghetti. Bake at 350° for 20 minutes. Top with triangles. Bake 3-5 minutes more or until cheese melts.

A pleasing combination and an economical main course.

CRAB CAKES SUPREME

Serves: 4

1 lb. fresh canned crab claw meat
2 eggs, beaten
1/4 cup minced onion
1/2 cup cracker meal
3 Tbsp. mayonnaise
1 Tbsp. prepared mustard
1/2 tsp. Worcestershire sauce
1/2 tsp. salt
1/4 tsp. freshly ground pepper
Oil for frying

Pick over crab meat and discard any shell. Mix together lightly with other ingredients except oil. Form into 8 round flat cakes. Pan fry in 1″ oil at 350° or over medium-high heat until golden.

For appetizer form into bite-size balls. Fry as above. Serve hot from chafing dish with cocktail picks and tartar sauce for dipping.

OVEN FRIED SCALLOPS

Serves: 3-4

1 egg
1 Tbsp. water
1/2 tsp. thyme
1/4 tsp. dill weed
1/4 tsp. salt
1/8 tsp. pepper
1 lb. scallops
1/2 cup Saltine cracker crumbs
4 Tbsp. butter
Chopped chives

Beat together first 6 ingredients. Dip scallops in egg mixture, then roll in cracker crumbs. Place in shallow baking pan. Drizzle butter over scallops. Bake sea scallops 15-18 minutes at 425°, turning once. Bake bay scallops 5-8 minutes at 425° without turning. Garnish with chopped chives to serve.

Be careful not to overcook or scallops will be rubbery and tough.

BAKED TROUT HEINTZELMAN

Serves: 6-8

6-8 small whole trout
1 cup chopped fresh mushrooms
1 Tbsp. dry minced onion, rehydrated
1 Tbsp. dry parsley
1 Tbsp. dry green onion
1 tsp. dry chervil
1/8 tsp. dry tarragon, crushed
1/8 tsp. thyme, crushed
3 Tbsp. butter, melted
1/2 tsp. salt
1/4 tsp. pepper
1 lemon, sliced paper thin
2 small onions, thinly sliced
Parsley sprigs

Rinse trout and wipe dry. Spread mushrooms in buttered 2-qt. shallow casserole. Combine next 6 ingredients and sprinkle over fish. Arrange fish over mushroom mixture. Top with 3 Tbsp. butter. Sprinkle with salt and pepper. Arrange and overlap alternate slices of lemon and onion on each fish. Cover with buttered brown paper. Bake at 400° for 15 minutes. Baste with pan juices. Bake uncovered 5 minutes more. Garnish with parsley sprigs and serve from baking dish.

Trout is perfect but any other small whole fish or fillets may be substituted.

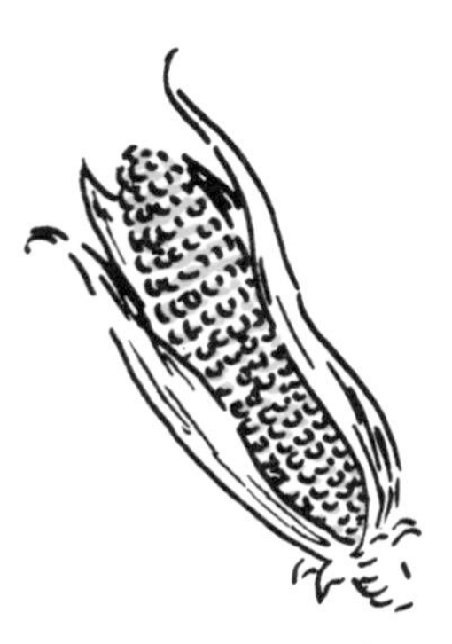

SCALLOPED OYSTERS AND CORN

Serves: 10-12

1 qt. oysters
1 17-oz. can cream style corn
1 17-oz. can whole kernel corn, drained
1/2 cup cream
1/2 tsp. salt
1/2 tsp. pepper
1/4 tsp. Tabasco sauce
2 sticks butter, melted
4 cups coarse cracker crumbs

Drain oysters and reserve 1 cup liquor. Chop oysters coarsely. Mix next 6 ingredients. Toss together butter and crumbs. Place 1/3 crumb mixture over bottom of 3-qt. shallow casserole. Spread over 1/2 corn mixture and 1/2 oysters. Sprinkle with 1/3 crumbs. Cover with rest of corn and oysters. Top with crumbs. Pour over reserved oyster liquor. Bake at 375° for about 45 minutes.

Prepare this casserole early in the day. Bake when ready. Add this dish to your Thanksgiving menu.

FLOUNDER FLORENTINE

Serves: 6-8

2 lb. flounder fillets
2 Tbsp. butter
2 tsp. lemon juice
1 tsp. dry parsley flakes
1 tsp. oregano
1 pkg. frozen spinach souffle, thawed
4 Tbsp. butter, melted
1/2 tsp. garlic salt
4 Tbsp. grated Parmesan cheese
Parsley sprigs
6-8 lemon wedges

If using frozen fillets, press out excess water. Place 1/2 fillets in 2-qt. shallow casserole coated with 2 Tbsp. butter. Sprinkle with 1/2 lemon juice, parsley and oregano. Spread spinach over fillets. Top with remaining fish, 2 Tbsp. butter and remaining lemon juice. Sprinkle with parsley, oregano, garlic salt and Parmesan. Bake at 400° for 20-30 minutes. Baste with remaining butter while baking. Garnish with parsley and lemon wedges.

Very easy to make and can be doubled. Also can be made in individual ramekins.

BAKED FILLET OF SOLE

Serves: 4

1 1/2 tsp. salad oil
1 1/2 tsp. flour
1/2 cup white wine
1/4 lb. mushrooms, sliced
1/2 cup thinly sliced green onions with tops
1 tsp. tarragon leaves
1/4 cup chopped fresh parsley
1-1 1/2-lb. fillet of sole
1/2 tsp. salt
1/4 tsp. pepper
1/4 tsp. paprika
1 Tbsp. butter, melted
1/2 cup soft bread crumbs
4 oz. Swiss cheese, grated

Pour oil into 8"x11" baking dish. Stir in flour. Stir in wine and spread over bottom of dish. Combine mushrooms, onions, tarragon and 2 Tbsp. parsley. Sprinkle evenly in dish. Arrange fillets over mushrooms. Season with salt, pepper and paprika. Stir together butter, crumbs and remaining parsley. Spinkle over fish. Bake uncovered at 350° for about 20 minutes. Cover with cheese and return to oven until cheese melts. Serve with pan juices.

Any good white fish may be used in this recipe.

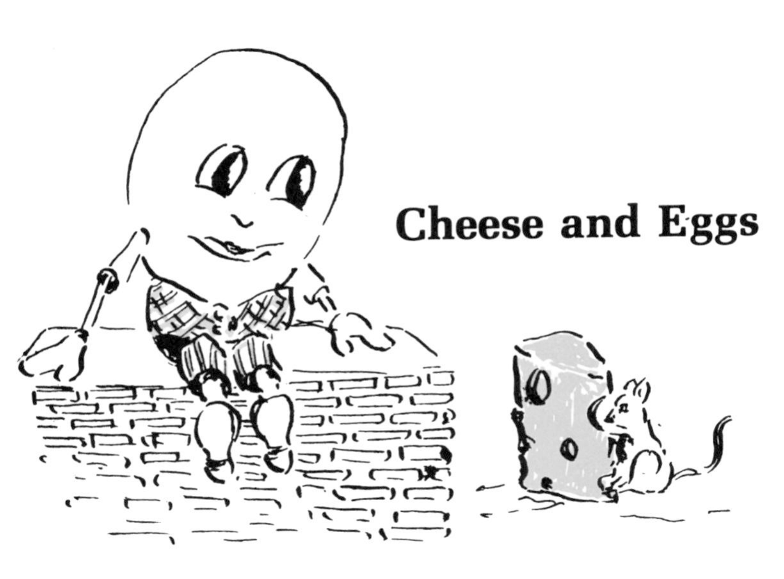

Cheese and Eggs

DO-AHEAD SCRAMBLED EGGS

Serves: 10-12

12 eggs
1 1/3 cups milk
2 Tbsp. flour
1/8 tsp. baking powder
1 tsp. salt
1/8 tsp. pepper
1 stick butter
2 Tbsp. pimento
2 Tbsp. chopped fresh parsley

In jar of blender combine first 6 ingredients. Blend on high 1 minutes. Melt butter in electric skillet set at 300°. Pour in eggs and cook, stirring 2 minutes. Mixture will be thin. Pour into serving dish. Place in 200° oven for 1-2 hours. To serve garnish with pimento and parsley.

While in the oven the eggs set perfectly and remain light and fluffy.

CHILE EGG PUFF

Serves: 12

10 eggs
1/2 cup flour
1 tsp. baking powder
1/2 tsp. salt
1/4 tsp. white pepper
1 pt. small curd cottage cheese
1 lb. Monterey Jack cheese, shredded
1 stick butter, melted
2 4-oz. cans diced green chiles, drained

Beat eggs until light and lemon colored. Add remaining ingredients and blend together well. Pour into buttered 9"x13" baking dish. Bake at 350° for 35 minutes or until top is golden and center appears firm.

There is a nice bite to this dish. If you wish, use pimento instead of green chiles.

BAKED DEVILED EGG CASSEROLE

Serves: 6

6 hard-boiled eggs
2 tsp. prepared mustard
3 Tbsp. sour cream
1/4 tsp. salt
2 Tbsp. butter
1/2 cup chopped onion
1/2 cup chopped green pepper
1 10 3/4-oz. can cream of mushroom soup
3/4 cup sour cream
1 Tbsp. flour
1/4 cup chopped pimento
1/2 cup shredded Cheddar cheese

Shell eggs and cut in half lengthwise. Mash yolks with next 3 ingredients. Fill whites and set aside. Melt butter and sauté onion and green pepper. Stir in soup. Mix sour cream and flour together. Stir in. Add pimento. Pour 1/2 soup mixture into shallow casserole. Arrange eggs yolk side up. Pour over remaining soup. Top with cheese. Bake at 350° for about 20 minutes.

Serve this at brunch, for lunch, or for a light and easy supper.

ASPARAGUS PIE

Serves: 6

1 8-oz. pkg. frozen asparagus spears or 1/2 lb. fresh
2 eggs
1 cup cottage cheese
4 Tbsp. butter, melted
1/4 cup flour
1/2 tsp. baking powder
1/4 tsp. salt
1 cup sour cream
1 tomato, peeled and thinly sliced
1/4 cup grated Parmesan cheese

Cook asparagus until just tender. Arrange in spoke fashion in bottom of buttered 9″ pie plate. Beat eggs until frothy. Add cottage cheese and butter. Beat until almost smooth. Stir flour, baking powder and salt into sour cream. Add to eggs. Pour carefully over asparagus. Arrange tomato slices on top. Sprinkle with Parmesan. Bake at 350° for 30 minutes or until center is firm. Let stand 10 minutes before serving.

For a brunch dish, consider placing very thin slices of ham in pie plate first, then continuing with recipe.

CRAB QUICHE

Serves: 6

1 1/2 cups fresh, frozen or canned crabmeat
2 Tbsp. chopped fresh parsley
2 Tbsp. dry vermouth
1/2 tsp. dry minced onion
1/2 tsp. salt
1/8 tsp. pepper
4 eggs
1 1/2 cups milk
1/4 tsp. rosemary
1/8 tsp. Cayenne pepper
1/4 cup grated Swiss cheese
Paprika
1 unbaked 9″ pastry shell

Mix crab, parsley, vermouth, onion, salt and pepper and place in pie shell. Beat eggs lightly, add milk, rosemary and cayenne pepper and beat again. Pour over crab, sprinkle with grated cheese and dust paprika over top. Place in 450° oven and bake 10 minutes. Reduce temperature to 350° and continue baking 20 minutes or until knife inserted near center comes out clean. This may be served as a lunch or brunch dish or cut in smaller pieces as an appetizer. The baked quiche may be frozen and reheated in a 250° oven for 20 minutes before serving.

The tasting committee unanimously rated this "10" — superb!

ITALIAN OMELET

Serves: 8-10

1 1/2 lb. bulk hot sausage
1/4 lb. bacon
1 10-oz. pkg asparagus
6 oz. Scamorza cheese
6 oz. Muenster cheese
6 oz. Ricotta cheese
6 eggs, beaten
1/2 cup chopped fresh parsley

Cook sausage until well browned. Drain. Dice bacon. Cook until crisp. Cook asparagus according to package directions using minimum time. Cut up Scamorza and Muenster cheeses, stir into sausage and return to heat until cheeses melt. Remove from heat. Stir in bacon and remaining ingredients. Pour into shallow casserole. Arrange asparagus spears in mixture. Bake at 400° for 10 minutes. Reduce heat to 225° and bake about 30 minutes more or until set.

This doubles easily. Freezes well wrapped in foil and remains moist when reheated.

BACON-TOMATO-CHEESE PUFF PIE

Serves: 6

1 lb. bacon
1 9″ unbaked pie shell
2 medium tomatoes, peeled and sliced
4 slices American cheese
3 eggs, separated
3/4 cup sour cream
1/2 cup flour
1/2 tsp. salt
1/4 tsp. pepper
Paprika

Fry bacon, drain and cut in 1″ pieces. Spread bacon in pie shell, cover with tomatoes and top with cheese. Beat yolks. Stir together sour cream, flour, salt and pepper. Stir into yolks. Beat egg whites until stiff. Carefully fold into yolk mixture. Pour into shell. Sprinkle with paprika. Bake at 350° for 35-40 minutes or until set.

This rises beautifully but falls quickly so serve immediately.

SCALLOPED BACON 'N EGGS

Serves: 4-6

1/4 cup chopped onion
2 Tbsp. butter
2 Tbsp. flour
1 1/2 cups milk
4 oz. Cheddar cheese, shredded
6 hard-boiled eggs, sliced
12 slices bacon, cooked and crumbled
1 1/2 cups crushed potato chips

Cook onion in butter in saucepan until crisp-tender. Add flour and cook, stirring 1 minute. Remove from heat and slowly add milk, stirring constantly. Return to heat. Cook, stirring until mixture bubbles. Stir in cheese until melted. In 1-qt. buttered casserole layer 1/2 eggs, 1/2 sauce, 1/2 bacon and 1/2 chips. Repeat. Bake at 350° for 15-20 minutes.

A perfect brunch dish that can be made ahead and easily doubled and doubled again for a crowd.

BLINTZE SOUFFLÉ

Serves: 6

12 frozen cheese blintzes
1 stick butter
4 eggs, slightly beaten
2 cups sour cream
1 tsp. vanilla
3 Tbsp. orange juice
1 1/2 tsp. grated orange rind
1 Tbsp. sugar

Completely defrost blintzes. Melt butter in 2-qt. shallow baking dish. Roll blintzes in butter and arrange side by side. Combine remaining ingredients and pour over. Cover and refrigerate overnight. Bake uncovered at 350° for about 45 minutes.

Serve these with extra sour cream or blueberry sauce as luncheon entrée or side dish for dinner.

CHEESE AND GREEN VEGETABLE PIE

Serves: 8

1/4 lb. mushrooms, sliced
1 small zucchini, diced
1 small green pepper, diced
3 Tbsp. butter
1 cup diced ham
1 lb. Ricotta cheese
4 oz. Mozzarella cheese, shredded
3 eggs, lightly beaten
1/2 cup chopped frozen spinach, thawed and drained
2 Tbsp. olive oil
1 Tbsp. dried dill weed
1 tsp. salt
1/2 tsp. pepper

Sauté first 3 vegetables in butter until tender. Add ham and sauté 2 minutes more. Cool. Mix together with remaining ingredients. Spoon into buttered 9″ pie plate. Bake at 350° for 45 minutes or until knife comes out clean. Let stand a few minutes before cutting.

The ham may be omitted. Crustless pies are a delight.

HERB CRÊPES BÉARNAISE

Serves: 8

Crêpes:
1 cup milk
3 eggs
6 Tbsp. flour
1/4 tsp. salt

Filling:
6 Tbsp. butter
1 1/2 lb. mushrooms, minced
2 Tbsp. minced onion
2 3-oz. pkg. cream cheese, softened
1 1/2 cups sour cream
2 Tbsp. grated Parmesan cheese
2 Tbsp. dried dill weed
2 Tbsp. chopped fresh parsley

For Crêpes: blend all ingredients in blender or food processor. Chill 1 hour. Liberally butter 5″-6″ crêpe pan. Over medium-high heat, cook crêpes using 2 Tbsp. batter. Cool, stack and set aside. For Filling: melt 1 Tbsp. butter. Sauté mushrooms and onion stirring occasionally until liquid evaporates. Beat together cream cheese and sour cream. Stir in mushroom mixture, Parmesan, dill and parsley. Divide filling among 16 crêpes, roll and place seam side down in 2 buttered 2-qt. shallow casseroles. Melt remaining butter and pour over crêpes. Bake at 325° for about 20 minutes.

If crêpes should tear while turning, don't despair. Tears will never show when filled and rolled.

BAKED EGGS IN PEPPER RINGS

Serves: 4

1 large green pepper
1 Tbsp. butter
4 eggs
1/4 tsp. salt
1/8 tsp. pepper
2 tsp. Parmesan cheese
1/8 tsp. oregano
1/8 tsp. basil
4 Tbsp. cream
4 Tbsp. fresh bread crumbs
2 Tbsp. butter, melted

Cut pepper into 4 rings 1/2" thick. Cook in lightly salted water 3-5 minutes. Drain Melt 1 Tbsp. butter in 1-qt. shallow casserole in oven. Place pepper rings in casserole. Break 1 egg in each ring. Sprinkle with seasonings. Pour 1 Tbsp. cream over each. Combine crumbs and butter. Sprinkle over. Bake at 350° for 15-20 minutes or until eggs are set.

This is very colorful. It would double, triple and more for a large brunch. Could easily be prepared ahead.

ALL-IN-ONE-BRUNCH

Serves: 8

2 Tbsp. butter
12 eggs, lightly beaten
1/2 cup sour cream
8 slices salami, chopped
6 green onions with tops, sliced
6 slices American cheese, chopped
12 cherry tomatoes, halved
1 4-oz. can sliced mushrooms, drained
1 tsp. salt
1/2 tsp. freshly ground pepper

Melt butter in 2-qt. rectangular baking dish. Combine remaining ingredients and blend well. Pour into prepared dish and bake at 350° for 30-40 minutes until puffed and golden. Serve immediately.

Served with fruit and a hot bread, this is truly complete.

CRAB-TOMATO-ALMOND QUICHE

Serves: 6

4 oz. Swiss cheese, shredded
1 9″ pie shell, unbaked
3 green onions with tops, sliced
1 small tomato, chopped
1/4-1/2 lb. backfin crabmeat
5 eggs, beaten
1 1/2 cups half and half
1/8 tsp. nutmeg
3 Tbsp. Dijon mustard
1/4 tsp. salt
1/4 tsp. pepper
1/2 cup almond slices

Evenly spread cheese into pie shell. Sprinkle over onions and tomatoes. Pick over crabmeat for shell and place over onions and tomatoes. Combine next 6 ingredients and carefully pour into shell. Spread almonds evenly over top. Bake at 375° for 30 minutes or until puffed and golden.

Backfin crabmeat is the best and also most expensive. Only slight loss of flavor will occur with a substitute.

MUSHROOM CRUST QUICHE

Serves: 6-8

3/4 lb. mushrooms, coarsely chopped
5 Tbsp. butter
1/2 cup finely crushed saltines
3/4 cup sliced green onions with tops
8 oz. Monterey Jack cheese, shredded
1 cup cottage cheese
3 eggs
1/4 tsp. pepper
1/4 tsp. paprika

Sauté mushrooms in 3 Tbsp. butter until limp. Add saltine crumbs. Spread into buttered 9″ pie plate. Sauté onions in remaining 2 Tbsp. butter 1 minute. Spread onions over mushrooms. Sprinkle shredded cheese over onions. Blend together next 3 ingredients until smooth. Carefully pour into pie plate. Sprinkle with paprika. Bake at 350° for 30 minutes or until knife inserted in center comes out clean.

This quiche is excellent served as a side dish for dinner, as a luncheon entrée or sliced slimly as an appetizer.

PARTY OMELET

Serves: 4-6

6 eggs, separated
1/4 tsp. cream of tartar
3/4 tsp. salt
1/4 tsp. pepper
1/2 tsp. dry mustard
1/3 cup milk
2 tsp. salad oil
2 Tbsp. butter

Sauce:
2 Tbsp. butter
2 Tbsp. flour
1/2 tsp. dry mustard
1/2 tsp. salt
1/8 tsp. pepper
1 cup milk
1 cup grated sharp Cheddar cheese
3 oz. crabmeat
Paprika
Parsley sprigs

Bring eggs to room temperature. In large bowl beat whites with cream of tartar until stiff peaks form. In small bowl beat yolks until thick and lemony, about 5 minutes. Add salt, pepper and mustard to yolks. Beat in milk to blend. Gently fold in egg whites until just combined. Heat oil and butter in 10″ skillet. Tilt pan to coat. Evenly spread in egg mixture. Cook over low heat 2 minutes without stirring. Place uncovered in oven and bake at 350° for 15 minutes or until golden. For Sauce: melt butter, stir in next 4 ingredients, cook, stirring for 1 minute. Remove from heat. Slowly stir in milk, return to heat and cook, stirring until thickened and bubbling. Stir in cheese to melt. Add crabmeat. Keep warm. To serve, cut omelet in wedges. Top with sauce. Dust with paprika. Garnish with parsley sprigs.

For an added touch to this excellent omelet, top with tomato slices before covering with sauce.

POTATO CRUST CHEESE PIE

Serves: 6-

3 medium potatoes
1 medium onion
1 egg, beaten
1/2 cup wheat sprouts
1 1/2 cups shredded Swiss or Cheddar cheese
3 eggs
1 1/4 cups milk
3 Tbsp. chopped fresh parsley
1 tsp. salt
1/4 tsp. pepper
1/4 tsp. dry mustard
1/2 tsp. paprika
1/8 tsp. cayenne pepper

Scrub but do not peel or cook potatoes. Shred potatoes and onion. Pat dry on paper towel. Mix with 1 egg. Press mixture on bottom and sides of buttered 9″ pie plate to form crust. Sprinkle in sprouts, then cheese. Beat together eggs and milk. Add remaining ingredients. Pour over cheese. Bake at 375° for 45 minutes or until knife inserted in center comes out clean.

The sprouts may be omitted but they do give a special flavor.

NIGHT BEFORE FRENCH TOAST

Serves: 8

4 Tbsp. butter
1 10-oz. loaf French or Italian bread
8 large eggs
3 cups milk
1 Tbsp. sugar
1/2 tsp. salt
1 1/2 tsp. vanilla

Use 2 Tbsp. butter to coat 9″x13″ baking dish. Cut bread into 1″ slices and arrange in pan. Beat eggs. Add next 4 ingredients. Pour over bread. Cover and refrigerate overnight. To bake dot with 2 Tbsp. butter. Bake uncovered at 350° for 45-50 minutes. Let stand 5 minutes before serving.

Cut in squares and top with maple syrup or your favorite jam or jelly.

SAUSAGE BRUNCH CASSEROLE

Serves: 6

2 1/2 cups herb seasoned stuffing mix
2 cups shredded sharp Cheddar cheese
1 1/2-lb. sausage, browned and well drained
4 eggs
2 1/4 cups milk
3/4 tsp. dry mustard
1 10 3/4-oz. can cream of mushroom soup
1/2 cup milk

In a buttered 9″x13″ baking dish, evenly spread stuffing mix, sprinkle with cheese, then sausage. Beat together next 3 ingredients and pour over sausage mixture. Refrigerate at least 6 hours or overnight. To bake, mix together soup and milk. Pour over casserole and bake at 350° for about 45 minutes.

For a crowd, double ingredients and divide between two 9″x13″ dishes.

SPINACH AND SAUSAGE SOUFFLÉ

Serves: 6

1 pkg. frozen spinach souffle
1/2 lb. hot or sweet Italian sausage
2 eggs
3 Tbsp. milk
2 tsp. chopped onion
1/2 cup canned sliced mushroms, drained
3/4 cup grated Swiss cheese
1 unbaked 9″ pastry shell

Thaw spinach soufflé. Cook sausage slowly, breaking up large pieces until thoroughly cooked. Drain off fat. Beat eggs with milk and onion. Stir in spinach soufflé, sausage, mushrooms and cheese. Pour into pastry shell. Bake at 375° for 25-30 minutes. Freezing not recommended, however, may be reheated if prepared ahead.

This is really a cross between a quiche and a soufflé.

SPINACH QUICHE

Serves: 8

3 Tbsp. salad oil
3/4 cup chopped green pepper
3/4 cup chopped onion
1 1/2 cups sliced mushrooms
1 1/2 cups chopped zucchini
1 1/2 tsp. minced garlic
5 eggs
1 lb. Ricotta cheese
1 tsp. salt
1 10-oz. pkg. fresh or frozen spinach, cooked and chopped
1 cup grated Cheddar cheese

Heat oil in skillet. Sauté green pepper, onion, mushrooms, zucchini and garlic until crisp-tender, 5-8 minutes. Cool. Beat eggs with Ricotta cheese and salt. Drain spinach thoroughly, squeezing out as much moisture as possible. Add to egg mixture with vegetables and Cheddar cheese. Spread evenly in greased 10″ spring-form pan. Bake at 350° for 1 hour or until knife inserted near center comes out clean. Cool 10 minutes before cutting.

Calorie counters note — this is a crustless quiche.

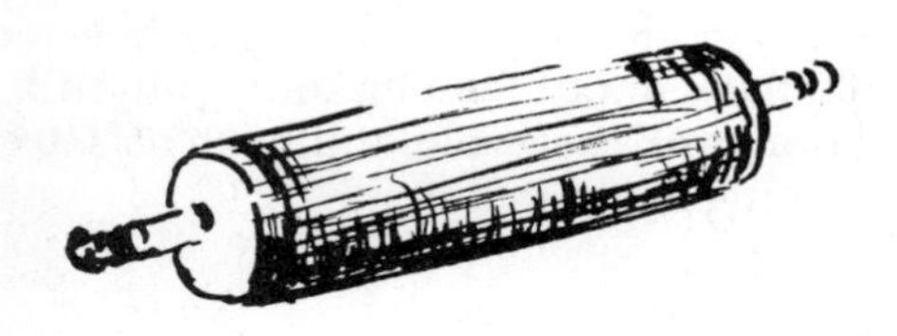

NEW ENGLAND CLAM QUICHE

Serves: 6-8

1 9″ pastry shell, unbaked
1/2 lb. bacon, crisply fried and crumbled
1 15-oz. can New England chowder
4 eggs, slightly beaten
1/2 cup finely chopped onion
1/2 cup sour cream
2 Tbsp. chopped fresh parsley
1/4 tsp. pepper
4 slices American cheese

Bake shell at 400° for 6 minutes. Combine next 7 ingredients and pour 2/3 into pie shell. Place cheese slices on top. Carefully pour over remaining clam mixture. Bake at 325° for 50-55 minutes. Let stand 15 minutes before cutting.

Add a can of well-drained clams for an even richer tasting quiche.

CHEESE CASSEROLE

Serves: 8

6 eggs
1 cup milk
1/2 cup flour
1 tsp. baking powder
1/2 tsp. salt
1 stick butter, melted
1 lb. Monterey Jack cheese, cubed
1 3-oz. pkg. cream cheese, cubed
1 8-oz. carton small curd cottage cheese
1 Tbsp. sugar

Beat eggs well. Stir in remaining ingredients. Pour into buttered 3-qt. rectangular baking dish. Bake at 350° for 1 hour. To garnish, sprinkle with paprika, chopped fresh parsley and/or chopped fresh chives.

Easy, good and recipe can be cut in half or doubled.

VERSATILE CHEESE STRATA

Serves: 6-8

12 slices white bread
1/2 lb. old English cheese, shredded
1/2 stick butter, melted
6 eggs, beaten
2 cups milk
1 tsp. parsley flakes
1/2 tsp. fines herbs
1/2 cup thinly sliced mushrooms
1 6-oz. can crabmeat

Cut crusts from bread. Place 6 slices in buttered 2-qt. shallow casserole. Mix together remaining ingredients. Pour 1/2 over bread. Top with remaining bread. Pour over remaining egg mixture. Cover and refrigerate overnight. Bake covered at 350° for 30 minutes. Remove cover and bake 30 minutes more. Serve immediately.

Options here are endless. For crabmeat substitute 3/4 cup chopped cooked shrimp, or ham, bacon, chicken or turkey. Add sautéed celery and onions. Choose your own combination.

Sandwiches

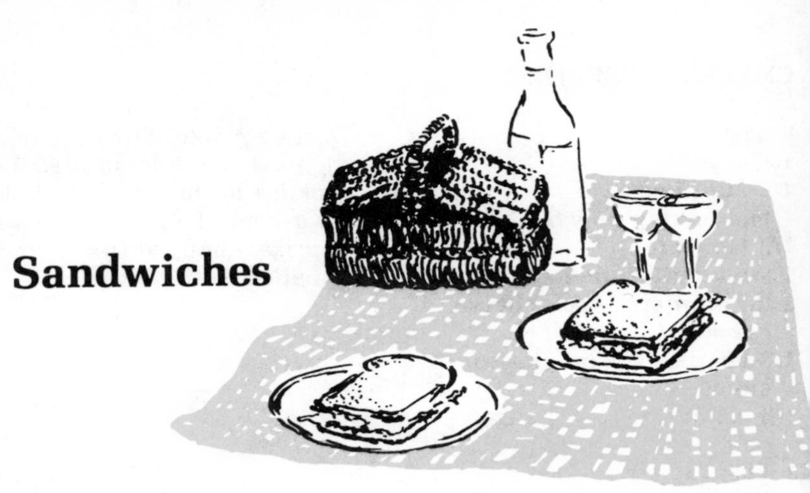

ITALIAN SANDWICH LOAF

Serves: 6-8

1 loaf Italian bread
1 lb. ground beef
1/3 cup Parmesan cheese
1/2 cup chopped onions
1 6-oz. can tomato paste
1/2 tsp. salt
1/2 tsp. oregano
1/2 tsp. basil
1/8 tsp. pepper
1 4 1/4-oz. can chopped ripe olives, drained
8 slices tomato
6 slices American cheese, sliced diagonally

Cut loaf of bread in half lengthwise. Combine next 9 ingredients, spread on bread halves and broil 5″ from heat for 10-12 minutes. Top with tomato slices, then cheese slices. Broil until cheese melts. Cut in serving size pieces.

If you choose, cut the bread in thick slices to begin with, spread with meat mixture and continue as recipe directs. Also, try Mozzarella or Provolone cheese.

BROILED VEGETABLE MEDLEY

Serves: 4

6 whole medium pita breads
1/2 head broccoli flowerets
2 small zucchini, sliced
3 whole green onions, sliced
10 fresh mushrooms, sliced
3 sprigs parsley, chopped
2 cloves garlic, minced
1/4 cup wheat germ
Good melting cheese

Lay whole pita breads on baking sheet. Combine next 6 ingredients, divide evenly and spread on breads. Stir garlic and wheat germ together and sprinkle over vegetables. Cover completely with slices of any good melting cheese such Monterey Jack or Jarlsberg. Place 4″-5″ beneath broiler and broil until cheese melts and is golden.

Eat with a knife and fork. The vegetables are warmed but not cooked.

TURKEY ALMOND DELIGHT

Yield: 2 cups

1 1/2 cups cooked finely minced turkey
2 hard-boiled eggs, chopped
1/2 cup chopped roasted almonds
1/2 cup mayonnaise
3 Tbsp. lemon juice
3/4 tsp. horseradish
1/2 tsp. salt
1 tsp. prepared mustard

Combine all ingredients with fork. Chill. Serve as sandwich filling or spread on crackers.

Chicken may be substituted for turkey with no loss of flavor.

HOT CHICKEN SANDWICH

Serves: 6

1 10 3/4-oz. can cream of chicken soup
1 cup sour cream
3 oz. chopped mushrooms
1 3-oz. jar capers
3/4 cup mayonnaise
1 hard-boiled egg, chopped
1 large stalk celery, chopped
12 slices sandwich bread
Soft butter
2 cups cooked chicken, sliced

Combine first 7 ingredients several hours ahead of time to blend flavors. Decrust bread and butter all sides. Lay 6 slices in 9″x13″ pan. Cover with chicken. Top with 6 other slices. Pour sauce over and bake at 350° for about 30 minutes.

Garnish with parsley sprigs and serve with a cranberry salad.

DOUBLE CHEESE MUFFINS

Serves: 6

12 oz. small curd cottage cheese
1/2 cup wheat germ
2 whole green onions, sliced
1/4 tsp. oregano
1/4 tsp. basil
1/4 tsp. salt
1/8 tsp. white pepper
3 whole wheat English muffins, halved and toasted
1 large tomato, cut in 6 slices
12 strips Cheddar cheese
3 Tbsp. minced fresh parsley

Combine first 7 ingredients and mound on toasted muffins. Top each with tomato slice and 2 strips of cheese, crisscrossed. Broil 3″-4″ from heat for 5 minutes or until cheese melts. Sprinkle with parsley.

This is mild but tasty, and a treat for children.

SANDWICH LOAF

Serves: 10

1 12 1/2-oz. can tuna, drained
2 stalks celery, diced
3 whole green onions, sliced
Mayonnaise
6 hard-boiled eggs
2 tsp. yellow mustard
3/4 tsp. salt
1/4 tsp. pepper
1 small onion, minced
2 4 1/4-oz. cans chopped black olives, drained
11 oz. cream cheese, softened
Milk
20 slices enriched bread, decrusted
Soft Butter

Combine tuna with celery, onion and enough mayonnaise to make good spreading consistency. Set aside. Mash eggs with fork and combine with mustard, salt, pepper, onion and enough mayonnaise for easy spreading. Set aside. Combine olives with 1/4 cup mayonnaise. Set aside. Beat cheese with enough milk to make a thick icing. To assemble: butter bread, lay 5 slices bread, butter up, lengthwise on serving platter. Spread on tuna mixture evenly. Lay 5 slices bread, butter up, firmly over tuna. Spread with egg mixture. Cover with 5 more slices bread. Spread with olives. Top with last 5 slices, butter down. Frost entire loaf with cream cheese. Chill. At serving time, decorate with parsley and pimento stars.

Though better prepared just a couple of hours before serving, this is still delicious the next day.

GRILLED CHEDDAR CHEESE SANDWICH

Serves: 2

4 slices bacon
2/3 cup shredded sharp Cheddar cheese
1 Tbsp. chopped green pepper
1 tsp. Worcestershire sauce
1/2 tsp. dry mustard
1 tsp. grated onion
2 tsp. butter, softened
2 slices rye bread
4 tomato slices
Parsley sprigs

Cook bacon until crisp, drain and set aside. Toss together next 5 ingredients. Butter bread, place 2 slices tomatoes on each, mound cheese on top. Broil 6" from heat for about 5 minutes or until cheese melts. Top with bacon. Garnish with parsley.

Basically the classic sandwich, it receives extra dash here. Yes, it can be made in large amounts.

ROAST BEEF SANDWICHES

Serves: 6

1 1/2-oz. Bleu cheese, crumbled
1/4 cup salad oil
1 1/2 Tbsp. lemon juice
1/2 tsp. salt
1/4 tsp. sugar
1/8 tsp. freshly ground pepper
Dash paprika
2 large onions, thinly sliced and separated into rings
3 whole large pita breads, cut in half
18 thin slices roast beef
Shredded lettuce
Shredded Swiss cheese

Combine first 7 ingredients and pour over onion rings. Marinate overnight. To assemble; press cut pitas open. Keep each half circle intact. Arrange 3 slices beef in each. Add marinated onions, lettuce and cheese.

These are easy to eat out-of-hand and a sandwich that men enjoy.

BAKED CHICKEN SANDWICHES

Serves: 6

1/2 lb. fresh mushrooms, sliced
1/4 cup sliced green onions with tops
4 Tbsp. butter
3 Tbsp. flour
3/4 cup milk
1 10 3/4-oz. can cream of mushroom soup
3 cups diced cooked chicken
1 2-oz. jar pimentos, chopped
12 slices sandwich bread
3 eggs, slightly beaten
1/3 cup milk
2 cups potato chips, crushed lightly
1/2 cup almonds, slivered

Sauté mushrooms and onions in butter until tender. Stir in flour. Blend 3/4 cup milk and soup and slowly stir in. Cook until thickened and bubbling. Add chicken and pimento. Place 6 slices bread in 9″x13″ pan. Spread with chicken mixture. Top with remaining bread. Cover and refrigerate at least 8 hours or overnight. Stir eggs and 1/3 cup milk together in shallow dish. Cut sandwiches in half. Dip both sides in egg mixture, then in potato chips. Place on buttered cookie sheet. Top with almonds. Bake at 350° for about 25 minutes.

Serve with asparagus spears and broiled tomatoes with cheese topping.

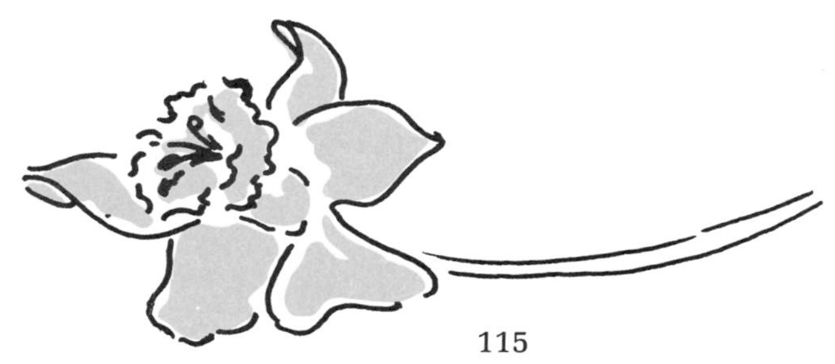

DILLED BEEF SANDWICHES

Serves: 6

3/4 cup sour cream
2 tsp. Poupon mustard
1 tsp. horseradish
2 Tbsp. dry onion soup mix
18 thin slices roast beef
12 slices rye bread
Soft butter
12 slices tomato
12 slices dill pickle, cut lengthwise
2 cups alfalfa sprouts

Combine first 4 ingredients. Let stand 30 minutes or more. Place 3 slices beef on each of 6 slices lightly buttered bread. Spread each with equal amounts sour cream mixture. Add 2 slices tomato and pickle. Top with 1/3 cup sprouts on each sandwich. Cover with remaining bread slices and cut diagonally in half.

These are grand sandwiches to have prepared for a late night crowd.

MUSHROOM SANDWICHES

Serves: 6

2 cups chopped mushrooms
2 medium onions, diced
4 Tbsp. butter
1/3 lb. sharp cheese, shredded
2 eggs, beaten
12 slices toast
12 thin slices tomato

Sauté mushrooms and onion in butter until tender. Stir in cheese and egg. Spread on toast and top with tomato slices. Broil 6″ from heat for about 5 minutes.

Served with a jello salad, these sandwiches would be a fine Sunday lunch for the family.

HOT CHEESE-SALAMI SANDWICH

Yield: 10 sandwiches

1 unsliced sandwich loaf
1/2 lb. American cheese, grated
1/4 cup mayonnaise
2 tsp. prepared mustard
1 tsp. grated onion
1 cup chopped ripe olives
20 thin slices salami
2 Tbsp. butter, melted

Cut crusts from top and sides of loaf. Cut to, but not through, bottom crust in 20 even slices. Combine next 5 ingredients. Spread facing sides of first cut with cheese filling. Repeat with every other cut. Place 2 slices salami inside each cheese sandwich. Spread remaining cheese mixture on top of loaf. Tie loaf together with string. Brush sides with butter. Place on baking sheet. Bake at 350° for 25-30 minutes. To serve, snip string and cut sections without filling through bottom crusts.

You will find this sandwich good for a tail-gate picnic. Wrap in foil and keep in a warming chest.

Add an Accompaniment

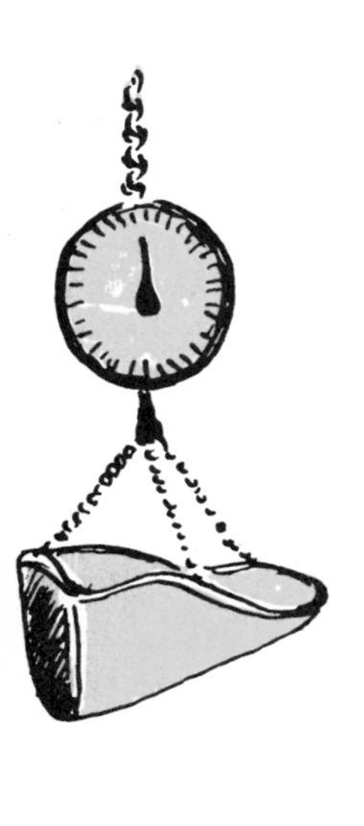

Vegetables

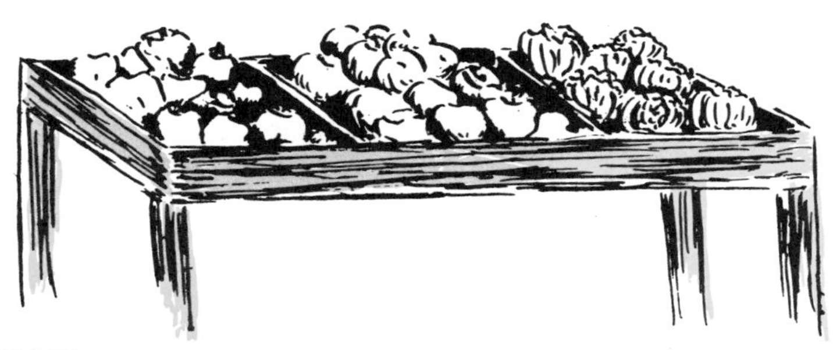

BEETS WITH PINEAPPLE

Serves: 4

2 Tbsp. brown sugar
1 Tbsp. cornstarch
1/4 tsp. salt
1 9-oz. can pineapple tidbits
1 Tbsp. butter
1 Tbsp. lemon juice
1 1-lb. can sliced beets, drained

Combine first 3 ingredients in saucepan. Stir in pineapple with syrup. Cook, stirring constantly until mixture thickens and bubbles. Add remaining ingredients and heat through.

This easily made, easily doubled recipe has grand eye appeal. Fresh beets make it even better.

LIMA BEAN AND CORN CASSEROLE

Serves: 6-8

2 cups fresh lima beans or 1 10-oz. pkg. frozen
2 cups fresh corn or 1 10-oz. pkg. frozen
1 cup sour cream
1 2 1/2-oz. can deviled ham
3 Tbsp. minced onion
1 tsp. salt
1 3-oz. can sliced broiled mushrooms, drained
1/2 cup dry bread crumbs
1 Tbsp. butter

Cook vegetables separately in small amount of water until just tender. Blend together sour cream, deviled ham, onions and salt. Combine drained vegetables and sour cream mixture. Spoon into buttered shallow 1 1/2-qt. baking dish. Top with mushrooms. Sprinkle with crumbs. Dot with butter. Bake at 350° for about 30 minutes.

A glorified version of succotash that can be prepared year round.

SAUTÉED CHERRY TOMATOES

Serves: 8

4 Tbsp. butter
1 qt. cherry tomatoes
1/2 tsp. sugar
1/2 tsp. salt
1/4 tsp. freshly ground pepper
1 tsp. basil leaves
2 Tbsp. chopped fresh parsley

Heat butter in large skillet over high heat until it foams, add tomatoes, toss, sprinkle with sugar and shake pan back and forth for 3 minutes to form a shiny glaze. Remove from heat, stir in remaining ingredients and serve immediately.

Use these as a garnish as well as a vegetable.

BAKED TOMATOES

Serves: 4-6

4-6 medium tomatoes
1 cup dry bread crumbs
1 tsp. seasoning salt
1/4 tsp. pepper
1/4 tsp. Cayenne pepper
1/2 tsp. white or brown sugar
1/4 tsp. fines herbs
2 Tbsp. finely chopped green onion
1 Tbsp. finely chopped green pepper
4 Tbsp. butter
1/4 cup grated sharp cheese
Paprika

Peel and slice tomatoes 1/2″ thick. Combine next 8 ingredients. Top tomato slices with crumb mixture. Dot with butter. Sprinkle with cheese and paprika. Layer tomatoes in shallow baking dish. Bake at 375° for 20-30 minutes.

This can be prepared up to baking point early in the day and refrigerated, covered, until dinner time.

PEAS WITH COINTREAU

Serves: 6

2 10-oz. pkg. frozen peas
1 tsp. salt
1/4 tsp. pepper
1/8 tsp. nutmeg
1 Tbsp. butter
1 Tbsp. Cointreau
Rind of 1 orange, grated

Cook peas without salt according to package directions. Drain well. Season with salt, pepper and nutmeg. Just before serving add butter and Cointreau. Pour into serving dish and sprinkle orange peel over peas.

Should you be lucky enough to have any left over, toss them in your next salad.

WHOLE STUFFED CABBAGE

Serves: 6-8

1 medium Savoy cabbage
1 large onion, chopped
1/4 lb. bacon, chopped
2 cloves garlic, minced
3 Tbsp. olive oil
1 cup fresh bread crumbs
1/4 cup milk
1/4 cup chopped fresh parsley
1 egg, lightly beaten
1/4 tsp. thyme
1/2 tsp. salt
1/4 tsp. pepper
1 cup chicken stock

Remove large outer leaves of cabbage and reserve. Trim core evenly with bottom of cabbage. Cook cabbage and outer leaves in 2″ boiling salted water for 15 minutes. Drain and run under cold water. Squeeze all water out of cabbage. Place on cheese cloth large enough to cover cabbage and to tie on top. Carefully open cabbage by separating each leaf 1 at a time. Cut out core and chop. Sauté with onion, bacon and garlic in 2 Tbsp. olive oil until onion is golden. Chop outer leaves and add. Mix bread crumbs, milk and parsley. Stir in bacon mixture. Add egg and seasonings. Distribute stuffing between cabbage leaves starting at center and reshaping cabbage. Brush with 1 Tbsp. olive oil, pull up cheese cloth and tie on top. Put in oiled deep 3-qt. casserole. Pour chicken stock over cabbage. Bake covered at 400° for 1 hour. Remove cheese cloth, place on small platter and cut in wedges to serve.

This takes time to prepare, but is truly lovely to look at when complete.

CHINESE CABBAGE IN CREAM SAUCE

Serves: 6

1 1/4 lb. Chinese or celery cabbage
1 medium onion
3 Tbsp. salad oil
1 tsp. sugar
1 tsp. salt
1 cup chicken stock
2 Tbsp. cornstarch
3 Tbsp. water
4 Tbsp. light cream
1 slice crisp bacon, crumbled

Cut cabbage crosswise in 1/4″ slices. Cut onion in half, then in 1/4″ slices. Heat oil in large skillet. Add cabbage and onion. Sauté 3 minutes, stirring to coat with oil. Cover and steam 5 minutes. Place in colander. Sprinkle with sugar and salt. In same skillet heat chicken stock. Mix cornstarch and water, add and cook, stirring until thick. Add cream, stir in cabbage, heat through. Turn into warm serving dish. Sprinkle with bacon.

Different and very good but should be served immediately to keep cabbage crisp.

SAUTÉED VEGETABLES

Serves: 6-8

2 medium zucchini, sliced
2 medium yellow squash, sliced
1 green pepper, halved and sliced
1 large onion, sliced
1/2 lb. mushrooms, sliced
4 Tbsp. butter
2 tomatoes, quartered
1 tsp. salt
1 tsp. ground ginger

Sauté first 5 ingredients in butter 5-6 minutes or until crisp-tender. Add tomatoes, salt, ginger and stir. Cover and simmer 3 minutes. Serve immediately.

A pleasing combination of vegetables and the secret is quick-cooking to keep them crisp.

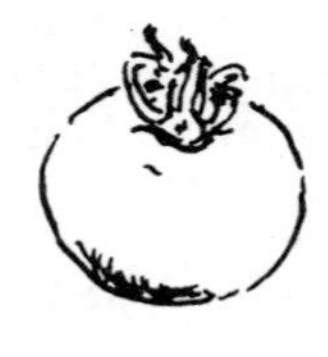
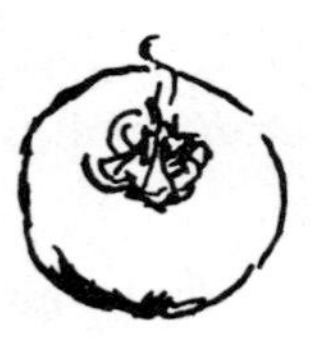
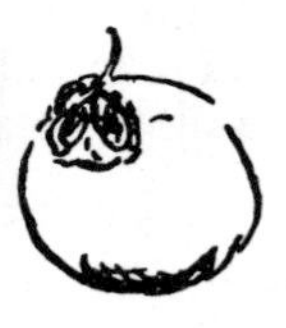

SPECIAL SPINACH

Serves: 12

4 10-oz. pkg. frozen chopped spinach
1/2 lb. fresh mushrooms
2 Tbsp. butter
1/2 cup mayonnaise
1/2 cup sour cream
1/2 tsp. salt
1/4 tsp. white pepper
1 8 1/2-oz. can artichoke hearts, drained and quartered
3 tomatoes
1/2 cup dry bread crumbs
4 Tbsp. butter
1/4 cup grated Parmesan cheese

Defrost and drain spinach. Sauté mushrooms in 2 Tbsp. butter. Combine next 4 ingredients and stir in spinach, mushrooms and artichoke hearts. Pour into buttered 3-qt. rectangular baking dish. Slice tomatoes 1/2″ thick and place on spinach mixture. Sauté crumbs in 4 Tbsp. butter until golden, stir in Parmesan cheese and sprinkle over casserole. Bake at 350° for 20-25 minutes.

Prepare ahead and bake when ready. With a light soup and hot bread, this could also be a meatless meal.

BROCCOLI WITH CREAM CHEESE SAUCE

Serves: 4-6

2 lb. fresh broccoli
3 Tbsp. butter
1/4 cup minced onion
3 Tbsp. flour
2 tsp. chicken-flavored instant bouillon
1 1/2 cups milk
4 oz. whipped cream cheese
1/2 cup plain yogurt
1 tsp. dill weed

Prepare broccoli, slash stems, and cook 8-10 minutes or until crisp-tender. Melt butter, sauté onion until golden, blend in flour and bouillon and cook 1 minute. Remove from heat, slowly stir in milk. Return to medium-high heat and cook, stirring constantly until sauce is thick and bubbling. Stir in cream cheese and blend in yogurt and dill. Just heat through. Pour over broccoli in serving dish.

Use the sauce over other freshly cooked vegetables — equally good.

SCALLOPED TOMATOES

Serves: 8-10

2 28-oz. cans peeled whole tomatoes
4 slices white bread, crusts removed and cut in 1/4″ cubes
1 stick butter
3/4 cup sugar
1 tsp. salt
1/4 tsp. pepper

Drain all but 1/2 cup juice from tomatoes. Place in 2-qt. shallow casserole. Cut tomatoes part way through, spread and place 1/2 bread cubes between wedges and around tomatoes. Melt butter and stir in remaining bread cubes. Sprinkle sugar, salt, pepper and buttered bread over tomatoes. Bake at 375° for about 45 minutes.

Fresh tomatoes may be used for canned. Increase the sugar slightly. Can be frozen after baking and goes particularly well with roast beef.

SWISS GREEN BEANS

Serves: 8

2 10-oz. pkg. frozen French style green beans
2 Tbsp. flour
2 Tbsp. butter
2 Tbsp. sugar
1 small onion, grated
4 oz. Swiss cheese, shredded
1 pt. sour cream
2 cups cornflakes
2 Tbsp. butter

Cook green beans 2 minutes. Drain well. In top of double boiler over hot water mix next 6 ingredients. Cook, stirring until cheese melts. Fold into beans. Place in buttered 2-qt. casserole. Crush cornflakes and toast in butter. Sprinkle over top. Bake at 350° for about 40 minutes.

Cut in half or doubled, this recipe easily adapts.

SAVORY SPINACH SQUARES

Serves: 8

4 eggs, beaten
2/3 cup milk
4 Tbsp. butter, melted
1/2 cup minced onion
4 Tbsp. minced fresh parsley
1 tsp. Worcestershire sauce
1 1/2 tsp. salt
1/2 tsp. thyme leaves
1/2 tsp. nutmeg
2 10-oz. pkg. frozen spinach, cooked and drained
2 cups cooked rice
2 cups shredded American cheese

Stir together first 9 ingredients. Combine remaining ingredients. Mix all together well. Pour into buttered shallow 2-qt. baking dish. Bake at 350° for 40-45 minutes. Cut in squares to serve.

If doubled, increase baking time by 10 minutes. May be prepared early in the day.

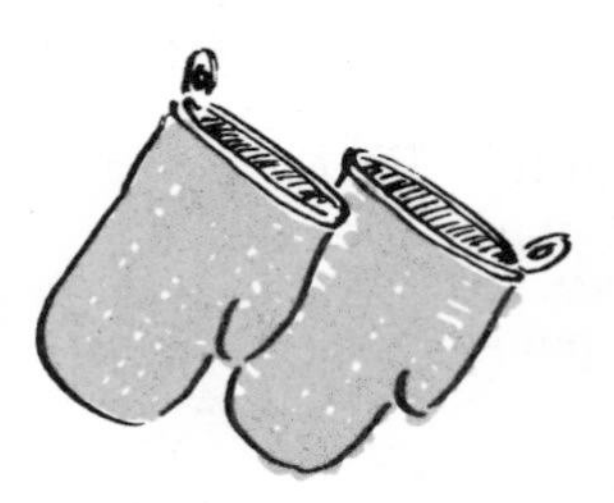

SPINACH SOUFFLÉ

Serves: 8-10

2 10-oz. pkg. frozen chopped spinach
4 eggs, well beaten
1 medium onion, minced
1/2 cup grated Parmesan cheese
1/2 cup grated Mozzarella cheese
1/2 tsp. salt
2 cups herb stuffing mix
1 1/2 sticks butter, melted
1/4 cup coarsely chopped walnuts

Cook spinach according to package directions. Drain well and cool. Mix with remaining ingredients and place in 2-qt. casserole or soufflé dish. Chill at least 1 hour. Bake at 350° about 20 minutes.

A make-ahead soufflé that can be kept in the refrigerator up to 8 hours before baking.

ZUCCHINI CASSEROLE

Serves: 8

2 lb. fresh zucchini
1/2 lb. bacon
3 large onions, sliced
1/2 tsp. salt
1/4 tsp. pepper
1 1/2 tsp. basil
1 cup catsup
2 cloves garlic, sliced
1/2 cup grated Parmesan cheese
1 cup croutons

Wash, trim ends and cut unpeeled zucchini into 1/4″ slices. Cut bacon in pieces. Sauté 2 minutes, pour off most fat, add onions and sauté until crisp-tender. In 2-qt. casserole cover bottom with zucchini, sprinkle on a little salt, pepper and basil. Dot with catsup. Add layer of bacon and onions. Sprinkle with few slices garlic and 1 Tbsp. Parmesan cheese. Repeat until all ingredients are used except Parmesan. Bake covered at 350° for 1 hour. Uncover, top with croutons and any remaining Parmesan. Bake 30 minutes more.

Smells wonderful while cooking and tastes the same. Bake pork chops or meat loaves in same oven.

STUFFED ZUCCHINI WITH CHEESE

Serves: 6

6 8″ zucchinis
1 cup minced onion
4 Tbsp. butter
2 tsp. minced onion
1 1/2 Tbsp. butter
1 1/2 Tbsp. flour
1 cup whipping cream, scalded
1/2 tsp. salt
1/4 tsp. pepper
1/8 tsp. nutmeg
1/4 cup fine bread crumbs
4 Tbsp. grated Parmesan cheese
2 Tbsp. butter, melted
Paprika
Parsley sprigs
Lemon wedges

Trim ends from zucchini. Cut off 1/3 zucchini lengthwise. Cook all zucchini in boiling salted water 8-10 minutes until just crisp-tender. With small spoon, scoop pulp out of tops and bottoms leaving 1/4″ shell in bottoms. Discard tops. Invert zucchini on paper towels to drain. Finely chop pulp. Using cloth towel squeeze out all moisture. Sauté onion in 4 Tbsp. butter. Add pulp and cook 5-6 minutes. Set aside. Cook 2 tsp. onion, butter and flour over low heat 3 minutes, stirring constantly. Add scalded cream, stirring constantly. Stir in seasonings, crumbs, 2 Tbsp. cheese and pulp mixture. Dry zucchini shells and heap in filling. Sprinkle with last 2 Tbsp. Parmesan, dribble with melted butter. Dust with paprika. Place in buttered baking dish and bake at 450° for 10-15 minutes. Garnish with parsley sprigs and lemon wedges to serve.

Though the directions are long, this is not hard to make. Prepare early in the day and assemble in late afternoon.

HARVARD CARROTS

Serves: 6

4 cups sliced carrots
1/2 cup sugar
1 1/2 Tbsp. cornstarch
6 Tbsp. water reserved from cooking carrots
2 Tbsp. vinegar
4 Tbsp. butter

Boil carrots until barely tender, drain and reserve 6 Tbsp. water. Combine sugar and cornstarch. Add carrot water and vinegar. Cook, stirring until thickened and clear. Add carrots and heat on low 5 minutes. Stir in butter and serve.

Add a sprinkle of freshly grated nutmeg or slivers of crystallized ginger for extra flavor.

SWEET POTATO-CASHEW BAKE

Serves: 6

1/3 cup brown sugar, packed
1/2 cup broken cashews
1/2 tsp. salt
1/2 tsp. ginger
4 medium sweet potatoes, cooked, and sliced
1 cup sliced canned peaches, drained
2 Tbsp. butter

In small bowl blend together first 4 ingredients. In buttered 1 1/2-qt. casserole, arrange 1/3 sweet potatoes, 1/3 peaches, 1/3 brown sugar mixture. Repeat twice. Dot with butter. Bake covered at 350° for 1/2 hour. Uncover, baste with liquid in casserole and bake 10 minutes more, basting twice.

Walnuts could be used for the cashews, but the peaches are what make this special.

POTATO CASSEROLE

Serves: 10-12

1 2-lb. pkg. frozen shredded hash brown potatoes
1 onion, chopped
1/2 cup chopped green pepper
1 10 3/4-oz. can cream of potato soup
1 10 3/4-oz. can cream of celery soup
8 oz. sour cream
1/2 tsp. salt
1/2 tsp. pepper
4 oz. sharp Cheddar cheese, shredded

Thaw potatoes. Dry on paper towels. Combine with remaining ingredients, except cheese. Spoon into buttered shallow 2-qt. casserole. Bake uncovered at 325° for 1 hour and 15 minutes. Sprinkle with cheese. Bake 15 minutes more.

This is very easy and goes together in minutes.

CAULIFLOWER CUSTARD

Serves: 4-6

1 head cauliflower
2 eggs, beaten
3/4 cup milk
1/2 cup shredded sharp cheese
3 Tbsp. butter, melted
3 Tbsp. chopped fresh parsley
1/2 tsp. instant onion
1/2 tsp. salt
1/8 tsp. pepper
1/2 cup buttered bread crumbs

Cut cauliflower into flowerets. Cook in boiling salted water 7-8 minutes. Drain well. Place in 1-qt. casserole. Combine next 8 ingredients. Pour over cauliflower. Top with crumbs. Bake at 350° for 30 minutes or until custard is set.

Two 10-oz. packages of frozen cauliflowerets, cooked and drained, may be used for fresh.

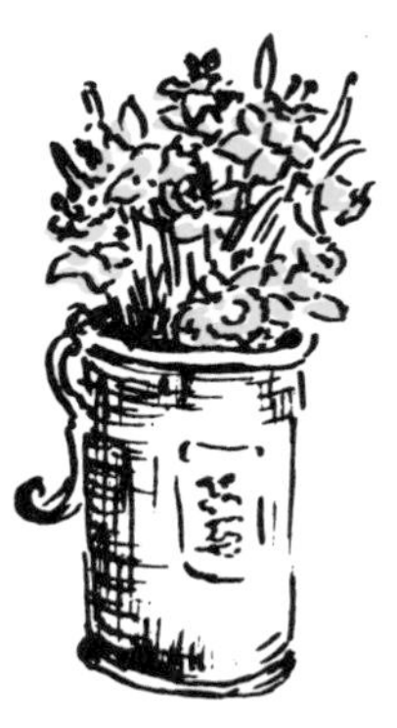

WEST COAST ZUCCHINI

Serves: 8

2 1/2-3 lbs. zucchini, cut in 1/2″ slices
6 green onions with tops, sliced
12 fresh mushrooms, sliced
1 6-oz. can pitted ripe olives
2 tomatoes, thickly sliced
1 clove garlic, crushed
1/4 tsp. salt
1/8 tsp. pepper
1 tsp. oregano or Italian seasoning
1 15-oz. can tomato sauce
8 oz. Monterey Jack cheese, sliced

Place first 5 ingredients in shallow 2 or 3-qt. casserole. Combine garlic, seasonings and tomato sauce. Pour over vegetables. Bake at 375° for 20-25 minutes. Cover top with cheese. Return to oven for 5 minutes more or until cheese melts.

For crisp zucchini cook the minimum time. This is a good meatless main dish.

CAULIFLOWER AU GRATIN

Serves: 8

1 large head cauliflower
5 Tbsp. grated Parmesan cheese
1 cup grated Gruyère cheese
1 1/4 cups bread cubes
4 Tbsp. butter, melted
Paprika

Béchamel Sauce:
2 Tbsp. butter
2 Tbsp. flour
1/8 tsp. thyme
1/8 tsp. nutmeg
1/8 tsp. salt
2 1/2 cups warm milk
1 bay leaf
1 dash Cayenne pepper

Break cauliflower into flowerets. Cook in boiling salted water 7-8 minutes until just crisp-tender. Drain and rinse under cold water. Drain again. Lightly stir together cauliflower, Béchamel sauce and cheeses. Spoon into buttered 2-qt. casserole. Combine bread cubes and butter. Sprinkle over flowerets. Dust with paprika. Bake at 350° for 15-20 minutes. For Béchamel Sauce: melt butter, add flour and cook, stirring for 3 minutes. Add remaining ingredients and bring to boil, stirring constantly. Reduce heat and simmer gently for 40-45 minutes or until sauce is reduced by 1/2. Remove bay leaf and strain.

If the cauliflower is overcooked it loses its color. Crisp-tender is the key.

SPINACH WITH WALNUTS

Serves: 6

2 10-oz. pkg. fresh spinach
3 Tbsp. olive oil
4 green onions with tops, sliced
1 cup coarsely chopped walnuts
1/2 tsp. salt
1/4 tsp. freshly ground pepper
Lemon wedges

Remove stems from spinach, wash, drain and tear in large pieces. Place in covered pan over high heat. At first sign of steam, remove lid and toss spinach with fork just until all pieces begin to wilt. Remove from heat. Heat oil, stir in onions and walnuts. Pour over spinach, add seasonings and toss lightly. Serve immediately. Garnish with lemon wedges.

This takes only a few minutes to prepare and is a change from the usual butter and lemon juice topping.

EASY POTATOES AU GRATIN

Serves: 12

1/2 clove garlic, crushed
2 Tbsp. butter
1 2-lb. pkg. frozen hash brown potatoes
2 tsp. salt
1/2 tsp. pepper
1/8 tsp. nutmeg
4 cups milk
8 oz. Swiss cheese, shredded
2 eggs, slightly beaten
4 Tbsp. butter

Combine garlic and butter and rub inside 2-qt. casserole. Break apart potatoes and stir together with salt, pepper, nutmeg, milk, 1 1/2 cups cheese and eggs. Pour into casserole. Dot • with butter. Bake at 350° for 1 1/2 hours. Sprinkle with remaining cheese and bake 15 minutes more.

There are many variations of this recipe using the convenient frozen hash browns. See our recipe for Potato Casserole.

SWEDISH POTATOES

Serves: 10-12

12 potatoes, cooked, peeled and diced
2 large onions, chopped
1 lb. American cheese, diced
2 4-oz. jars pimentos, sliced
2 green peppers, diced
6 slices fresh bread, cubed
2 sticks butter, melted
1/2 cup milk

Mix together first 5 ingredients. Spoon 1/2 mixture in buttered 3-qt. shallow casserole. Cover with cubed bread. Top with remaining potato mixture. Combine butter and milk and pour over potatoes. Bake covered at 350° for 1 hour.

These potatoes go particularly well with ham.

CREAMED CORN

Serves: 8

2 10-oz. pkg. frozen corn, thawed
1 cup whipping cream
1 cup milk
1 tsp. salt
1 Tbsp. sugar
1/8 tsp. white pepper
2 Tbsp. butter, melted
2 1/2 Tbsp. flour
1 Tbsp. grated Parmesan cheese

Combine first 6 ingredients, bring to boil, simmer 5 minutes. Blend butter and flour, add to corn, bring to simmer, stirring, remove from heat and serve. Or pour into shallow casserole, sprinkle with cheese and place under broiler until golden.

This is a recipe every one must try for it is so easy and absolutely delicious.

MONTEREY POTATOES

Serves: 6-8

1 medium onion, diced
1/2 green pepper, diced
1 1/2 Tbsp. butter
1 1/2 Tbsp. olive oil
2 1-lb. cans sliced potatoes
1 10 3/4-oz. can cream of celery soup
2 Tbsp. lemon juice
1 tsp. salt
1/4 tsp. white pepper
6 oz. Monterey Jack cheese, shredded
2 Tbsp. chopped fresh parsley
Paprika

Sauté onion and green pepper in butter and olive oil until tender. Stir potatoes in well. Add next 6 ingredients. Mix carefully. Turn into buttered 1 1/2-qt. casserole. Dust with paprika. Bake at 350° for 40 minutes.

Convenient with canned potatoes, but even better when made with freshly boiled potatoes.

ROASTED POTATOES

Serves: 8

4 large baking potatoes
1 tsp. seasoned salt
6 Tbsp. butter

Scrub potatoes. Do not peel. Cut in half lengthwise. Score in diamond design on cut side. Sprinkle with seasoned salt. Melt butter in shallow baking pan. Place potatoes cut side down. Bake at 400° for 1 hour.

Nothing could be easier. Having 20 people for dinner? Prepare 10 potatoes.

MUSHROOMS FLORENTINE

Serves: 6-8

1 lb. fresh mushrooms
2 Tbsp. butter
2 10-oz. pkg. frozen chopped spinach
1 tsp. salt
1/2 cup chopped onion
4 Tbsp. butter, melted
6 oz. Cheddar cheese, shredded

Slice stems off mushrooms. Wipe mushroom caps clean with damp paper towel. Sauté in 2 Tbsp. butter, browning lightly, cap side first. Line shallow 10" square casserole with spinach that is thawed, drained and seasoned with salt, onion and melted butter. Sprinkle with 1/2 cup cheese. Arrange mushrooms, stem side down, over spinach and sprinkle with remaining cheese. Bake at 350° for 20 minutes.

This is easily doubled and a good vegetable dish for a large crowd. May be prepared ahead.

ARTICHOKE CASSEROLE

Serves: 4-6

8 1/2-oz. can artichoke hearts
3/4 lb. fresh mushrooms
2 Tbsp. butter
1 cup Hellman's mayonnaise
6 oz. Cheddar cheese, shredded
6 oz. Mozzarella cheese, shredded
1/4 tsp. garlic powder
2 Tbsp. grated Parmesan cheese
2 Tbsp. seasoned bread crumbs
Paprika

Quarter artichoke hearts. Slice mushrooms and sauté in butter until they release their moisture. Drain. Arrange artichoke hearts and mushrooms in 1 1/2-qt. shallow baking dish. Combine next 4 ingredients. Spread over vegetables. Sprinkle with remaining ingredients. Bake at 350° for about 1/2 hour.

The topping is delicious and should work well over other vegetable combinations.

BROCCOLI LOAF

Serves: 8

1 bunch broccoli
1/4 cup chopped green onions
1/4 cup chopped shallots
2 Tbsp. butter
2 eggs, beaten
1 tsp. tarragon leaves
1/8 tsp. garlic powder
1/2 tsp. salt
1/3 cup grated Parmesan cheese
1 1/2 cups cooked rice

Mushroom Sauce:
1/2 lb. mushrooms, sliced
3 Tbsp. butter
1 Tbsp. sherry
1 Tbsp. cornstarch
1/3 cup water

Cook broccoli in salted water until barely tender. Drain, cool and chop coarsely. Sauté onions and shallots in butter. Combine next 6 ingredients. Stir in onions, shallots and broccoli. Pour into well-buttered bundt pan. Bake at 350° for 30 minutes. To serve, unmold on large platter. Pour mushroom sauce into center and over loaf. For Mushroom Sauce: sauté mushrooms in butter 5 minutes. Add sherry. Combine cornstarch and water. Add to mushrooms. Cook, stirring 5 minutes on low heat.

Use 1/2 cup more green onions if shallots are not available.

RATATOUILLE CASSEROLE **Serves: 6**

1 medium eggplant
2 medium zucchini
1 large onion
2 green peppers
1/4 cup olive oil
2 cloves garlic, minced
1 tsp. minced fresh thyme, or 1/2 tsp. dried
1 bay leaf
1 tsp. salt
1/4 tsp. pepper
4 medium tomatoes, peeled
1 cup chopped fresh parsley
1/2 cup pitted ripe olives
2 cups grated Fontina cheese
3/4 cup grated Parmesan cheese

Peel eggplant. Cut in 1 1/2″ cubes. Cut zucchini in 1/2″ slices. Chop onion coarsely. Cut green peppers in 1 1/2″ squares. Heat oil in large heavy pan. Add eggplant and sauté 5 minutes. Stir in onion, zucchini, green pepper and seasonings and cook 4 minutes. Cut tomatoes in 1″ wedges. Add to pan with parsley. Simmer 20 minutes, stirring occasionally. Stir in olives and remove from heat. Cool. Layer 1/3 vegetables in casserole, 1/3 Fontina and 1/3 Parmesan cheese. Repeat. Bake at 425° for 30 minutes.

Good late summer picnic dish that uses garden vegetables to advantage.

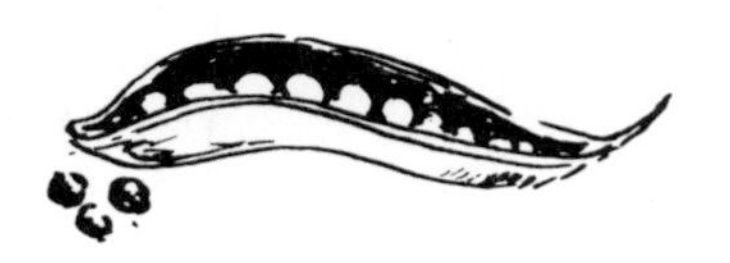

MIXED VEGETABLES WITH SAUCE **Serves: 20**

2 10-oz. pkg. frozen green beans
2 10-oz. pkg. frozen peas
2 10-oz. pkg. frozen lima beans
1 tsp. salt
2 cups mayonnaise
4 Tbsp. olive oil
1 Tbsp. Worcestershire sauce
1 small onion, grated
1 tsp. prepared mustard
Dash Tabasco sauce

Cook vegetables separately as packages direct. Drain, stir together and add salt. Combine remaining ingredients and heat. Spoon over vegetables.

The sauce can be prepared early in the day and heated at serving time.

CARROTS WITH HERBS

Serves: 4-6

3 Tbsp. butter
1 lb. carrots, thinly sliced
3 Tbsp. water
1/4 tsp. salt
3 Tbsp. cream
1/2 tsp. sugar
1/2 tsp. marjoram
1 Tbsp. chopped fresh parsley

In frying pan, melt butter, add carrots, water and salt. Simmer covered for 3 minutes. Carrots should be crisp. Add next 3 ingredients. Simmer uncovered 3 minutes more or until liquid is absorbed. Sprinkle with parsley.

A food processor slices the carrots perfectly in seconds.

LIMA BEANS WITH MUSHROOMS AND CELERY

Serves: 6-8

2 10-oz. pkg. frozen baby lima beans
1 medium onion, minced
5 stalks celery, thinly sliced
1 stick butter
1 1/2 lb. mushrooms, sliced
2 Tbsp. flour
1/2 tsp. pepper
2 cups whipping cream
Paprika

Cook lima beans according to package directions. Drain and set aside. Sauté onions and celery in butter until crisp-tender. Add mushrooms. Cook 5 minutes. Stir in flour and pepper until blended. Remove from heat and slowly stir in cream. Return to heat and cook, stirring until mixture bubbles. Add lima beans. Garnish with paprika.

Prepare this any time ahead and just reheat to serve.

MUSHROOM SOUFFLÉ CASSEROLE

Serves: 6-8

1 lb. fresh mushrooms, coarsely chopped
4 Tbsp. butter
1/2 cup chopped onion
1/2 cup chopped green pepper
1/2 cup chopped celery
1/2 cup mayonnaise
3/4 tsp. salt
1/4 tsp. pepper
8 slices white bread, buttered
2 eggs
1 1/2 cups milk
1 10 3/4-oz. can cream of mushroom soup

Sauté mushrooms in butter 5 minutes. Add next 6 ingredients. Cut 3 slices bread in cubes. Place in buttered 2-qt. casserole. Pour mushroom mixture over bread cubes. Top with 3 more slices bread, cubed. Beat eggs with milk. Pour over casserole. Cover and refrigerate at least 1 hour or up to 24 hours. Spoon undiluted soup over top of casserole. Top with remaining 2 slices bread, cubed. Bake at 325° for 50-60 minutes.

If you like, top casserole with grated cheese for last 10 minutes of baking.

SCALLOPED MUSHROOMS AND ALMONDS

Serves: 6

3 lb. small mushrooms
1/3 cup butter
2 cups light cream
4 Tbsp. flour
1/2 tsp. salt
1/4 tsp. white pepper
1/3 cup toasted almonds
2 Tbsp. snipped fresh parsley
Paprika

Sauté mushrooms in butter 5 minutes. Stir 1/2 cup cream into flour. Add remaining cream to mushrooms. Stir in flour mixture and cook, stirring until sauce bubbles. Simmer 3 minutes. Add salt, pepper and almonds. Pour into casserole. Bake at 350° for about 15 minutes. Sprinkle with parsley and paprika to serve.

A marvelous side dish to serve with any roast or ham.

CARAWAY BRUSSELS SPROUTS

Serves: 8

1 1/2 lb. fresh brussels sprouts
2 cups chicken broth
6 Tbsp. butter, melted
1 1/2 Tbsp. fresh lemon juice
1 Tbsp. caraway seeds
1/2 tsp. salt
1/4 tsp. freshly ground pepper
3 Tbsp. fresh bread crumbs
2 Tbsp. butter

Trim stems, discard blemished outer leaves and rinse sprouts in cold water. Cook in broth over medium-high heat 5-7 minutes or until just tender. Drain and toss with next 5 ingredients. Place in baking dish, sprinkle with bread crumbs and dot with butter. Place under broiler until crumbs are crisp and golden. Serve immediately.

Two 10-oz. pkg. frozen Brussels sprouts may be substituted.

FESTIVE ONIONS

Serves: 6

4 cups sliced onions
5 Tbsp. butter
2 eggs
1 cup cream
1/2 tsp. salt
1/4 tsp. white pepper
2/3 cup grated Parmesan cheese

Sauté onions in butter until clear. Spread in 10″ square baking dish. Beat eggs until light. Add cream, salt and pepper. Pour over onions. Sprinkle with Parmesan cheese. Bake at 425° for 15 minutes.

For color, add chopped green or red pepper or fresh snipped parsley.

ACORN SQUASH WITH SLICED APPLES

Serves: 6

3 fresh acorn squash
1/2 cup boiling water
1/2 tsp. salt
3 tart apples, peeled, cored and cut in wedges
6 Tbsp. butter
6 Tbsp. brown sugar
Nutmeg and cinnamon
1/2 cup boiling water

Cut squash in half and remove seeds. Place cut side down in buttered baking dish. Pour in 1/2 cup boiling water. Bake at 350° for 20 minutes. Remove from oven, pour off liquid, turn squash upright, sprinkle with salt. Fill squash with apples, dot with butter and brown sugar, sprinkle with nutmeg and cinnamon. Pour 1/2 cup boiling water into dish and bake 30 minutes more or until squash and apples are tender.

Eat the whole thing. You will find the skin of the squash tender and tasty.

SWEET POTATO SOUFFLÉ

Serves: 6

3 medium sweet potatoes, cooked
2 eggs, separated
3/4 cup sugar
4 Tbsp. butter, melted
1 tsp. vanilla
1/2 tsp. cinnamon
1 13-oz. can evaporated milk
1/2 cup chopped nuts

Cool, peel and mash potatoes. Beat egg yolks and stir in with next 5 ingredients. Beat egg whites until stiff and fold into potato mixture. Fold in nuts. Spoon into buttered 1 1/2-qt. soufflé dish or casserole. Bake at 350° for about 30 minutes.

Prepare ahead up to beating and adding egg whites. Complete just before baking.

BROCCOLI SOUFFLÉ

Serves: 8

1 10-oz. pkg. frozen chopped broccoli
3 Tbsp. butter
3 Tbsp. flour
1 cup milk
1 cup mayonnaise
1/2 tsp. salt
1 small onion, minced
6 eggs, separated
1/8 tsp. salt

Cook broccoli in 1/2 time given on package. Drain and set aside. Melt butter, stir in flour and cook until bubbling. Remove from heat, slowly stir in milk, return to heat, stirring until thick. Combine broccoli with sauce, mayonnaise, salt and onion. Beat egg yolks and stir in. Beat egg whites with 1/8 tsp. salt until stiff. Fold into broccoli mixture. Spoon into buttered 10″ × 12″ baking dish. Place in pan of hot water. Bake at 325° for about 45 minutes.

Here is one soufflé that can be held in the oven on warm indefinitely.

HOT CAULIFLOWER WITH SHRIMP SAUCE

Serves: 4-6

4 Tbsp. butter
1/4 cup flour
1 cup milk
1 cup light cream
1/2 tsp. salt
1/4 tsp. white pepper
1/2 cup whipping cream
1 large head cauliflower
2 cups chopped cooked shrimp
12 whole cooked shrimp

Melt butter, stir in flour and gradually add milk and cream, stirring constantly. Cook and stir until mixture thickens and bubbles. Remove from heat. Stir in salt and pepper. Whip cream and fold in. Trim stem and leaves from cauliflower and cook in boiling salted water until crisp-tender, about 15 minutes. Drain, place on hot platter and keep warm. Add chopped shrimp to sauce and heat through. Pour sauce over cauliflower and garnish with whole shrimp.

Sherry may be used for part of the milk; 1/4 cup and 3/4 cup milk works well.

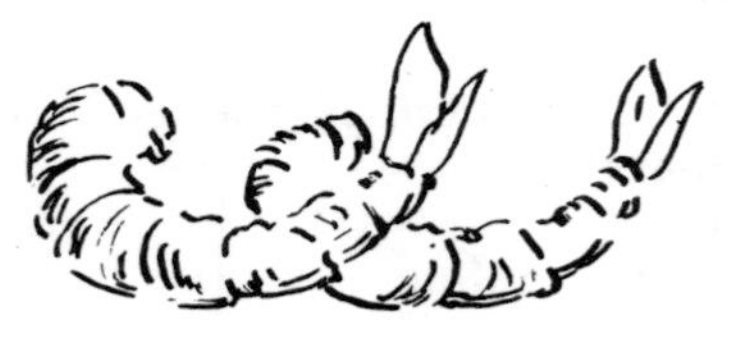

VEGETABLE MEDLEY

Serves: 10-12

2 lb. fresh spinach
1/4 tsp. salt
1/8 tsp. pepper
1 lb. mushrooms, coarsely chopped
2 lb. tomatoes, peeled, seeded, chopped and cut in chunks
3 cloves garlic, minced
2-3 shallots, minced
1 cup chopped fresh parsley
1 tsp. dried thyme
1 cup beef or chicken stock
1/4 tsp. nutmeg
1/4 tsp. salt
1/8 tsp. pepper
2 Tbsp. butter

Trim stems from spinach, wash well and steam until spinach just wilts. Rinse under cold water and squeeze out all moisture. Chop coarsely, lightly salt and pepper. Set aside. Over medium heat cook and stir mushrooms until they release their moisture. Add tomatoes, increase heat to medium-high and cook, stirring until 1/2 liquid evaporates. Add remaining ingredients except butter. Lightly salt and pepper. Heat through. Spoon 2/3 spinach into buttered 9″ pie plate. Pour mushroom mixture over spinach. Mask top with remaining spinach. Dot with butter. Bake at 400° for 15-20 minutes.

Four 10-oz. pkg. frozen spinach may be used for fresh. Cook according to directions and drain well.

MUSHROOM STUFFED TOMATOES

Serves: 8

8 firm ripe tomatoes
1 lb. mushrooms, sliced
4 Tbsp. butter
8 oz. sour cream
5 tsp. flour
3 oz. Bleu cheese, crumbled
1/2 tsp. leaf oregano
1/2 tsp. basil
2 Tbsp. chopped fresh parsley
2 Tbsp. dry sherry
1/2 tsp. salt
1/4 tsp. white pepper
Paprika

Cut slice from top of each tomato, scoop out pulp, invert and drain. Sauté mushrooms in butter until tender, drain and set aside. Combine next 9 ingredients, cook over low heat, stirring constantly until thickened and smooth. Stir in drained mushrooms. Stuff tomatoes, place in shallow baking pan and sprinkle with paprika. Bake at 375° for 15 minutes.

This would be a dish to enjoy year round if only lovely red, ripe tomatoes were always available.

MIXED VEGETABLE CASSEROLE

Serves: 12

4 Tbsp. butter
3/4 cup chopped green pepper
1 clove garlic, crushed
1/4 cup flour
1 cup milk
3/4 tsp. salt
1/8 tsp. pepper
1/8 tsp. basil
1/8 tsp. oregano
1/4 tsp. sugar
4 oz. Cheddar cheese, grated
1 28-oz. can tomatoes, well drained
1 10-oz. pkg. frozen whole kernel corn, defrosted
1 16-oz. can whole small onions, drained

Melt butter and sauté green pepper and garlic for 5 minutes. Stir in flour. Slowly add milk, stirring until thickened and bubbling. Stir in seasonings, sugar and 1/2 cheese until melted. Remove from heat. Add vegetables. Turn into shallow 2-qt. baking dish. Sprinkle with remaining cheese. Bake at 350° for 45 minutes.

Three and a half cups of fresh tomatoes, peeled, cut in wedges and seeded may be used for the canned.

Rice and Pasta

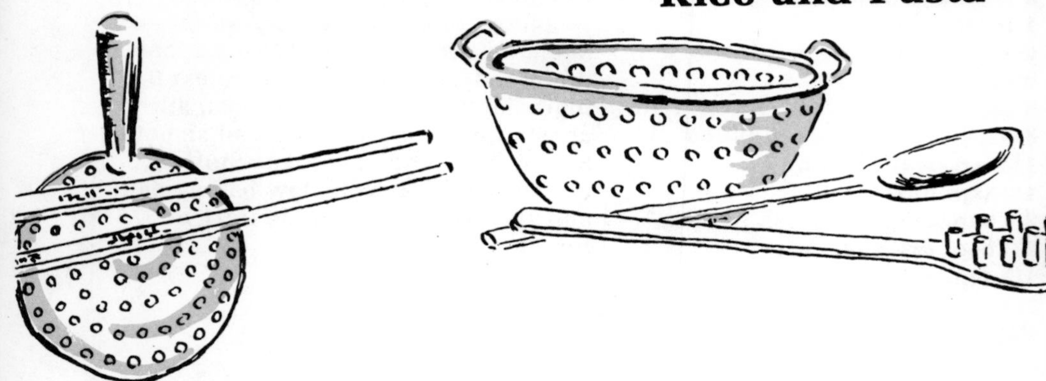

BROWNED WHITE RICE

Serves: 6

1/4 cup butter
1 cup uncooked rice
1/3 cup chopped almonds
1 tsp. salt
1/4 tsp. pepper
1 10 1/2-oz. can beef consommé
1 cup water

Melt butter in skillet over medium heat. Add rice and almonds. Stir until golden brown. Stir in remaining ingredients. Place in 1 1/2-qt. casserole. Bake covered at 300° for 1 hour and 30 minutes.

Sprinkle top generously with chopped fresh parsley just before serving.

RICE WITH PINE NUTS

Serves: 6-8

2 Tbsp. chopped onion
4 Tbsp. butter
1 cup uncooked long grain rice
1/3 cup vermicelli, broken in 1″ pieces
1/2 cup pine nuts
1/3 cup golden raisins
2 cups chicken stock
1 tsp. salt
1 tsp. chervil, crumbled
1/8 tsp. pepper

In large saucepan sauté onion in butter until soft. Stir in next 3 ingredients. Sauté, stirring often until golden. Add remaining ingredients, bring to boil, cover and simmer 20-25 minutes.

This may also be called Risotto Pignolia.

CALICO RICE

Serves: 12

1 1/2 cups uncooked rice
3 eggs, beaten
2 cups grated Cheddar cheese
2 1/2 cups chicken broth
1 stick butter, melted
1/2 cup chopped fresh parsley
3 pimentos, chopped
3 green onions with tops, chopped
1/2 tsp. salt
1/4 tsp. white pepper

Cook rice, then combine with remaining ingredients. Pour into buttered 2 1/2-qt. casserole. Bake uncovered at 350° for 40-45 minutes.

The parsley, pimentos and green onions hold their color, lending this dish eye appeal.

BARLEY AND MUSHROOM CASSEROLE

Serves: 6-8

1 cup pearl barley
1 stick butter
1 large onion, chopped
1 lb. mushrooms, sliced
2 cups beef broth
1/4 tsp. salt
1/4 tsp. pepper
1/2 cup toasted almonds

Wash barley well, drain and pat dry. Brown barley lightly in 5 Tbsp. butter. Add onion and 1/2 lb. mushrooms Sauté until tender. Pour into buttered 2-qt. casserole. Add 1 cup broth, salt and pepper. Bake covered at 350° for 20 minutes. Add remaining broth, cover and bake 20 minutes. If barley begins to dry out, add about 1 cup water. Bake 20 minutes more or until liquid is absorbed. Sauté remaining mushrooms in 3 Tbsp. butter until very dark. Mix in almonds and spread over casserole just before serving.

Barley becomes hard if it is allowed to dry out while cooking. Usually found in soups, barley is delicious served this way.

RUSTY RICE

Serves: 6

6 Tbsp. butter
1 large onion, chopped
1 cup dry red wine
1 cup chicken broth
1 cup brown rice
1/2 tsp. salt

Melt butter and sauté onion until crisp-tender. Slowly add wine and broth. Bring to boil. Add rice, stir, cover and simmer 50-60 minutes.

For a more exciting flavor and rustier rice use 2 cups red wine instead of 1 cup wine and 1 cup chicken broth.

RICE RING

Serves: 12

6 cups cooked rice
8 oz. Monterey Jack cheese, shredded
1 4-oz. can peeled green chili peppers, chopped
1 tsp. salt
1 tsp. pepper
2 cups sour cream
1 pimento, cut in thin strips
Celery leaves
Tomato wedges

Combine first 5 ingredients, tossing lightly to mix. Fold in sour cream. Spoon into buttered 8-cup ring mold packing lightly. Bake at 350° for about 30 minutes. Cool on rack 5 minutes. Loosen edge and center. Carefully unmold on serving platter. Place pimento strips on ring. Fill center with celery leaves and tomato wedges.

This may be baked and served in a buttered casserole, if preferred.

RICE AND MUSHROOM BAKE

Serves: 6

1 cup uncooked rice
1 10 3/4-oz. can cream of mushroom soup
1 10 1/2-oz. can beef broth
4 Tbsp. butter, melted
1 4-oz. can mushroom pieces, drained

Combine all ingredients in 2-qt. casserole. Bake covered at 350° for 1 hour, stirring once.

This is very easy and reheats well.

MACARONI-CHEDDAR PUFF

Serves: 6-8

1 cup uncooked elbow macaroni
6 Tbsp. butter
6 Tbsp. flour
2 tsp. dry mustard
1 tsp. salt
1 1/2 cups milk
1 Tbsp. Worcestershire sauce
6 oz. Cheddar cheese, shredded
6 eggs, separated

Cook macaroni according to package directions. Drain and cool. Melt butter, add next 3 ingredients and cook, stirring until bubbling. Remove from heat. Slowly stir in milk and Worcestershire sauce. Return to heat and cook, stirring until mixture thickens and boils 1 minute. Stir in cheese until melted. Set aside. Beat egg whites until soft peaks form. In large bowl beat egg yolks until thick and lemony. Very slowly beat cheese sauce into yolks. Fold in egg whites, then macaroni. Spoon into buttered 2-qt. soufflé dish. Gently form deep circle in mixture 1″ from edge. This creates the high crown. Bake at 300° for about 1 hour. Serve at once.

A very royal version of the ordinary macaroni and cheese.

GOLDEN RICE SQUARES

Serves: 6

1/4 cup chopped onion
3 cups shredded carrots
1/2 cup water
2 cups cooked rice
2 eggs, beaten
1 1/2 cups shredded sharp cheese
1/2 tsp. salt
1/4 tsp. pepper
1 Tbsp. dried green pepper or 2 Tbsp. fresh green pepper
1 cup cooked peas
1 10 3/4-oz. can cream of mushroom soup
1 4-oz. can mushroom stems and pieces, drained
2/3 cup milk
1 cup cubed cooked ham

Combine first 3 ingredients. Bring to boil, remove from heat and drain well. Add next 6 ingredients. Spoon mixture into buttered 6″x10″ baking dish. Bake at 325° for 45 minutes or until firm. Combine remaining ingredients and heat through. Cut rice in squares and serve with sauce.

An economical dinner that uses leftover ham to good advantage.

SPINACH AND LINGUINE CASSEROLE

Serves: 4

1 10-oz. pkg. frozen chopped spinach
1 egg, beaten
1/2 cup sour cream
1/4 cup milk
3 Tbsp. grated Parmesan cheese
2 tsp. dried onions
1/2 tsp. salt
1/8 tsp. pepper
8 oz. Monterey Jack cheese, shredded
4 oz. linguine, cooked and drained
3 Tbsp. grated Parmesan cheese

Cook spinach according to package directions. Drain well. Combine next 8 ingredients and mix well. Stir in spinach and linguine. Turn into 10″x6″ baking dish. Sprinkle with Parmesan. Bake covered at 350° for 15 minutes. Uncover and bake 20 minutes more.

This is another very good "complete in itself" meatless meal.

CREAMY MACARONI-CHEESE BAKE

Serves: 6

2 cups elbow macaroni
1/3 cup salad dressing
1/4 cup chopped green pepper
2 Tbsp. chopped fresh parsley
1/4 cup minced onion
1 10 3/4-oz. can cream of mushroom soup
1/2 cup milk
1 cup shredded American cheese

Cook macaroni according to package directions. Drain. Combine macaroni with next 4 ingredients. Blend soup, milk and 1/2 cup cheese. Stir into macaroni. Place in 1-qt. casserole. Top with remaining cheese. Bake uncovered at 400° for 25 minutes.

Bake this casserole with Lemon Barbecued Meat Loaves. Just increase the baking time to 40-45 minutes.

NOODLES WARSAW

Serves: 6

8 oz. broad noodles
2 cups cottage cheese
2 cups sour cream
1 clove garlic, minced
1 medium onion, minced
1 tsp. Worcestershire sauce
2 drops Tabasco sauce
1/2 cup grated Parmesan cheese
1/2 tsp. salt
1/4 tsp. pepper

Cook noodles according to package directions. Combine with remaining ingredients. Turn into buttered shallow 2-qt. casserole. Bake covered at 350° about 45 minutes.

This is very easy. Consider adding a teaspoon or 2 of dillweed and garnish with parsley or paprika.

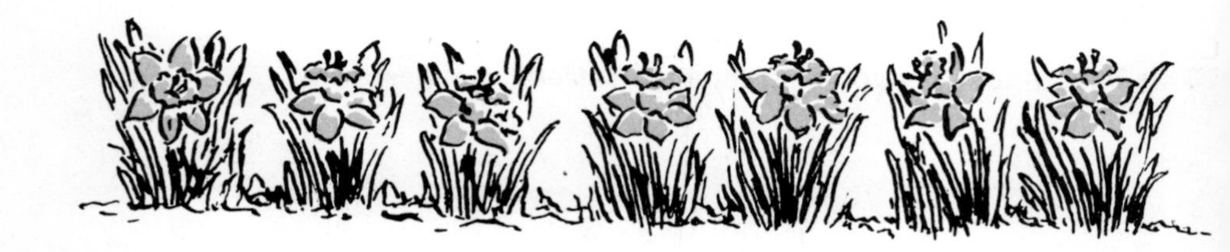

SUMMER PASTA

Serves: 4

1/2 cup olive oil
1/4 cup red wine vinegar
1/4 cup tomato puree
3 hard-boiled eggs, finely chopped
3 green onions with tops, sliced
1 large clove garlic, minced
1/8 tsp. oregano
3 Tbsp. minced fresh parsley
1 carrot, thinly sliced
8 black olives, sliced
1/2 tsp. salt
1/4 tsp. pepper
1 lb. pasta
Parmesan cheese

Combine oil and vinegar, add puree and mix well. Stir in next 9 ingredients. Let stand at room temperature 2 hours or refrigerate overnight. Bring back to room temperature before serving. Prepare favorite pasta, top with sauce and sprinkle with Parmesan.

Here is another opportunity for imagination. Slice zucchini instead of carrot. Add more olives and parsley.

PASTA WITH ARTICHOKE SAUCE

Serves: 6

4 Tbsp. olive oil
4 Tbsp. butter
2 Tbsp. flour
1 cup chicken broth
2 cloves garlic, crushed
Juice of 1 lemon
1 Tbsp. minced fresh parsley
2 Tbsp. grated Parmesan cheese
8 1/2-oz. can artichoke hearts, cut in half
1 lb. fetuccini or linguine
2 Tbsp. olive oil
1 Tbsp. grated Parmesan cheese
1 Tbsp. butter

Heat together 4 Tbsp. olive oil and butter, add flour and cook, stirring for 3 minutes. Slowly stir in chicken broth, add next 3 ingredients and cook, stirring 5 minutes more. Add 2 Tbsp. Parmesan and artichoke hearts and heat through. Cook pasta as package directs. Drain and toss with remaining oil, Parmesan and butter. Serve with sauce.

Compliments will abound when you serve this recipe.

MEATLESS MANICOTTI

Serves: 4

12 manicotti shells
3 cups diced zucchini
2 Tbsp. butter
1 1/2 cups cottage cheese
1 1/2 cups shredded Cheddar cheese
1 1 1/2-oz. pkg. Sloppy Joe seasoning mix
1 12-oz. can tomato paste
2 1/4 cups boiling water

Cook shells according to package directions. Drain, rinse in cold water, drain again. Cook zucchini in butter 3-4 minutes. Add cottage cheese, 1 cup Cheddar and mix well. Stuff shells. Arrange in single layer in shallow baking dish. Stir together next 3 ingredients and spoon over shells. Cover and bake at 375° for 30 minutes. Uncover, sprinkle with remaining 1/2 cup cheese and bake 10 minutes more.

A medium onion, diced, could be added and cooked with the zucchini or add a carrot, grated.

CANNELLONI WITH RICOTTA CHEESE

Serves: 4

Crêpes:
3/4 cup flour
1/8 tsp. salt
1 egg + 1 yolk
1 1/4 cups milk
1 Tbsp. butter, melted
1/4 cup grated Parmesan cheese

Filling:
2 cups Ricotta cheese
2 egg yolks, beaten
1 cup grated Parmesan cheese
2 Tbsp. chopped fresh parsley
1/8 tsp. nutmeg
1/4 tsp. salt
1/8 tsp. white pepper
1/4 cup diced onion
1/4 cup diced green pepper
1 Tbsp. butter
2 cups tomato puree
1/2 tsp. oregano
1/2 tsp. basil leaves
2 Tbsp. chopped fresh parsley
2 Tbsp. Parmesan cheese
2 Tbsp. butter, melted

For Crêpes: place ingredients in jar of blender. Blend 10 seconds. Cook in 5″-6″ crêpe pan over medium-high heat, using 3 Tbsp. batter for each crêpe. Lightly butter pan after each. Set 8 crêpes aside. Freeze others for another use. For Filling: stir together first 7 ingredients. Set aside. Sauté onion and pepper in butter until crisp-tender. Stir in next 4 ingredients. Simmer together 5-10 minutes. Place 3 Tbsp. tomato sauce in bottom of shallow 2-qt. casserole. Divide Ricotta mixture evenly among 8 crêpes, fill, roll and place seam side down in casserole. Spoon over remaining tomato sauce. Sprinkle with Parmesan cheese. Pour over melted butter. Bake at 400° for about 20 minutes.

For 8, double Riccota filling and increase tomato sauce ingredients by 1/2.

Salads and Dressings

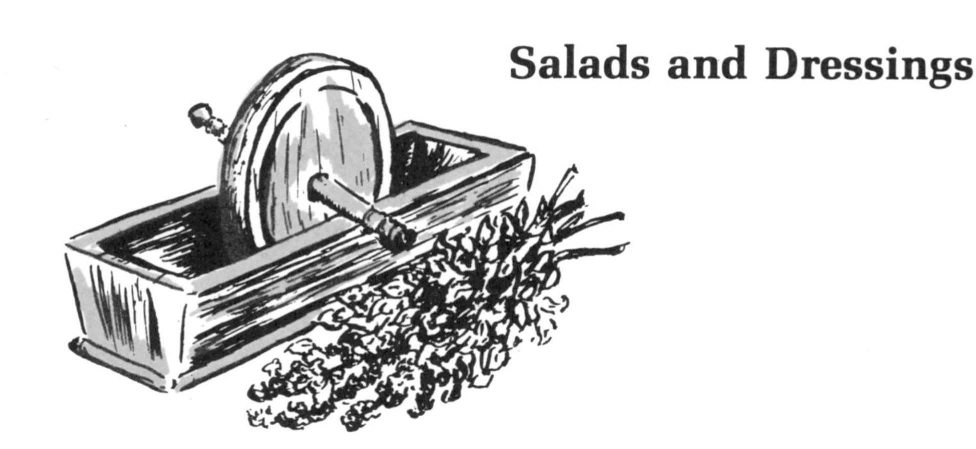

VEGETABLE SALAD VINAIGRETTE

Serves: 16

1 small head cauliflower
4 medium carrots
2 10-oz. pkg. frozen asparagus spears
1/2 lb. green beans
2 medium tomatoes, wedged
8 oz. fresh mushrooms, sliced
1 8-oz. can artichoke hearts, drained
Paprika
Parsley sprigs

Vinaigrette Dressing:
2 cups salad oil
1 cup white wine vinegar
2 Tbsp. sugar
2 Tbsp. prepared horseradish
2 Tbsp. grated onion
2 Tbsp. Dijon mustard
2 Tbsp. chopped pimento
1 1/2 tsp. salt
1 tsp. celery salt
1 tsp. fines herbs
1/2 tsp. pepper
1 clove garlic, crushed

Cook whole cauliflower covered in 1″ boiling salted water until crisp-tender, about 8 minutes. Drain. Rinse with cold water. Cut carrots into 1 1/2″x1/4″ strips. Cook as above until crisp-tender, about 3 minutes. Rinse in cold water. Cook asparagus 3 minutes. Rinse as above. Snap ends from beans, cook until crisp-tender, about 8 minutes. Rinse. Pat vegetables dry. Place cauliflower in center of serving platter. Arrange carrots around cauliflower. Decoratively place all remaining vegetables on platter. Cover and chill several hours. To serve, sprinkle cauliflower with paprika. Garnish platter with parsley sprigs. Serve vinaigrette dressing in separate bowl. For Dressing: combine all ingredients in large jar. Cover, shake well, and refrigerate.

This is lovely enough to serve as an edible centerpiece.

POTATO SALAD WITH HERRING

Yield: 2 quarts

8 medium potatoes
1/2 cup salad oil
1/4 cup white vinegar
2 tsp. seasoned salt
1 cup sour cream
1/2 cup mayonnaise
2 3-oz. cans Kingli herring, drained and chopped
1 cup chopped red onions
1 tsp. dill weed
Red onion rings
Parsley sprigs

Cook potatoes in jackets in boiling salted water until done. While still warm, peel, dice and add oil, vinegar and seasoned salt. Cover and chill 1 hour. Add next 5 ingredients. Chill to blend flavors. At serving time, garnish with onion rings and sprigs of parsley.

If Kingli herring, available in specialty stores and some super markets, cannot be found, use 4 oz. of luncheon herring.

SEAFOOD SALAD WITH SAFFRON DRESSING

Serves: 4-6

3 cups shrimp or langostinos, cooked
1 1/2 cups potatoes, cooked and cubed
1 1/2 cups peas, cooked
1 cup head lettuce
1 cup romaine lettuce
Black olives

Saffron Dressing:
1 cup mayonnaise
1/4 cup lemon juice
1/3 tsp. powdered saffron or 6 threads
1 Tbsp. water
2 tsp. salt
1/4 tsp. white pepper
4 drops liquid red pepper seasoning
2 Tbsp. minced onion
1 tsp. prepared mustard

Cut seafood in bite-sized pieces and chill with potatoes and peas. Wash and chill greens. An hour before serving tear greens and toss all salad ingredients together lightly with saffron dressing. Chill 1 hour. Garnish with black olives to serve. For Dressing: mix mayonnaise and lemon juice together. Dissolve saffron in water and add. If using threads, mash well in water and just use liquid. Stir in remaining ingredients, mix well and chill.

A very special salad and an excellent luncheon selection.

FROZEN WALDORF SALAD

Serves: 8

1/2 cup sugar
1/2 cup pineapple juice
1/8 tsp. salt
1/4 cup lemon juice
1/2 cup diced celery
1/2 cup crushed pineapple, well-drained
2 medium apples, diced
1/2 cup walnuts, broken
1 cup whipping cream
8 maraschino cherries

In a saucepan combine first 4 ingredients. Cook, stirring constantly over medium-high heat until thick. Cool. Stir in next 4 ingredients. Whip cream and fold in. Spoon into 8″ square pan. Freeze. To serve, remove from freezer 5 minutes before serving, cut in squares and garnish with cherries.

Serve this salad with stuffed pork chops in place of applesauce.

BAY SHRIMP WITH MELON CRESCENTS

Serves: 6-8

2 lb. bay shrimp
1 cup mayonnaise
1/2 cup catsup
1 tsp. lemon juice
1 tsp. dill weed
1 cantaloupe

Cook and clean shrimp. Mix together next 4 ingredients. Stir in shrimp. Chill. Cut cantaloupe into 6-8 wedges. Place on salad plates. Spoon shrimp over each.

For another way to serve, cut melon in cubes. Place in large glass bowl in layers with shrimp. Garnish with fresh dill.

MACARONI SALAD

Serves: 10

1 1-lb. box small elbow macaroni
3/4 cup sugar
2 Tbsp. flour
1/2 tsp. salt
1 20-oz. can pineapple chunks
2 cans mandarin oranges
1 10 1/2-oz. jar maraschino cherries
2 eggs, beaten
1 pt. whipping cream, whipped

Cook macaroni in salt water for 8-10 minutes. Drain. Cool. In saucepan stir together sugar, flour and salt. Drain all fruits and slowly stir juice into sugar mixture. Add eggs. Cook, stirring until mixture just boils and is thickened. Cool. Stir into macaroni and chill overnight. Next morning, cut up pineapple, oranges and cherries, reserving 3-4 for garnish. Add to macaroni. Stir in whipped cream. Decorate with cherries. Chill until serving time.

A very unusual and surprisingly good combination. 2 8-oz. cartons of Cool Whip may be substituted for whipped cream.

TURIN 'N TUNA

Serves: 4

1 7-oz. can tuna
2 cups cooked shell macaroni
3/4 cup diced sweet pickle
1/2 cup diced pineapple
2 hard-boiled eggs, chopped
1/2 cup diced celery
1/4 cup diced green pepper
2 Tbsp. chopped onion
3/4 cup mayonnaise
1 tsp. salt
1/8 tsp. pepper

Drain and flake tuna. Stir together with remaining ingredients. Chill.

When tomatoes are in season, cut 1 or 2 in wedges and use as a garnish.

VEGETABLE SALAD

Serves: 12

1 small cauliflower
1 bunch broccoli
1 10-oz. pkg. frozen peas, defrosted and uncooked
8 oz. Cucumber dressing
1 purple onion
3 cups shredded lettuce

The day before, wash, dry and cut cauliflower and broccoli into bite-size flowerets. Place in bowl. Toss with peas and cucumber dressing. Cover lightly. Chill overnight. 4 hours before serving add purple onion sliced in thin rings. At serving time add shredded lettuce.

Good salad to serve in place of a vegetable.

DRESSED POTATO SALAD

Serves: 6-8

5 large potatoes
1 cup chicken broth
2/3 cup French dressing
1 bunch green onions with tops, sliced
2 Tbsp. chopped fresh parsley
1 Tbsp. celery seed
3/4 cup mayonnaise

Boil potatoes in skins. Peel and cube while hot. Pour over broth and dressing. Chill 2-3 hours or overnight. Drain off liquid, if any. Stir in remaining ingredients. Let stand 1 hour.

Can be made a day or two ahead. Marvelous with ham or broiled chicken.

ANTIPASTO SALAD

Serves: 12

2 7-oz. cans tuna, drained and chunked
1/2 lb. mushrooms, sliced
1 5-oz. jar stuffed green olives, drained and cut in half
1 6-oz. can pitted black olives, drained and cut in half
1 8-oz. can artichoke hearts, drained and cut in quarters
4 oz. tiny sweet pickles, sliced in half lengthwise
2 1/2-oz. cocktail onions
1 2-oz. jar sliced pimentos, drained

Dressing:
2 8-oz. cans tomato sauce
1/2 cup salad oil
4 Tbsp. vinegar
Juice of 1 lemon

Combine all ingredients and toss gently with dressing. Cover and refrigerate at least 24 hours. Serve on bed of shredded lettuce. For Dressing: shake together well all ingredients.

The perfect salad to have on hand during the hot days of summer.

FROZEN PEA SALAD

Serves: 6-8

2 10-oz. pkg. frozen peas, partially thawed
1/4 cup sliced green onions with tops
1/4 cup diced celery
1/2 tsp. salt
1/2 tsp. pepper
8-oz. sour cream
10 slices bacon, cooked crisp, crumbled
1/2 cup cashew halves

Mix together first 6 ingredients. Refrigerate. At serving time, stir in bacon and cashews.

Slivered almonds could be substituted for cashews. To double, use only 1 1/2 cups sour cream.

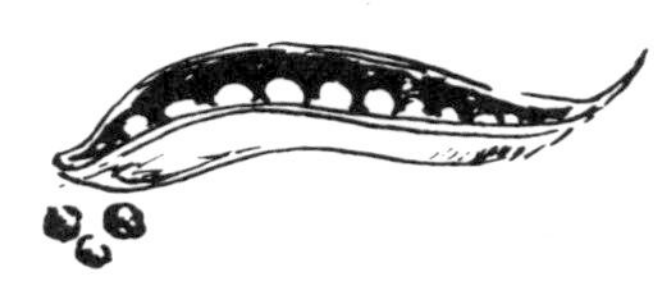

BUFFET SALAD

Serves: 12-16

1 8-oz. can artichoke hearts, rinsed and drained
1 1-lb. can green asparagus, drained
1 1-lb. can white asparagus, drained
1 head cauliflower, steamed 3 mins. and separated into pieces
1 1-lb. can miniature whole beets, drained
1 avocado, sliced and sprinkled with lemon juice
2 tomatoes, peeled and sliced
1 cucumber, partially peeled and sliced
1/4 lb. fresh mushrooms, sliced
3 cups Italian dressing
Lettuce leaves
Chopped pimento
Grated hard-boiled egg yolks
Fresh or dried dill weed
Fresh parsley
Capers

Place each vegetable in separate container. Pour 1/3 cup dressing over each. Place in refrigerator several hours or overnight. Near serving time, line large platter with lettuce leaves. Attractively arrange vegetables on lettuce. Garnish cauliflower with pimento, green asparagus with egg yolk, cucumber with dill, tomatoes with parsley, mushrooms with capers.

There are many more vegetable combinations that can be added or used instead. Be creative!

OLD-FASHIONED CHICKEN SALAD

Serves: 6

1 3-lb. chicken
1 cup water
1/2 tsp. salt
1/4 tsp. pepper
1/4 cup French dressing
1 cup thinly sliced celery
1/2 cup mayonnaise
2 Tbsp. capers or chopped sweet pickle
6 slices pineapple
Lettuce leaves
1 hard-boiled egg, sliced

Place chicken in Dutch oven. Pour in water. Season with salt and pepper. Bake covered at 350° for 2 1/2 hours. Cool. Remove enough meat from chicken to make 2 cups diced. Pour on French dressing and chill 2-3 hours. Pour off dressing. Add celery, mayonnaise and capers or pickles. Toss just to mix. Top each pineapple slice evenly with salad. Garnish with egg and extra capers.

This is easily doubled. Place on individual plates covered with shredded lettuce or arrange attractively on a large platter.

CRUNCHY HAM SALAD

Serves: 4

1/4 head iceberg lettuce, torn in bite-size pieces
2 medium slices baked ham, cut in bite-size pieces
3/4 cup lo-cal cottage cheese
1 medium carrot, sliced
2 stalks celery, cut up
1 Tbsp. sunflower seeds
3 Tbsp. soynuts
3 Tbsp. creamy Bleu cheese dressing
4 Tbsp. creamy Italian dressing
1 Tbsp. bacon bits
1/4 tsp. garlic salt
1/4 tsp. salad seasoning

Layer ingredients in large bowl in order given. Toss together lightly. Use more or less dressing to suit.

Substitute chunks of tuna or salmon for ham.

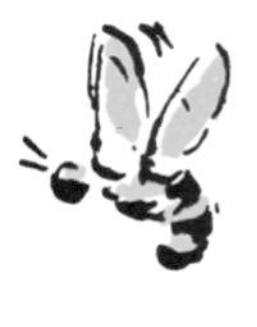

ORIGINAL CAESAR SALAD

Serves: 6-8

3 medium heads romaine lettuce
1 egg, room temperature
Juice of 1 1/2 fresh lemons
1/8 tsp. salt
1/8 tsp. Worcestershire sauce
1 1/2 Tbsp. wine vinegar
1 cup croutons
1/3 cup garlic flavored salad oil
6 Tbsp. Parmesan cheese
Freshly ground pepper

Wash, dry and chill lettuce until crisp. Tear into pieces and place in large wooden bowl. Push to 1 side. In other side, break in egg and add next 4 ingredients. Whisk together until well combined. Gently toss in lettuce. Spinkle over next 3 ingredients. Gently toss again. Top with freshly ground pepper.

Soak 2 cloves garlic, peeled, sliced and threaded on a toothpick in oil for 1 week. Anchovies are an optional addition.

KOREAN SALAD

Serves: 8-10

1 lb. fresh spinach
1 1-lb. can bean sprouts, drained
1 8-oz. can water chestnuts, sliced
2 hard-boiled eggs, sliced
5 strips bacon, cooked crisp and crumbled

Dressing:
1 cup salad oil
2/3 cup sugar
1/3 cup catsup
1 medium onion, cut up
1 tsp. salt
1/4 cup cider vinegar
1 Tbsp. Worcestershire sauce

Wash and dry spinach. Tear into bite-size pieces. Sprinkle over next 4 ingredients. For Dressing: combine all ingredients in blender until well mixed. Carefully toss salad with desired amount of dressing. Serve immediately.

Spinach in salads bruises easily, so use fewest tosses necessary to just barely combine.

RICE AND MINT SALAD

Serves: 8-10

2 Tbsp. olive oil
2 Tbsp. tarragon vinegar
1/2 tsp. salt
1/2 tsp. nutmeg
3 cups warm cooked rice
1 6-oz. can pitted black olives, cut in half
1 cup Calamata olives, pitted and cut in half
1/4 cup minced fresh mint
1/2 cup chopped green and sweet red peppers
Tomato wedges

Whip together first 4 ingredients. Stir in remaining ingredients except tomatoes. Chill. Mound on plate and garnish with tomatoes.

A nice accompaniment to lamb. Also is refreshing to serve with highly seasoned foods. If Calamata olives can't be found, substitute a similar greek olive.

MARINATED BROCCOLI

Serves: 16

3 bunches fresh broccoli
1 cup cider vinegar
1 1/2 cups salad oil
1 Tbsp. dill weed
1 Tbsp. sugar
1 tsp. salt
1 tsp. pepper
1 tsp. garlic salt

Wash, peel tough skin and cut broccoli into bite-size pieces, including sliced stems. Place in large jar. Shake together remaining ingredients. Pour over broccoli and refrigerate 24 hours or longer, turning jar occasionally. Remove from marinade to serve. Marinade may be reused.

Substitute other vegetables instead of 1 or 2 bunches broccoli, such as cauliflowerets, zucchini strips, barely cooked carrots and small mushrooms.

POACHED CHICKEN CURRY SALAD

Serves: 8

4 whole chicken breasts
1 small onion, chopped
1 Tbsp. salad oil
2 tsp. curry powder
1/4 cup tomato juice
1/4 cup red wine
2 Tbsp. apricot jam
1 1/2 cups mayonnaise

Cut in half, skin and bone chicken breasts. Poach until tender. Refrigerate. Sauté onion in oil until soft. Add curry powder and cook, stirring 1 minute. Add juice and wine. Simmer until reduced by half. Add jam and cool. Press through strainer and add to mayonnaise. Arrange breasts on platter, top each with sauce and chill.

To serve, garnish platter with watermelon pickles and preserved kumquats, parsley or watercress.

TOSSED FRESH FRUIT SALAD

Serves: 6-8

1 cantaloupe
1 honeydew melon
1 fresh pineapple
1 pt. strawberries
2 oranges
1 head iceberg lettuce

Dressing:
1/3 cup light corn syrup
3/4 cup Hellman's mayonnaise
1/4 cup orange juice
1/8 tsp. grated onion

Peel and cut melons in bite-size chunks. Cube pineapple. Wash and hull strawberries. Peel and slice oranges. Refrigerate fruit. Wash, spin dry and crisp lettuce. To serve, cut lettuce in 1" cubes, add fruit and lightly toss with dressing. For Dressing: slowly stir corn syrup into mayonnaise. Stir in orange juice and onion. Chill.

For individual servings, heap the fruit and lettuce on chilled salad plates and top with dressing.

CRÈME DE MÊNTHE MOLDED SALAD

Serves: 8

1 3-oz. pkg. lime jello
3/4 cup boiling water
1 8 1/4-oz. can crushed pineapple
3 Tbsp. Crème de Mênthe
1/2 cup sour cream
1 cup diced pears
1/2 cup yogurt
1/2 cup sour cream
1 tsp. lime juice
Lime slices

Dissolve jello in boiling water. Drain pineapple and combine juice and Crème de Mênthe with water to make 3/4 cup. Add to jello. Chill until slightly thickened. Add 1/2 cup sour cream and beat until light and creamy. Fold in pears and pineapple. Pour into oiled 4-cup ring mold and chill until set. Combine yogurt, sour cream and lime juice and serve in separate bowl. Garnish salad and dressing with lime slices.

A refreshing salad that is easy and attractive.

SPINACH SALAD

Serves: 8-10

1 10-oz. pkg. fresh spinach
4 slices bacon, cooked and crumbled
1/2 cup diced green pepper
1/2 cup sliced celery
1 cup sliced mushrooms
1 tsp. dried oregano leaves
2 Tbsp. chopped fresh parsley
1/2 tsp. salt
Juice of 1/2 lemon
1/4 cup Creamy Italian dressing
1/4 cup Sweet and Sour dressing
1/4 cup Creamy Bacon dressing
2 hard-boiled eggs, grated
1/2 red onion, sliced
1/2 cup grated Parmesan cheese

Croutons:
10 slices bread
1 stick butter
1 tsp. oregano
1 tsp. dried parsley
1/2 tsp. garlic powder
1/2 tsp. celery salt
1 Tbsp. Italian seasoning

Wash, dry, tear spinach and place in chilled salad bowl. Add next 8 ingredients. Toss. Combine dressings. Toss lightly. Sprinkle eggs, onion, Parmesan and croutons on top in order given. Serve immediately. For Croutons: cut bread into 1/2″ squares leaving on crusts. Melt butter in large skillet. Toss bread in butter quickly to coat evenly. Add remaining ingredients. Mix well. Cook over low heat stirring occasionally for 1 1/2-2 hours or until toasty. Use 1/2 in salad. Cool and store remainder in air-tight container.

This is an excellent salad to serve for lunch. You may use more or less of any ingredient given.

TOMATO BROCCOLI SALAD

Serves: 12-16

2 lb. broccoli, trimmed and cut into flowerets
1/3 cup butter
2 Tbsp. olive oil
2 medium onions, chopped
2 cloves garlic, crushed
4 medium tomatoes, peeled and chopped
2 tsp. sugar
1 tsp. dried basil
1 tsp. dried oregano
1 cup mayonnaise
Cherry tomatoes

Place broccoli in 3″ boiling salted water. Simmer uncovered 5 minutes. Drain. Rinse in cold water. Drain again. Sauté onion and garlic in butter and oil until crisp-tender. Stir in next 4 ingredients. Simmer uncovered over medium heat 10 minutes, stirring occasionally. Cool. Stir in mayonnaise. Fold in broccoli. Chill several hours. Garnish with cherry tomatoes to serve.

Serve this salad on a bed of torn fresh spinach leaves for a special flavor and added nutrition.

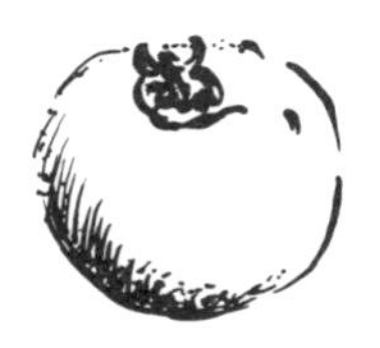

MARINATED ZUCCHINI SALAD

Serves: 8

1 1-lb. can whole baby carrots, drained
2 medium zucchini, thinly sliced
1 14-oz. can hearts of palm, drained and thickly sliced
2/3 cup salad oil
1/4 cup vinegar
1 small clove garlic, minced
1 tsp. sugar
3/4 tsp. salt
3/4 tsp. dry mustard
1/8 tsp. pepper
Bibb lettuce leaves
2 oz. Bleu cheese, crumbled

In shallow dish, combine carrots, zucchini and hearts of palm. In jar, combine next 7 ingredients. Shake well and pour over vegetables. Cover. Chill several hours or overnight. To serve, drain marinade and arrange on plates of lettuce and top with cheese.

Easy, colorful, can be doubled and will keep many days.

SEVEN LAYER JELLO

Serves: 12-16

1 3-oz. pkg. each cherry, lemon, lime and orange jello
2 cups milk
2 envelopes unflavored gelatin
1/2 cup boiling water
2 cups sour cream
1 cup sugar
2 tsp. vanilla

Make each package jello separately by dissolving in 1 cup boiling water and stirring in 1/2 cup cold water. Cool to room temperature. Pour cherry jello into 9″x13″ pan. Refrigerate to set. Heat milk. Dissolve gelatin in boiling water. Stir into milk. Stir in remaining ingredients until smooth. Pour 1 1/2 cups white layer over cherry jello. Refrigerate to set. Repeat with lemon, white, lime, white and orange, refrigerating each layer until set. Cut in squares to serve.

Though somewhat time-consuming to make, the result is very colorful.

MOLDED BEET SALAD

Serves: 12

3 12-oz. cans shoestring beets
1 6-oz. pkg. lemon jello
1/2 cup sugar
1/2 cup cider vinegar
2 Tbsp. prepared horseradish
1/2 cup mayonnaise
1 Tbsp. prepared horseradish
1/4 tsp. salt

Drain beets, save juice and add enough water to make 3 cups liquid. Bring to boil. Pour over gelatin and sugar. Stir until dissolved. Add beets, vinegar and horseradish. Pour into 6-cup mold. Chill until firm. Mix mayonnaise, horseradish and salt together in separate bowl as topping.

A tart and not-too-sweet salad that men enjoy.

HEARTY CORNED BEEF SALAD

Serves: 8

1 3-oz. pkg. lemon jello
1 cup boiling water
3 Tbsp. vinegar
1 12-oz. can corned beef
1 cup chopped celery
1 cup chopped green pepper
1 small onion, finely chopped
3 hard-boiled eggs, chopped
1 cup mayonnaise
1 1/2 Tbsp. horseradish
1/2 tsp. salt
Salad greens

Dissolve jello in boiling water. Add vinegar. Refrigerate until slightly thickened, about 1 hour. Break up corned beef with fork. Stir beef and next 7 ingredients into jello mixture. Pour into 6-cup ring mold. Chill until set. Unmold on salad greens.

This can be made up to 2 days ahead and can be a meal in itself.

CELERY NUT ASPIC

Serves: 10-12

1 6-oz. pkg. strawberry jello
1/2 tsp. salt
1 3/4 cups boiling water
2 8-oz. cans tomato sauce
3 Tbsp. vinegar
1/8 tsp. pepper
1 cup chopped nuts
1 cup chopped celery
1/2 tsp. grated onion
2 tsp. Worcestershire sauce
2 tsp. horseradish

Dissolve jello and salt in boiling water. Stir in remaining ingredients. Pour into 6-cup mold. Chill until set.

An aspic with a bit of bite that is a good addition to summer patio meals.

MOLDED CHICKEN SALAD

Serves: 8

1 3-oz. pkg. lemon jello
1 10 3/4-oz. can chicken rice soup
1 cup chopped celery
1 cup chopped walnuts
1 Tbsp. grated onion
1/2 cup mayonnaise
1 1/2 cups finely chopped cooked chicken
1/2 tsp. salt
1 cup whipping cream

Dissolve jello in undiluted soup brought to boil. Chill until slightly thickened. Whip jello. Fold in remaining ingredients. Pour into 6-cup mold or 7″x11″ dish. Chill. To serve unmold or cut in squares.

This is rich enough to be the entrée for a lovely luncheon.

JELLO CHIFFON MOLD

Serves: 12

1 6-oz. pkg. strawberry jello
1 envelope unflavored gelatin
2 cups boiling water
1 8-oz. pkg. cream cheese, softened
1 10-oz. pkg. frozen strawberries, defrosted
1 8-oz. carton Cool Whip, defrosted

Stir jello and gelatin together. Add boiling water and stir extra well to thoroughly dissolve. Place cream cheese and strawberries with juice in blender jar. Blend well. Pour into jello. Fold in Cool Whip. Pour into 9″x13″ pan. Chill until set.

One 13-oz. can crushed pineapple with juice plus lemon jello or 1-lb. can peeled apricots with juice and apricot jello may be used instead of strawberry.

VEGETABLE RELISH SALAD

Serves: 8

1 cup chopped celery
1 cup chopped green onion
1 cup chopped white onion
1 12-oz. can white shoe peg corn, drained
1 1-lb. can small green peas, drained
1 1-lb. can French cut green beans, drained
3/4 cup vinegar
1 cup sugar
1 tsp. salt
1/2 tsp. pepper
1 Tbsp. water
1/2 cup salad oil

Combine first 6 ingredients. Bring remaining ingredients to boil, cool and stir into vegetables. Marinate 24 hours.

A three-bean type of salad with only 1 type of bean.

CRANBERRY SALAD

Serves: 12

1 qt. fresh cranberries
3 1/2 cups water
2 cups sugar
2 Tbsp. unflavored gelatin
1 cup cold water
1 cup chopped nuts
2 8-oz. cans crushed pineapple, drained

Bring cranberries and 3 1/2 cups water to boil. Reduce heat to medium-high and cook 10 minutes. Remove from heat, add sugar. Stir until sugar dissolves. Dissolve gelatin in 1 cup cold water, stir in and let stand until cool. Add nuts and pineapple, pour into 8-cup mold and chill.

One cup grapes, halved and seeded, are an optional addition.

CHERRY SALAD

Serves: 12

1 6-oz. pkg. cherry jello
2 cups boiling water
1/2 cup cold water
1 21-oz. can cherry pie filling
1 pkg. Dream Whip
1 3-oz. pkg. instant vanilla pudding
1 1/2 cups milk

Dissolve jello in boiling water. Stir in cold water and cherry pie filling. Pour into 2-qt. shallow casserole. Chill until set. Beat together last 3 ingredients. Spread on top of jello. Chill. Cut in squares to serve.

A very sweet salad that could also be served as a dessert.

PORT WINE CRANBERRY SALAD MOLD

Serves: 12

1 6-oz. pkg. strawberry gelatin
2 cups boiling water
1 1-lb. can whole cranberry sauce
1 8 1/2-oz. can applesauce
1/2 cup ruby port
1/4 cup chopped walnuts

Dissolve gelatin in boiling water. Add next 3 ingredients. Chill until syrupy. Fold in walnuts. Pour into 6-cup mold and chill until firm.

Now that you have opened the bottle of port wine, you must sip some after dinner.

GINGER ALE SALAD

Serves: 8

1 3-oz. pkg. lemon jello
1/2 cup boiling water
1 1/2 cups ginger ale
1/2 cup chopped walnuts
1/2 cup diced celery
1 8 3/4-oz. can fruit cocktail, well drained
1 Tbsp. finely chopped crystallized ginger

Dissolve jello in boiling water and stir in ginger ale. Chill until slightly thickened. Fold in remaining ingredients. Pour into 4-cup mold and chill until firm.

Consider using individual molds and turning them out onto a bed of freshly shredded lettuce.

TUNA FRUIT SALAD

Serves: 4

1 11-oz. can mandarin oranges
1 cup pineapple chunks
3/4 cup thinly sliced celery
2 Tbsp. minced onion
1/2 cup chopped walnuts
1 7-oz. can solid pack tuna
3/4 cup mayonnaise
1 Tbsp. lemon juice
1 tsp. prepared mustard
Lettuce leaves
4 cups lettuce, shredded
Paprika

Drain fruit, reserving 2 tsp. pineapple juice. Combine fruit and next 4 ingredients. Mix together mayonnaise, lemon juice, mustard, reserved pineapple juice and stir into tuna. Arrange lettuce leaves on 4 serving plates. Place 1 cup shredded lettuce on each. Top with salad. Garnish each with dollop of mayonnaise and a dash of paprika.

For a salad luncheon, these servings could be arranged on the same platter with Old-Fashioned Chicken Salad.

POTATO SALAD

Serves: 12-16

12 medium baking potatoes
1/4 cup cider vinegar
2 tsp. salt
1 tsp. pepper
2 tsp. celery seed
3 medium onions, finely chopped
3 large stalks celery, diced
1 1/2 cups Hellman's mayonnaise
2 Tbsp. French's mustard
1 4-oz. jar pimento, diced
4 hard-boiled eggs, sliced

Boil unpeeled potatoes until just tender. Hold potatoes in folded paper towel and peel while hot. Into large bowl coarsely slice 3 potatoes or cut in uneven small chunks. Sprinkle with 1 Tbsp. vinegar, 1/2 tsp. salt, 1/4 tsp. pepper, 1/2 tsp. celery seed. Repeat, using up these ingredients. Cover and set aside 1 hour. Add remaining ingredients in order listed. Stir together well. Chop through mixture with wooden spoon about 12 times. Taste and add more salt if necessary. Chill.

Best if made a day ahead so flavors meld. You may wish to add more mayonnaise before serving.

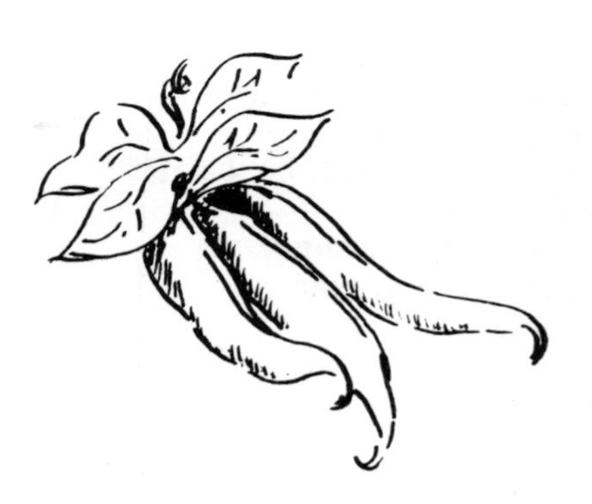

RANCH STYLE DRESSING

Yield: 1/3 cup

3 Tbsp. salt
4 tsp. dried parsley
2 tsp. garlic powder
2 tsp. black pepper
1 tsp. onion powder

Dressing:
1 cup buttermilk
1 cup mayonnaise
1 Tbsp. dry mix

Stir together first 5 ingredients. Store in airtight jar. For Dressing: slowly stir buttermilk into mayonnaise. Stir in 1 Tbsp. dry mix. Will keep in refrigerator for several days.

A delicious dip for vegetables can be made by using sour cream instead of the buttermilk.

POPPY SEED SALAD DRESSING

Yield: 2 cups

1 cup salad oil
1/2 cup cider vinegar
6 Tbsp. sugar
1 small onion, diced
1 tsp. dry mustard
1 tsp. salt
1 tsp. poppy seeds
2 Tbsp. lemon juice

Place all ingredients in jar of blender. Blend just to mix. Store in covered jar in refrigerator. Shake vigorously before using.

This is a perfect dressing for spinach salads made with mandarin orange sections, mushroom slices and rings of purple onion.

OLIVE NUT DRESSING

Yield: 3 cups

1 8-oz. pkg. cream cheese, softened
1/2 cup mayonnaise
2 Tbsp. sour cream
3 Tbsp. milk
1/2 cup chopped pecans
1 cup chopped salad olives
1/8 tsp. pepper

Mash cheese with fork, add next 3 ingredients and blend well. Stir in remaining ingredients. Add more milk if thinner dressing is desired.

Serve over lettuce wedges. Omit milk and sour cream and use as a spread for sandwiches or crackers.

ROQUEFORT DRESSING

Yield: 2 cups

1 clove garlic, crushed
3 Tbsp. fresh chives, minced
1 Tbsp. lemon juice
1/2 cup sour cream
1 cup mayonnaise
1/4 tsp. salt
1/4 tsp. pepper
1/2 cup crumbled Roquefort cheese

Stir together all ingredients. Store covered in refrigerator.

If you have been experimenting to find the best Roquefort dressing, be pleased. This is it! Naturally, American Bleu may be used.

BACON SALAD DRESSING

Yield: 3 cups

1/2 cup sugar
1/4 cup cider vinegar
1/4 cup water
1/4 lb. bacon
1 small onion, chopped
2 cups mayonnaise

Bring sugar, vinegar and water to boil. Cool. Fry bacon until crisp. Drain on paper towels. Crumble. Sauté onion until golden in bacon fat. Remove with slotted spoon and add with bacon to cooled syrup. Beat slowly into mayonnaise. Use hot or cold.

Splurge and serve this dressing over watercress.

RUSSIAN DRESSING

Yield: 3 cups

2/3 cup salad oil
1/4 cup white vinegar
2/3 cup catsup
1/2 cup sugar
1 tsp. salt
1 tsp. paprika
1 Tbsp. chopped onion
1 clove garlic, crushed
Juice of 1 lemon

Place all ingredients in jar of blender. Blend just to mix. Store in covered jar in refrigerator.

This is a good basic dressing, easy to keep on hand, and so much less expensive than buying the bottled kind.

FRENCH DRESSING

Yield: 3 1/2 cups

1 cup salad oil
1 cup vinegar
1 cup catsup
1 cup sugar
1 tsp. salt
1/2 tsp. pepper
1 medium onion, minced
1 garlic clove, quartered

Shake together well first 7 ingredients. Thread garlic on toothpick and drop in. Cover and set aside. Use as needed over salad greens.

This dressing is very good served over shredded lettuce topped with slices of orange and purple onion.

CHUTNEY DRESSING

Yield: 3 cups

1 cup mayonnaise
1 cup chili sauce
1/4 cup chutney, chopped
2 tsp. grated onion
1/2 cup whipping cream

Mix ingredients together in order listed, stirring cream in slowly. Will dress 3-qt. salad greens or make enough to top 6 chef-style salads.

Using a little less cream, this is a good dip for fresh vegetables.

CELERY SEED DRESSING

Yield: 1 1/2 cups

1/2 tsp. paprika
1/2 cup sugar
1 tsp. salt
1 1/2 tsp. dry mustard
1/2 tsp. celery seed
1 1/2 tsp. grated onion
1/4 cup cider vinegar
1 cup salad oil

Blend together first 7 ingredients. Slowly beat in oil. Store in covered jar.

A versatile dressing to use on avocado, fresh spinach or tossed salads.

LO-CAL SALAD DRESSING

Yield: 1 cup

1 Tbsp. sugar
1 Tbsp. flour
1 tsp. dry mustard
1/2 tsp. salt
1/8 tsp. paprika
Dash red pepper
3/4 cup skim or low-fat milk
2 egg yolks, lightly beaten
3 Tbsp. vinegar

Combine first 6 ingredients in saucepan. Add milk. Cook, stirring constantly until mixture thickens and bubbles. Stir small amount into egg yolks, stir yolks into pan. Cook, stirring 2 minutes more. Cover surface with wax paper. Cool 10-15 minutes. Stir in vinegar. Refrigerate in covered jar. There are 18 calories per Tbsp.

For a diet tartar sauce, stir in chopped pickle, parsley and green onion.

Breads, Rolls and Coffee Cakes

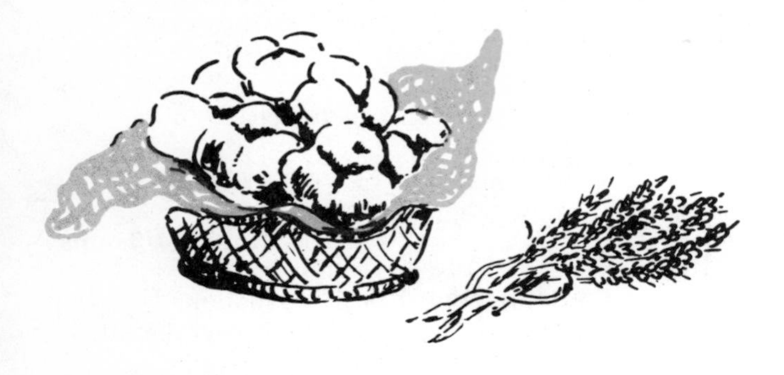

PRUNE BREAD

Yield: 1 loaf

1/4 cup sherry
8 oz. finely chopped dried prunes
1/2 cup sugar
2 cups flour
1/2 tsp. salt
3 tsp. baking powder
1 tsp. cinnamon
2 eggs
1 cup buttermilk

Pour sherry over chopped prunes. Cover and let stand at room temperature for 24 hours. Combine dry ingredients. Add eggs and buttermilk and mix well. Stir in prunes and sherry. Turn into well greased 9″ × 5″ loaf pan. Bake at 350° for 40-50 minutes until toothpick inserted near center comes out clean.

Moist and delicious.

APPLE BREAD

Yield: 1 loaf

1/4 cup shortening
2/3 cup sugar
2 eggs, well beaten
2 cups sifted flour
1 tsp. baking powder
1 tsp. baking soda
1 tsp. salt
6 gratings fresh nutmeg
2 cups coarsely grated raw apple
1 Tbsp. grated lemon peel
1 cup chopped walnuts

Cream shortening and sugar until light and fluffy. Beat in eggs. Mix together dry ingredients. Add alternately with apple to egg mixture. Stir in lemon peel and walnuts. Batter will be stiff. Pour into greased and floured 8″ × 4″ loaf pan and bake at 350° for 50-60 minutes. Cool on rack. Slice when cold.

This bread is moist and delicious when toasted.

ZUCCHINI CHEESE BREAD

Yield: 1 loaf

3 cups flour
1/3 cup sugar
5 tsp. baking powder
1 tsp. salt
2 Tbsp. grated onion
1 cup grated zucchini
3 Tbsp. grated Parmesan cheese
1/2 tsp. baking soda
1/3 cup butter, melted
2 eggs, beaten
1 cup buttermilk

Combine first 9 ingredients. Add eggs and buttermilk and mix well. Turn into greased and floured 9″ × 5″ loaf pan. Bake at 350° for 55-60 minutes.

Food processor may be used for grating onion and zucchini.

PUMPKIN BREAD

Yield: 3 loaves

4 cups sifted flour
4 cups sugar
2 tsp. baking powder
1 1/2 tsp. salt
1 tsp. baking soda
1 tsp. cinnamon
1 tsp. nutmeg
1 tsp. allspice
1/2 tsp. ground cloves
1 cup salad oil
1 1 lb.-13 oz. can pumpkin
2/3 cup water
1 cup coarsely chopped nuts
4 eggs, beaten

Stir together dry ingredients. Add oil, pumpkin and water, blending well. Stir in nuts and eggs. Pour into 3 greased 9″ × 5″ loaf pans. Bake at 350° for 1 hour. Test with toothpick. Continue baking, if necessary, until toothpick comes out clean. Cool on racks.

This is rich, moist and very flavorful.

RICH BATTER BREAD

Yield: 2 loaves

1 pkg. active dry yeast
1/2 cup warm water
1/8 tsp. ginger
3 Tbsp. sugar
1 13-oz. can evaporated milk
1 tsp. salt
2 Tbsp. salad oil
4-4 1/2 cups flour
1 Tbsp. butter, melted

Grease 2 1-lb. coffee cans with plastic lids. Grease underside of lid and set aside. Dissolve yeast in water. Stir in ginger and 1 Tbsp. sugar. Let stand in warm place until bubbly, about 15 minutes. Stir in remaining 2 Tbsp. sugar, milk, salt and oil. On low speed of mixer, beat in flour 1 cup at a time, adding only enough to make stiff but sticky dough. Place in prepared cans. Place lids on top tightly. At this time, batter may be frozen for later baking. If baking now, place cans in warm place until lids pop off, 1-2 hours. Frozen bread will take up to 5 hours to pop lids. Bake at 350° on next to lowest oven rack for 45 minutes. Remove from oven. Brush tops with melted butter. Cool 5-10 minutes in upright position before removing from cans. Finish cooling on racks.

This is delicious toasted.

PROCESSOR YEAST BREAD

Yield: 1 loaf

1 cup water
1 Tbsp. honey
1 Tbsp. butter
1 pkg. active dry yeast
1 1/2 cups flour
1 cup whole wheat flour
1/4 cup wheat germ
1/3 cup instant dry milk powder
2 tsp. salt
1 egg, beaten
1 Tbsp. wheat germ

Heat water, honey and butter until butter melts. Cool to lukewarm. Add yeast and let stand until foamy. Place 1 cup flour, 1/2 cup of whole wheat flour, wheat germ, dry milk and salt in processor bowl fitted with steel blade. Blend on and off 3 times. With processor running add 1/2 yeast mixture through feed tube. Process 30 seconds. Let rest 2 minutes. Add remaining flours. With processor running add remaining yeast mixture through feed tube until dough forms ball. Place in greased bowl, turn greased side up, cover and let rise until doubled in bulk, about 1 1/2 to 2 hours. Punch down. Roll out on lightly floured surface into 12″ × 8″ rectangle. Beginning at short side roll tightly. Seal seam. Fold ends under. Place seam side down in greased loaf pan. Cover and let rise until double again, 45-60 minutes. Brush with egg and sprinkle with 1 Tbsp. wheat germ. Bake at 375° for 35 minutes or until loaf sounds hollow when tapped. Cool on rack.

If you have not yet made bread in your processor, this is a foolproof first time recipe.

BEST EVER ZUCCHINI BREAD

Yield: 1 loaf

2 cups shredded, unpeeled zucchini
3 eggs, beaten
2 cups sugar
1 cup salad oil
2 tsp. vanilla
3 cups flour
1 tsp. salt
1 tsp. baking soda
3 tsp. baking powder
1/4 tsp. nutmeg
3/4 cup chopped walnuts

Combine first 5 ingredients. Mix together dry ingredients and stir in. Add walnuts. Pour into buttered loaf pan. Bake at 350° for 1 hour 15 minutes or until toothpick comes out clean.

Well named, this bread will be a favorite recipe.

CORNBREAD

Serves: 8

1 1/2 cups self-rising corn meal
2 eggs, slightly beaten
3/4 cup salad oil
1 cup sour cream
1 8-oz. can cream style corn
1 Tbsp. grated onion
1 tsp. Sweet'n Low

Stir together all ingredients until just barely mixed. Bake in greased 8″ square pan at 400° for 20-25 minutes.

Regular corn meal plus 1/2 tsp. salt and 1/2 tsp. baking soda may be used in place of self-rising corn meal.

MEXICAN CORN BREAD

Serves: 6-8

2 eggs, beaten
1 cup cream style corn
1 Tbsp. baking powder
1 cup sour cream
2/3 cup melted shortening or salad oil
1 cup cornmeal
1 1/2 tsp. salt
1 3 1/2-oz. can green chilies
1 cup grated Cheddar cheese

Mix eggs, corn, baking powder, sour cream, shortening, cornmeal and salt. Pour half the batter into greased 9″ square baking pan. Drain chilies, open out flat and arrange evenly over batter. Sprinkle with half the cheese. Add remaining batter and top with remaining cheese. Bake at 350° for 1 hour.

Perfect bread to serve with chili.

HERB BREAD

Yield: 4 French loaves

1/2 cup warm water
1 tsp. sugar
1/4 tsp. ground ginger
2 pkg. active dry yeast
1 1/2 cups lukewarm chicken stock
2 Tbsp. sugar
1 tsp. thyme leaves
1 tsp. savory
1 tsp. crushed rosemary
3 cups flour
1 stick butter, softened
3 1/2-4 cups flour
1 egg white
1 Tbsp. water

Combine first 4 ingredients. In large bowl combine next 6 ingredients. Add yeast mixture and butter. With mixer, beat 30 seconds on low, 3 minutes on high. By hand stir in remaining flour. Knead until smooth and elastic. Place in greased bowl, turn to grease top, cover. Let rise until doubled in bulk. Punch down. Divide and form into 4 loaves. Place 2 crosswise on 2 greased cookie sheets. Cover and let rise until doubled again. Bake at 350° for 20 minutes. Combine egg white and 1 Tbsp. water. Brush glaze over loaves. Bake 15-20 minutes more. Cool on racks.

Two long Italian loaves may be made from this dough. Also can be made into rolls, brushing before baking with glaze. Or make a combination.

HERB PARMESAN CASSEROLE BREAD

Yield: 1 loaf

2 pkg. active dry yeast
2 cups warm water
2 Tbsp. sugar
1 Tbsp. salt
2 Tbsp. soft butter
1/2 cup + 1 Tbsp. grated Parmesan cheese
1 Tbsp. dried oregano leaves
4 1/4 cups sifted flour

In large mixer bowl, sprinkle yeast over water and let stand 10 minutes. Add sugar, salt, butter, 1/2 cup cheese, oregano and 3 cups of the flour. Beat on low speed until blended. Beat 2 minutes on medium speed until smooth. Scrape bowl and beaters. With wooden spoon beat in remaining flour. Cover bowl with towel and let rise 45 minutes in warm place free from drafts until more than doubled. Preheat oven to 375°. Lightly grease a 1 1/2-2 qt. casserole. With wooden spoon stir batter down and beat vigorously 25 strokes. Turn batter into prepared casserole. Sprinkle with 1 Tbsp. cheese. Bake at 375° for 55 minutes until browned. Remove from casserole to cool on rack. Serve slightly warm, cut in wedges.

This flavorful bread is a good accompaniment for soup or salad.

CINNAMON NUT BREAD WITH STRAWBERRIES

Yield: 2 loaves

3 cups flour
1 tsp. baking powder
1 tsp. salt
1 Tbsp. cinnamon
2 cups sugar
4 eggs, beaten
1 1/4 cups salad oil
2 cups fresh or frozen sliced strawberries
1 cup chopped pecans

Stir together dry ingredients. Add remaining ingredients, beating well. Pour into 2 greased and floured 9″ × 5″ loaf pans. Bake at 350° about 1 hour or until toothpick comes out clean. Let stand 5 minutes. Turn out of pans and cool on racks.

This versatile bread can be served at breakfast, at a coffee or a tea party.

VEGETABLE BREAD

Yield: 3 loaves

2 Tbsp. active dry yeast
1/2 cup warm water
1 stalk celery
2 large carrots
1″ wedge cabbage
1 cup chopped fresh parsley
1/2 cup salad oil
2 eggs
1 13-oz. can evaporated milk
3 Tbsp. honey
8-9 cups whole wheat flour
1 Tbsp. salt

Dissolve yeast in water. Cut celery, carrots and cabbage in chunks. Place in blender or food processor with next 5 ingredients and puree. Stir into yeast. Beat in flour and salt. Knead 10 minutes. Divide in thirds and form loaves. Place in greased loaf pans. Let rise until doubled. Bake at 400° for 20 minutes. Reduce heat to 350° and bake 15 minutes more or until hollow sounding when tapped. Remove from pans and cool on racks.

This was a favorite among all the breads tested. It freezes well and toasts perfectly.

WHOLE WHEAT CORN BREAD

Yield: 2 loaves

1 pkg. active dry yeast
1 Tbsp. sugar
1/4 cup hot water
1 3/4 cup hot water
1 Tbsp. salt
2 Tbsp. butter, melted and cooled
4 cups flour
1 cup whole wheat flour
1/2 cup white corn meal
1 egg, beaten

Dissolve yeast with sugar in 1/4 cup of hot water in large bowl. Add the additional water, salt and cooled butter. Mix flours and corn meal together and add cup by cup to the yeast mixture. Incorporate as much flour as needed to have a firm dough. Knead dough until smooth and elastic and no longer sticky. Form into a ball and place in a buttered bowl. Cover lightly and put in a warm place to rise until doubled in bulk. Remove from bowl and punch down well. Divide in 2 and place each ball of dough under a bowl to rest for 10-20 minutes. Remove bowls. Punch dough down again to eliminate air. Form into 2 balls and place in buttered loaf pans sprinkled with white corn meal. Return to warm place to rise again. When loaves have risen, slash 2 or 3 times across top and coat with beaten egg. Bake at 350° for 55-60 minutes.

Slice and freeze the second loaf for later use.

ROUND ONION LOAVES

Yield: 2 loaves

3/4 cup milk
1 envelope onion soup mix
1/2 cup sugar
1 stick soft butter
2 pkg. active dry yeast
1/2 cup warm water
1 egg, beaten
4 cups unsifted flour
4 Tbsp. melted butter

Scald milk, stir in onion soup mix and blend well. Stir in sugar and butter until butter melts. Cool until lukewarm. Stir yeast into lukewarm water until dissolved. Add to milk mixture with egg and 1/2 of flour and beat with a wooden spoon until smooth. Add remaining flour. Batter will be stiff. Cover tightly and refrigerate 2-24 hours. Cut dough in half, flatten, and press evenly into 2 greased 1 1/2-qt. casseroles. Brush with melted butter and let rise until doubled in bulk. Bake at 375° for 35 minutes or until done. Loaves should sound hollow. Turn out on racks, brush with more melted butter and cool.

These would be good baked in miniature pans for a shorter time and served individually.

BROWN SUGAR COFFEE CAKE **Yield: 2 cakes**

2 cups brown sugar, packed
1/4 cup white sugar
1/2 cup shortening
1 tsp. cinnamon
1/2 tsp. nutmeg
1/2 tsp. allspice
2 cups flour
1 tsp. baking powder
1 cup sour milk
1/2 tsp. baking soda
2 eggs

Combine sugars, shortening, spices, flour and baking powder. Mix until crumbly. Remove 1 cup and set aside for topping. Stir soda into sour milk and add to dry ingredients with eggs. Mix until well blended. Divide batter evenly between 2 8″ round greased and floured cake pans. Sprinkle reserved topping over the batter. Bake at 350° for 30-35 minutes.

Stays moist and freezes well.

SCONES **Serves: 8**

2 cups flour
3 Tbsp. sugar
1 tsp. baking soda
1 tsp. salt
1 tsp. cream of tartar
3 Tbsp. shortening, melted
1 cup buttermilk

Sift together dry ingredients. Stir in shortening and buttermilk. Dough will be soft. Make 2 balls. On lightly floured surface roll each 1″ thick. Cut in quarters. Bake in skillet set at 350° or over medium-high heat for 12 minutes on 1 side, 10 minutes on the other.

Serve these moist scones hot with lots of butter.

RAISIN CASSEROLE BREAD **Yield: 2 loaves**

1 cup scalded milk
1/2 cup sugar
1 tsp. salt
1/4 cup butter
1/2 cup warm water
2 pkg. active dry yeast
1 egg, beaten
4 1/2 cups unsifted flour
1 cup seedless raisins

Mix first 4 ingredients. Cool to lukewarm. Pour water into large warm bowl. Add yeast and stir until dissolved. Stir in milk mixture, egg and 3 cups flour. Beat until smooth. Stir in enough remaining flour to make stiff dough. Cover and let rise for about 1 hour or until doubled in bulk. Stir down. Stir in raisins and turn into 2 greased 1-qt. casseroles. Do not let rise again. Bake at 350° for 40-45 minutes. Cool on racks.

A bread that beginning bakers will find a pleasure to make.

BISCOTTA

Serves: 12

1 stick butter
1/2 cup sugar
1 egg
1 tsp. almond extract *or*
1/2 tsp. anise extract
1 tsp. vanilla
2 cups flour
2 tsp. baking powder
1/2 tsp. baking soda
1/2 cup milk
1/4 cup chopped candied cherries
1/2 cup chopped nuts
1 cup confectioners' sugar
2 Tbsp. milk

Cream butter and sugar until mixture is light and fluffy. Add egg and extracts and mix well. Add flour which has been mixed with baking powder and soda alternately with milk, stirring well after each addition. Stir in cherries and nuts. On lightly greased cookie sheet, shape batter into 12″ circle with hole in center. Bake at 350° for about 20 minutes. When cool, frost with glaze made with confectioners' sugar and milk. Or, slice 1/2″ thick and toast lightly on cut sides. Then frost tops with glaze.

So good with coffee for that mid morning break!

QUICK APRICOT PASTRIES

Serves: 8-12

1 8-oz. can crescent rolls
1/2 cup apricot jam
1 large egg, beaten
1 cup sour cream
1 Tbsp. sugar
1/2 tsp. vanilla

Unroll crescent rolls and pat evenly on bottom of 9″x13″ baking pan. Spread with jam. Bake at 425° for 15 minutes. Remove from oven. Reduce oven temperature to 325° Combine remaining ingredients. Spread evenly over rolls. Bake 5-7 minutes more. Serve warm.

Pastry is flaky and best when freshly made. For variety, use cherry or blueberry jam.

CINNAMON STICKS

Serves: 4

1 cup flour
1 cup sugar
2 tsp. cinnamon
1 1/2 sticks butter, softened
1 egg, separated
1/2 tsp. vanilla
1 cup coarsely chopped pecans

Sift together flour, sugar and cinnamon. Beat in butter, egg yolk and vanilla. Spread 1/4″ thick on ungreased cookie sheet. Briskly stir egg white 3-4 times and brush on dough to glaze. Sprinkle with nuts. Bake at 325° for 30 minutes. Cool 10 minutes, cut in sticks and serve warm.

Surely these can be eaten with the fingers! Wrap sticks in a napkin and serve in a basket.

CORNMEAL BATTER ROLLS

Yield: 1 dozen

3/4 cup flour
3/4 cup yellow cornmeal
1 pkg. active dry yeast
1 tsp. baking powder
3/4 cup milk
1/3 cup shortening
3 Tbsp. sugar
1 tsp. salt
1 egg
3/4 cup flour

Combine first 4 ingredients in mixing bowl. Stir together next 4 ingredients and heat until warm and shortening melts. Pour into dry ingredients. Add egg. Beat on low 1/2 minute, scraping bowl. Beat 3 minutes on high. Add remaining flour. Beat 2 minutes on low. Cover and let rise 1 hour. Stir down. Drop into greased muffin cups. Cover and let rise 45 minutes. Bake at 325° for 20-25 minutes.

Batter may be refrigerated overnight. To bake, stir down, let rest 10 minutes, drop into greased muffin cups. Cover and let rise 1 hour. Bake.

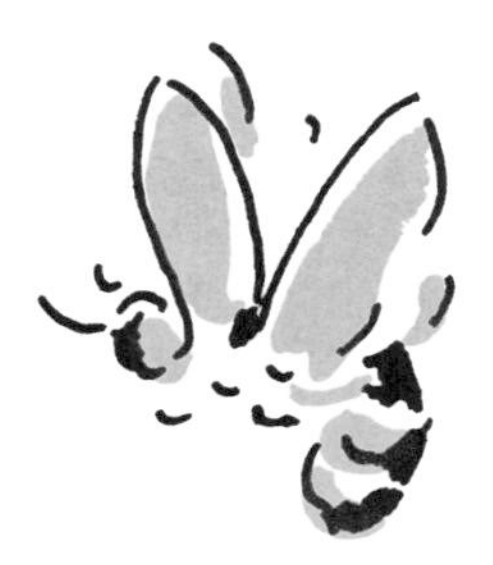

WEEKEND YEAST ROLLS

Yield: 3 dozen

3 pkg. active dry yeast
1 1/2 cups water
5 cups flour
1 tsp. salt
1/3 cup sugar
1/2 cup salad oil
1 egg

Dissolve yeast in water. If planning to bake immediately, water should be lukewarm. If for later use, dissolve yeast in 1/4 cup lukewarm water and add 1 1/4 cups cold water. Add remaining ingredients. Mix until well blended. Continue stirring until elastic strands form when spoon is pulled from bowl. Dough is sticky. Place in greased bowl and cover. If using immediately, let rise 30 minutes, punch down, form rolls, place in greased pan, let rise 45 minutes and bake. If for later use, refrigerate. To bake, remove amount needed, form rolls, place in greased pan, let rise 45 minutes. Either way, bake at 450° for 15 minutes or until golden. 8″ square pan holds 1/3 of dough.

Perfect for weekend guests. Make dough Thursday, use 1/3 for Parkerhouse rolls Friday night, 1/3 for butterhorns on Saturday and the rest for cinnamon buns on Sunday morning.

SWEDISH KRINGLER

Serves: 12

Pastry:
1 cup flour
1/2 cup butter
1 Tbsp. water

Topping:
1 cup water
1 stick butter
1 cup flour
3 eggs at room temperature
1/2 tsp. almond extract

Icing:
1 cup confectioners' sugar
1 Tbsp. butter, melted
1/2 tsp. almond extract
Cream

For Pastry: mix first 2 ingredients, cutting butter into flour until crumbly. Add water and combine until dough gathers together. Divide in half and pat each portion into long strip 3" wide on cookie sheet. For Topping: in saucepan over medium-high heat combine water and butter and heat to boiling. Add flour all at once, remove from heat and stir until smooth. Add eggs one at a time beating well after each. Stir in almond extract. Divide mixture in 2 parts and spread 1 part on each strip of pastry. Bake at 350° for 55 minutes. For Icing: combine confectioners' sugar, melted butter, almond extract and enough cream to make spreading consistency. Spread over warm kringler.

For special occasions, garnish with toasted sliced almonds or candied cherries.

PROTEIN BREAD

Yield: 3 loaves

3 cups rolled oats
3 tsp. salt
3 Tbsp. shortening
3 cups boiling water
2 pkg. active dry yeast
1 cup lukewarm water
1/2 cup molasses
1/2 cup brown sugar
3/4 cup wheat germ
1 cup All Bran
1 cup whole wheat flour
8-9 cups white flour

In large bowl combine first 4 ingredients and let cool. Dissolve yeast in warm water and stir in. Add next 5 ingredients to bowl plus 2 cups white flour and beat well. Slowly add several more cups flour. When dough can be handled, begin to knead. Add flour as needed until dough becomes smooth and elastic and does not stick to hands or kneading surface. Knead a total of 20 minutes. Place in greased bowl, cover and let rise until doubled, 1 1/2-2 hours. Punch down, divide in 3 parts, shape loaves and place in greased loaf pans. Cover and let rise again until doubled. Bake at 350° for 45-50 minutes or until hollow-sounding when tapped.

Though somewhat sweet as a sandwich bread, this slices well and makes wonderful toast.

DATE NUT BREAD

Yield: 3 loaves

2 cups boiling water
1 lb. dates, coarsely cut
1 cup orange juice
3 Tbsp. fresh grated orange rind
1 1/2 cups broken nuts
7 cups flour, sifted
2 tsp. baking powder
2 tsp. baking soda
1 1/2 tsp. salt
4 cups brown sugar, packed
7 Tbsp. butter, softened
2 eggs
2 tsp. vanilla

Pour boiling water over dates and let stand until cool. Add orange juice, orange rind and nuts to dates. Sift together flour, baking powder, soda and salt. Set aside. Cream butter and brown sugar. Add eggs and beat well. Add vanilla and date-nut mixture, then sifted dry ingredients, mixing gently until batter is smooth, but do not over mix. Pour batter in 3 greased and floured 9″ × 5″ loaf pans. Bake at 325° for 45-60 minutes, or until toothpick inserted near center comes out dry. Remove from oven and turn out of pans onto cake racks to cool.

Bake in 1-lb. fruit or vegetable cans for attractive tea breads.

CRANBERRY NUT BREAD

Yield: 2 loaves

1 stick butter, softened
1 1/4 cups sugar
2 eggs
3 cups flour
3 tsp. baking powder
1 tsp. salt
1/2 tsp. baking soda
3/4 cup water
1/3 cup orange juice
2 cups cranberries, cut in half
1 cup chopped pecans
1 Tbsp. grated orange rind

Cream together butter and sugar. Sift together dry ingredients and add alternately in thirds with water and orange juice. Fold in remaining ingredients. Pour into 2 greased loaf pans. Bake at 350° for about 1 hour.

This slices nicely and also freezes well.

SPOON BREAD

Serves: 4-6

2 1/4 cups milk
2 Tbsp. butter
1 tsp. salt
2/3 cup cornmeal, white or yellow
3 eggs, separated

Scald milk. Add butter and salt. Slowly stir in cornmeal. Cook 2 minutes, stirring constantly. Stir small amount into 3 well beaten egg yolks. Stir egg yolk mixture into cornmeal. Cook and stir 2 minutes more. Cool 5 minutes. Beat egg whites until stiff. Fold in cornmeal mixture. Pour into buttered 2-qt. casserole. Bake at 375° for about 35 minutes. Serve immediately.

This doubles easily. Increase baking time to 45 minutes.

LEMON NUT BREAD

Yield: 1 loaf

1 stick butter
1 cup sugar
2 eggs
1 1/2 cups flour
1/2 tsp. salt
2 tsp. baking powder
1/2 cup milk
Rind of 1 lemon, grated
1/2 cup chopped nuts

Glaze:
Juice of 1/2 lemon
1/4 cup sugar
1 Tbsp. water

Cream butter and sugar. Add eggs and beat well. Sift dry ingredients together and add alternately with milk. Stir in lemon rind and nuts. Pour into greased loaf pan. Let stand at room temperature 20 minutes. Place in cold oven. Turn temperature to 350°. Bake 40-45 minutes. Remove from oven. Cool on rack 15 minutes. Remove from pan. Drizzle glaze over bread. For Glaze: combine ingredients and beat well.

This is an elegant addition to a tea table.

GOLD NUGGET BISCUITS

Yield: 2 Dozen

2 cups unsifted flour
4 tsp. baking powder
3/4 tsp. salt
1/3 cup shortening
3/4 cup milk
1 Tbsp. dried minced onion
1/3 cup grated raw carrots
3 Tbsp. chopped fresh parsley

Mix together flour, baking powder and salt. Cut in shortening until mixture resembles coarse meal. Add remaining ingredients and stir with fork just until soft dough forms. Pat out into 1/2″ thickness on floured board. Cut with 1″ cutter. Place on ungreased baking sheet with sides touching. Bake at 450° for 12-15 minutes.

A versatile biscuit that may be served for breakfast, lunch or dinner.

ANYTHING BREAD

Yield: 2 loaves

2 pkg. active dry yeast
1/2 cup warm water
1 cup milk
1/2 cup shortening
3 eggs, beaten
1/2 cup sugar
6-7 cups flour
1 1/2 tsp. salt

Combine yeast and water. Let stand 5 minutes. Scald milk, add shortening and cool. Stir in eggs, sugar and yeast. Beat in 2 cups flour and salt. Continue beating in flour until dough doesn't stick. Knead 20 minutes. Place in greased bowl, cover and let rise until doubled, 1 1/2-2 hours. Punch down, make dinner rolls, sweet rolls, 2 loaves bread or pizza crust. Let rise again 40 minutes and bake as follows: for bread 375° for 35 minutes, for pizza 375° for 15-20 minutes, for dinner rolls 375° for 15-20 minutes, for sweet rolls 350° for 20 minutes.

Make cinnamon bread by rolling out dough, sprinkling with cinnamon and sugar and rolling up. For Kolatches, after first rising, roll out 1/2" thick, cut circles, let rise, spoon pie filling in center and bake at 350° for about 20 minutes.

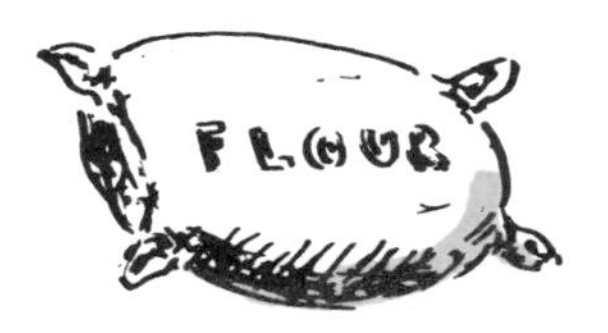

SEASONED ITALIAN BREAD

Serves: 8

1 loaf Italian Bread, unsliced
1 stick butter, softened
1 1/2 tsp. poppy seeds
1 Tbsp. Dijon mustard
4 green onions with tops, thinly sliced
1/8 tsp. salt
1/8 tsp. pepper
5 slices Mozzarella cheese, cut in thirds
3 slices bacon, cut in thirds

Slice bread every inch 3/4 of the way through. Mix together next 6 ingredients. Spread between slices. Place piece of Mozzarella between each slice. Fold foil tightly around sides and ends of loaf, leaving top free. Place bacon strips evenly across top. Bake at 350° for 20 minutes or until cheese melts and bacon is crisp.

For ease in serving, cut through each slice after baking. Replace foil boat.

BUTTERMILK MUFFINS

Yield: 7 dozen

2 cups 100% Bran
2 cups boiling water
1 qt. buttermilk
4 cups All Bran
3 cups sugar
4 eggs, beaten
2 sticks butter
5 cups flour
5 tsp. baking soda
1 tsp. salt

Pour boiling water over 100% Bran and cool. Add buttermilk and All Bran. In mixing bowl beat together butter, sugar and eggs. Stir in bran mixture. Combine dry ingredients and stir in until blended. Bake in greased muffin cups at 375° for 18-20 minutes. Batter will keep for 2 months in refrigerator in covered container. Use as desired to make quick hot muffins. Delicious as is or for variation add dates, blueberries, nuts, apples, etc.

This is a real convenience since it keeps unfrozen. Date lid of container.

CINNAMON BUNS

Serves: 12

2 loaves frozen bread dough, thawed
1 tsp. cinnamon
3/4 cup chopped walnuts
1 cup brown sugar, packed
1 stick butter
2 Tbsp. milk
1 5-oz. pkg. vanilla pudding

Pinch dough into walnut-sized pieces. Place 1/2 in buttered angel food cake pan. Sprinkle with cinnamon and nuts. Stir together remaining ingredients and heat until sugar dissolves and butter melts. Pour over dough. Top with remaining pieces of dough. Let rise until doubled in size. Bake at 350° for 30-40 minutes. Turn out of pan onto serving plate.

Good as, but less costly than bakery buns. Any leftover may be frozen and easily reheated.

JAM MUFFINS

Yield: 1 dozen

1 egg
1 cup milk
1/4 cup salad oil
2 cups sifted flour
1/4 cup sugar
3 tsp. baking powder
1 tsp. salt
12 tsp. jam

Grease 12 muffin tins or line with paper baking cups. Beat egg with fork. Add milk and stir. Add oil and stir. Sift dry ingredients into liquid. Stir until just moistened. Fill prepared tins 1/3 full. Drop 1 tsp. jam on top. Add more batter and fill cups 2/3 full. Bake at 400° for 20-25 minutes.

These freeze nicely and can be served for breakfast, lunch or dinner.

BLUEBERRY MUFFINS

Yield: 1 1/2 dozen

1/2 cup shortening
1/2 cup sugar
3 eggs
2 cups flour
3 tsp. baking powder
1/2 tsp. salt
1 cup milk
Fresh or frozen blueberries
2 Tbsp. sugar
1/2 tsp. cinnamon

Cream together shortening, sugar and eggs. Sift dry ingredients and add alternately in thirds with milk. Beat until fluffy. Fill greased muffin cups 2/3 full. Press about 5 well dried blueberries into batter of each muffin. Mix sugar and cinnamon. Sprinkle over. Bake at 400° for 15-20 minutes.

Quite good served plain, but butter is a nice addition.

SPICY APPLE MUFFINS

Yield: 1 dozen

1 1/2 cups flour
1/2 cup sugar
1/2 tsp. cinnamon
2 tsp. baking powder
1/2 tsp. salt
1/4 cup shortening
1 egg, slightly beaten
1/2 cup milk
1 cup chopped peeled apples

Topping:
1/3 cup brown sugar
1/2 tsp. cinnamon
1/2 cup coarsely chopped nuts

Sift together dry ingredients. Add shortening. Blend in egg and milk. Fold in apples. Fill greased muffin cups 2/3 full. For Topping: mix together ingredients and sprinkle over muffins. Bake at 375° for about 25 minutes.

These are a good dinner muffin as well as for breakfast or brunch

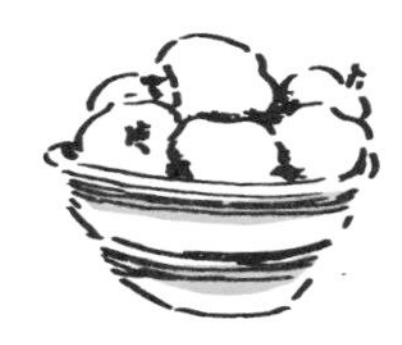

RUM-RAISIN ROLLS

Yield: 2 1/2 dozen

1 cup raisins
1/3 cup light rum
1 cup milk
2 pkg. active dry yeast
3/4 cup shortening
1/2 cup sugar
1 tsp. salt
1 cup boiling water
2 eggs, beaten
5 gratings fresh nutmeg
5 cups flour

Glaze:
1 1/2 cups confectioners' sugar
3 Tbsp. milk
1 tsp. rum extract

Soak raisins in rum 4 hours. Scald milk and cool to lukewarm. Sprinkle in yeast and stir to dissolve. Cream shortening, sugar and salt in large bowl. Add boiling water and stir until shortening melts. Stir in yeast mixture, eggs, raisins, rum and nutmeg. Gradually add flour and mix well. Cover and refrigerate overnight. Grease hands and shape dough into 2″ balls. Place on greased baking sheets and let rise covered in warm place about 1 hour or until doubled in bulk. Bake at 425° for 10-15 minutes. Glaze while warm. For Glaze: combine ingredients and mix well.

These freeze well and are good served hot or cold.

ORANGE COFFEE CAKE

Serves: 8-12

1 egg, beaten
1/2 cup milk
1/2 cup sugar
1/3 tsp. salt
2 Tbsp. grated orange rind
1 stick butter, melted
2 cups flour
4 tsp. baking powder
1/2 cup orange juice

Topping:
2 Tbsp. soft butter
1/2 cup brown sugar
1 tsp. cinnamon
1 tsp. nutmeg
1/2 cup chopped nuts

Mix together first 6 ingredients. Sift together flour and baking powder and add to egg mixture alternately with orange juice. Pour into well greased 9″x9″ pan. For Topping: mix ingredients and spread over batter. Bake at 375° for about 30 minutes.

A quick and easy solution for a coffee, brunch or special breakfast.

SOUR CREAM COFFEE CAKE

Serves: 8

1 cup sugar
1 stick butter
2 eggs, beaten
1/2 pt. sour cream
2 cups sifted cake flour
1 tsp. baking powder
1 tsp. baking soda
1 tsp. vanilla

Topping:
1/4 cup sugar
1/2 tsp. cinnamon
1/2 cup chopped nuts

Cream butter and sugar. Add eggs and sour cream. Beat until smooth. Sift together dry ingredients and add to egg mixture. Add vanilla. Blend thoroughly. Pour 1/2 into a greased 8″ × 8″ pan. Mix together topping ingredients and sprinkle with 1/2 of topping mixture. Add remaining batter and sprinkle with remainder of topping. Bake at 350° for 35-40 minutes.

Light in texture and easy to make, this also freezes well.

GOOD FOR YOU BRAN MUFFINS

Yield: 1 1/2 dozen

1 cup whole wheat flour
1 cup unprocessed bran
2 Tbsp. wheat germ
1/8 tsp. salt
3 tsp. baking powder
3/4 cup raisins
3/4 cup broken walnuts
1 egg, lightly beaten
1/4 cup salad oil
1/3 cup honey
2 Tbsp. orange juice
1 cup milk

Stir together dry ingredients with raisins and nuts. Combine all liquid ingredients and add to dry ingredients. Stir just enough to moisten. Spoon into 18 greased muffin cups. Bake at 400° for 15 minutes.

So good hot from the oven with butter and honey.

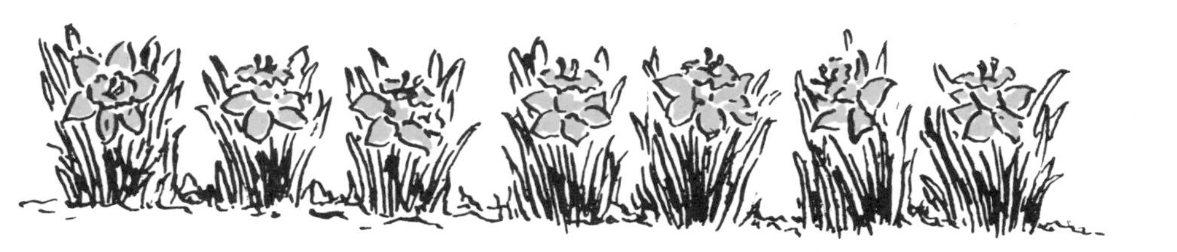

ORANGE HONEY MUFFINS

Yield: 1 dozen

1 cup flour
3 tsp. baking powder
1/2 tsp. salt
1/2 tsp. baking soda
1 cup rolled oats
1 cup orange juice
1/3 cup honey
1 egg, beaten
3 Tbsp. salad oil
1 Tbsp. grated orange peel

Sift dry ingredients. Add oats. Combine remaining ingredients. Stir into dry ingredients until just mixed. Fill greased muffin cups 2/3 full. Bake at 425° for 15 minutes or until golden.

Serve hot with lots of butter and honey.

HUSHPUPPIES

Yield: 5 dozen

2 cups stone ground yellow cornmeal
1 cup flour
2 Tbsp. baking powder
2 Tbsp. sugar
2 tsp. salt
2 tsp. baking soda
1 3/4 cups buttermilk
1 egg
1 cup minced onion
1/4 tsp. crushed red pepper
Oil for deep frying

Mix together first 6 ingredients in large bowl. Add buttermilk and egg. Beat well. Batter will be thick. Stir in onions and red pepper. Cover and let stand at room temperature 1 hour. Or refrigerate for up to 14 hours. Heat 1 1/2″ oil in heavy skillet to 325°. Drop in batter by tablespoonsful. Do not crowd. Cook about 3 minutes, turning twice, or until golden brown. Drain on paper towel.

These will hold for 30 minutes at 200° with oven door ajar.

SWISS CHEESE PANCAKES

Yield: 2 dozen

6 oz. Swiss cheese, grated
3/4 cup sour cream
3 egg yolks, slightly beaten
2 Tbsp. + 1 tsp. flour
1/4 tsp. salt
Dash pepper
1 tsp. dried thyme leaves, crumbled
1/2 tsp. dry mustard
2 Tbsp. butter

Beat together cheese, sour cream and egg yolks. Stir in next 5 ingredients and mix well. Melt 1/2 Tbsp. butter in skillet over medium heat. Drop batter by teaspoonsful and cook on each side until lightly browned. Repeat, adding butter as necessary. Serve immediately.

Sausages and applesauce are good accompaniments.

JAMES RIVER WAFFLES

Serves: 6

3 eggs, separated
2 cups buttermilk
2 cups flour
1/2 tsp. salt
2 tsp. baking powder
1 tsp. baking soda
6 Tbsp. butter, melted

Beat egg yolks until light. Stir in 1 cup buttermilk. Sift together dry ingredients and beat into yolk mixture. Stir in remaining buttermilk and butter. Beat egg whites until stiff and fold in. Bake in hot waffle iron.

Wherever you are, James River, these waffles bearing your name are delicious.

MAPLE WAFFLES

Serves: 4

1 3/4 cups flour
3 tsp. baking powder
1/2 tsp. salt
2 egg yolks, beaten
1 cup milk
1/2 cup maple-flavored syrup
1/2 tsp. maple flavoring
1/4 cup salad oil
2 egg whites, stiffly beaten

Sift together dry ingredients. Combine next 5 ingredients and stir into dry ingredients. Carefully fold in egg whites. Bake in hot waffle iron.

These richly colored waffles are soft when taken from the iron, but become crisp on the plate. Serve with melted butter and confectioners' sugar.

GOLDEN DELIGHT PANCAKES

Serves: 4

1 cup cream-style cottage cheese
4 eggs
1/2 cup flour
1 tsp. baking powder
1/4 cup salad oil
1/2 tsp. vanilla

Place all ingredients in jar of blender. Cover and blend on high for 1 minute, stopping once to stir down. Pour from large spoon onto hot griddle, turning once when bubbles break on surface. Cook until golden.

This batter also makes excellent waffles. Freeze any leftover and reheat in toaster.

EASY SOURDOUGH PANCAKES

Yield: 2 dozen

1 pkg. active dry yeast
1/4 cup warm water
1 egg, beaten
2 cups milk
2 cups biscuit mix

Soften yeast in water. Beat together remaining ingredients with whisk or rotary beater until blended. Stir in yeast. Let batter stand 1-1 1/2 hours at room temperature. Do not stir. Pour from large spoon onto hot griddle. When bubbles break on surface, turn and cook until golden.

Thin and light, these pancakes could pass for the ones started in the Yukon.

SWEDISH PANCAKES

Yield: 14

1 cup flour
3 Tbsp. sugar
1/2 tsp. salt
3 Tbsp. butter, melted
1 1/2 cups milk
2 eggs, beaten

Combine dry ingredients. Add remaining ingredients and stir to mix. Lightly butter a 6″ or 7″ heavy skillet and place over medium-high heat. Pour in enough batter to just cover bottom of skillet. Cook about 1 minute or until under side is golden, turn and cook other side. Remove to serving plate and keep warm. Cook remaining pancakes. Spread with butter and syrup, roll up and cut in slices.

Fill these pancakes with lingonberries, found in specialty food stores, for an authentic Swedish treat.

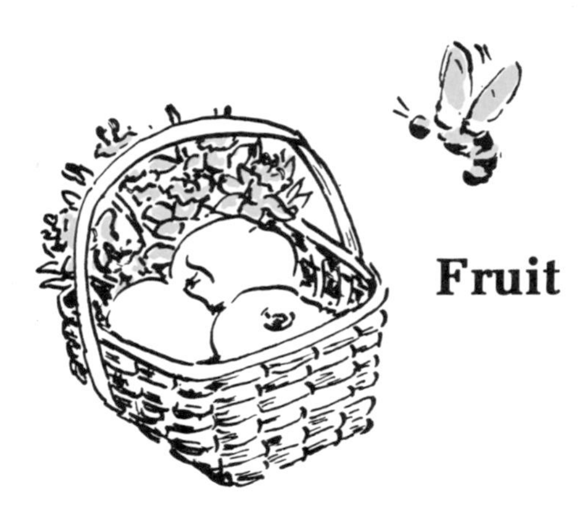

Fruit

HOT FRUIT COMPOTE

Serves: 12

1 1-lb. can sliced pineapple
1 1-lb. can peach halves
1 1-lb. can apple rings
1 1-lb. can pear halves
1 1-lb. can apricots
1 1-lb. can cherries or blueberries
1 stick butter
1/2 cup brown sugar, packed
2 Tbsp. flour
1 cup sherry

Drain fruits well. Cut if necessary and arrange in buttered 9″x13″ baking dish. In small saucepan combine remaining ingredients. Cook, stirring constantly over low heat until thickened and smooth. Pour over fruit. Refrigerate overnight. Bake at 350° for 30-40 minutes.

This accompanies ham well and is the perfect dish to serve at a brunch.

FRUIT SORBET

Serves: 6-8

1 3-oz. pkg. lemon jello
2 oranges, peeled, seeded and coarsely chopped
2 cups fresh or canned fruit, coarsely chopped
2 Tbsp. lemon juice
1 egg white
3 Tbsp. honey
1/8 tsp. cinnamon

Prepare jello according to package directions. Refrigerate until set. Combine jello and remaining ingredients in blender or processor. Blend or process until light and foamy. Pour into shallow pan. Freeze until nearly set. Blend or process again until slushy. Pour back into pan. Cover and freeze. Remove from freezer 15-20 minutes before serving.

Try interesting combinations for fresh fruit such as pineapple and peaches, or apricots and cantaloupe, or seeded cherries and cranberries.

BANANA FRITTERS

Serves: 6

6 bananas
1/2 cup white rum
2 eggs, lightly beaten
1 cup corn flake crumbs
Oil for deep frying

Peel bananas. Cut in 1″ pieces. Place in bowl and pour rum over bananas. Add more if needed to cover. Let stand 1 hour turning occasionally. Dip in egg, then crumbs. Deep fry 2 minutes at 375° or use 1″ oil in skillet. Drain and serve immediately.

These may be served on picks as an appetizer or used in place of potatoes for a main course. Use the rum for banana daiquiris.

BLACKBERRY SURPRISE

Serves: 4-6

8 slices bread
1 1/2 sticks butter, melted
4 cups blackberries
1 cup sugar
3 Tbsp. flour
1 Tbsp. lemon juice

Cut crusts from bread. Cut in strips. Dip in butter. Line 8″ deep dish pie pan or casserole with 1/2 of bread. Lightly toss together remaining ingredients. Pour into pie pan. Top with remaining butter dipped breadstrips. Bake at 325° for 30 minutes. Raise heat to 400° and bake 10 minutes more.

Flash frozen berries may be used for fresh. A pitcher of cream is a must. This is a favorite Sunday night farm supper.

BROILED GRAPEFRUIT WITH PORT

Serves: 6

3 large grapefruit
1 small seedless orange
3 Tbsp. frozen orange juice concentrate
2 Tbsp. light brown sugar
3 Tbsp. port
Cinnamon

Cut grapefruit in half. Carefully cut fruit from rind and membrane. Score orange and cut in 6 slices. Place 1 slice on each grapefruit half. Whip together juice, sugar and port. Pour 1 Tbsp. over each grapefruit half. Sprinkle each with cinnamon. Place on baking sheet. Broil about 5″ from heat for just a few minutes or until golden.

Medium dry sherry may be used instead of port, in which case this would be called broiled grapefruit with sherry.

ORANGE COTE D'AZURE

Serves: 4

4 navel oranges
2 Tbsp. mixed candied fruit
1 Tbsp. Kirsch or Grand Marnier
1 pt. vanilla ice cream
2 egg whites
1/4 tsp. cream of tartar
4 Tbsp. sugar
Confectioners' sugar

Cut tops off oranges. Scoop out pulp and freeze shells. Chop candied fruit and mix with Kirsch or Grand Marnier. Fold fruit with liquid into slightly softened ice cream. Fill orange shells and freeze again. To serve, beat egg whites with cream of tartar until stiff. Gradually add 4 Tbsp. sugar and beat until stiff peaks form. Spread over top of each orange. Place under broiler just long enough to brown meringue. Dust with confectioners' sugar.

These are easy, most attractive and shells can be prepared and filled days ahead.

BAKED PINEAPPLE

Serves: 6-8

2 eggs
2 Tbsp. cornstarch
1 cup sugar
1/4 cup water
1 20-oz. can crushed pineapple
Cinnamon
1/4 cup dry bread crumbs

Beat eggs. Beat in cornstarch, sugar and water. Stir in undrained pineapple. Pour into buttered 1 1/2-qt. shallow casserole. Sprinkle lightly with cinnamon. Bake covered at 350° for 45 minutes. Sprinkle with bread crumbs. Bake uncovered 15 minutes more.

This is an old recipe, as sweet as ever, but an ever-good side dish for ham or roast chicken.

BROILED MIXED FRUIT

Serves: 6-8

2 bananas
2 oranges
1 grapefruit
8 slices pineapple
1/4 tsp. cardamom
1/4 cup honey
1/4 cup orange juice

Peel bananas. Halve lengthwise and slice crosswise. Peel oranges and slice 1/4″ thick. Repeat with grapefruit, removing white pulp. Place fruit in well-buttered shallow casserole. Sprinkle with cardamom. Warm honey and juice, pour over fruit. Broil 3″-4″ from heat until edges are golden. Serve hot.

To prepare for broiling ahead of time, just dip bananas in lemon juice and water. Beautiful dish for a brunch.

SCALLOPED RHUBARB

Serves: 6-8

1 stick butter, melted
1 cup stale bread cubes
3 cups rhubarb, fresh or frozen
3/4 cup sugar

Melt butter in 1 1/2-qt. shallow baking dish. Stir in bread cubes. Cut rhubarb in small pieces and add with sugar. Bake at 325° for about 30 minutes.

A most quick and simple way to prepare this marvelous fruit.

CRANBERRY APPLE RELISH

Serves: 8

1 lb. fresh cranberries
3/4 cup sugar
1 1/2 cups boiling water
1 3-oz. pkg. lemon jello
1 cup applesauce

Combine cranberries, sugar and water. Bring to boil and boil rapidly for 5 minutes or until berries pop. Pour hot mixture over jello in 2-qt. casserole. Stir until jello dissolves. Stir in applesauce. Chill overnight.

A welcome change from the regular cranberry with oranges and nuts relish.

BAKED ORANGE SLICES

Serves: 8

2 medium oranges
1 cup sugar
1/2 cup water
1/16 tsp. cream of tartar
1 cinnamon stick

Cut unpeeled oranges into 1/4″ slices and arrange in shallow 1 1/2-qt. casserole. Combine remaining ingredients in saucepan and simmer for 5 minutes. Remove cinnamon stick. Pour hot syrup over oranges. Bake at 300° for 1 hour, turning slices once. Cool. Refrigerate overnight.

Use these as a garnish for meat or poultry or to add color whenever needed.

MINTED FRUIT COMPOTE

Serves: 4

2 cups cantaloupe or honey-dew melon
2 nectarines, sliced
1 cup green seedless grapes
1/4 cup mint jelly
1 Tbsp. water

Cut melon in 1/2″ cubes. Stir in nectarines and grapes. Melt jelly with water, stirring until smooth. Pour over fruit and toss to coat. Serve at room temperature.

Wonderfully easy. Other fruit combinations would be just as refreshing.

PEACHES FLAMBÉE

Serves: 6

6 canned peach halves
1/3 cup brandy
1/2 cup peach syrup
Rind of 1 orange, shredded
1/3 cup currant jelly
1 1/2 pt. vanilla ice cream
Toasted almonds

Drain peaches, reserving 1/2 cup syrup. Pour 1/2 brandy over peaches and let stand. Combine reserved syrup and rind, boil until reduced by 1/2. Stir in jelly until melted. Heat remaining brandy, ignite and pour over peaches. Place peaches on ice cream, pour over syrup and sprinkle with nuts.

Flame the peaches at the table for a dramatic effect.

GOURMET STRAWBERRIES

Serves: 6-8

1 pt. sour cream
4 Tbsp. brown sugar
1/4 tsp. cinnamon
1/4 cup brandy
1/2 cup white raisins
1 qt. fresh strawberries, washed and stemmed

Combine first 3 ingredients. Refrigerate. Bring brandy and raisins to boil. Cool. To serve, carefully fold all ingredients together, reserving 6-8 strawberries for garnish.

Leave strawberries whole unless quite large. Serve in stemmed sherbet glasses.

PEARS WITH MINT CUSTARD SAUCE

Serves: 8

1/4 cup sugar
1 Tbsp. cornstarch
1/4 tsp. salt
2 cups skimmed milk
2 egg yolks
1/4 tsp. peppermint extract
2 29-oz. cans pear halves, drained
1/2 cup toasted coconut

Combine sugar, cornstarch, salt, milk and egg yolks in heavy 2-qt. saucepan. Cook over medium heat, stirring with wire whip until sauce is slightly thickened, 5-10 minutes. Remove from heat. Stir in peppermint extract. Cover surface of sauce with plastic wrap or wax paper. Chill. To serve, place pear halves in dessert dishes. Pour sauce over and sprinkle with toasted coconut.

Nice light dessert and only 165 calories per serving. Garnish with fresh mint sprigs when available.

Sauces and Et Ceteras

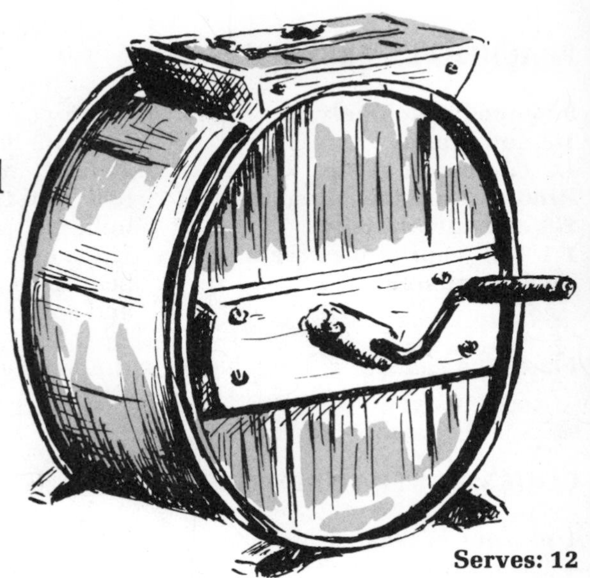

MUSHROOM SAUCE

Serves: 12

2 lb. mushrooms
6 Tbsp. butter, softened
5 Tbsp. flour
2 tsp. salt
2 tsp. prepared mustard
1/4 tsp. nutmeg
1/4 tsp. white pepper
1 pt. sour cream
1/4 cup minced fresh parsley
1/4 cup dried onions

Trim stems and wipe mushrooms clean with damp paper towel. Slice and set aside. Cream together remaining ingredients. Butter 2 1/2-qt. casserole and alternate layers of sliced mushrooms and sour cream sauce. Bake uncovered at 325° for 1 hour, stirring once or twice.

Excellent served with roast beef. Heat strips of leftover roast and stir into sauce for an easy stroganoff.

QUICK BORDELAISE SAUCE

Serves: 6

1 Tbsp. shallots or green onions, minced
4 Tbsp. butter
1 10 1/2-oz. can beef broth
1/2 tsp. thyme
1 1/2 Tbsp. cornstarch
1 4-oz. can sliced mushrooms, drained
1/2 cup dry red wine

Sauté shallots or green onions in butter 3 minutes. Add 3/4 can of broth and thyme. Stir cornstarch into remaining broth. Add to pan and cook, stirring until thickened and clear. Strain out shallots or onion. Add mushrooms and wine. Heat through. Serve with steaks or sliced roast beef.

This accompanies Steak Montrose. Any juices released by steaks while preparing may be stirred in.

HOLLANDAISE SAUCE

Yield: 3/4 cup

1 stick butter
3 egg yolks
1 Tbsp. lemon juice
1/16 tsp. Cayenne pepper
1/8 tsp. salt

Béarnaise Sauce:
3/4 cup Hollandaise sauce
2 Tbsp. white wine
1 Tbsp. tarragon vinegar
1 tsp. tarragon leaves
2 tsp. chopped onion
1/4 tsp. freshly ground black pepper

Heat butter until melted and hot. Place remaining ingredients in jar of blender. Turn blender on medium speed and slowly pour in hot butter. Turn blender off. For Béarnaise Sauce: leave Hollandaise sauce in blender. In small pan combine remaining ingredients. Bring to boil and boil rapidly until most liquid evaporates. Stir into Hollandaise, cover and blend 10 seconds. Keep both sauces warm over hot water.

Here are 2 classic sauces, the Hollandaise to serve over green vegetables, the Béarnaise to dress steaks and roasts.

DOUBLE ORANGE SAUCE

Yield: 2 cups

Rind of 1 orange, cut in strips
1/2 cup fresh orange juice
1/2 cup brown sugar, packed
1 cup orange marmalade
1 Tbsp. sherry
Butter

Cover orange strips with water and boil 15 minutes. Drain. Add juice and sugar to orange strips and simmer 10 minutes. Add marmalade and stir until melted. Stir in sherry, pour in pint jar and store in refrigerator. To use, add 1 stick butter to each cup sauce. Spoon over crêpes or pancakes.

Beyond several days the flavor of orange becomes strong.

STEAK SAUCE SUPREME

Yield: 2 cups

1 1/2 sticks butter
2 cloves garlic, minced
2 cups chopped onion
1 medium green pepper, chopped
8 oz. fresh mushrooms, sliced
1/8 tsp. dried rosemary
1/3 cup bottled diable meat sauce
1/3 cup dry red wine

In heavy skillet melt butter. Sauté onion and garlic 3 minutes. Add next 3 ingredients. Cook over medium heat until vegetables are tender. Add meat sauce and wine. Bring to a boil. Boil, stirring occasionally until most liquid evaporates. Skim off fat. Serve with grilled or broiled steaks.

The sauce may be made ahead, refrigerated and reheated to serve.

MUSTARD SAUCE

Yield: 1 2/3 cups

2 eggs
1/2 cup sugar
1/2 cup light cream
3 Tbsp. dry mustard
3 Tbsp. butter
1/2 cup vinegar, heated
1/4 tsp. salt

In top of double boiler, beat together eggs and sugar. Stir cream slowly into mustard, then stir into egg mixture. Add remaining ingredients, place pan over boiling water and cook, stirring until thick.

This is the perfect sauce to serve with ham loaf or with baked ham.

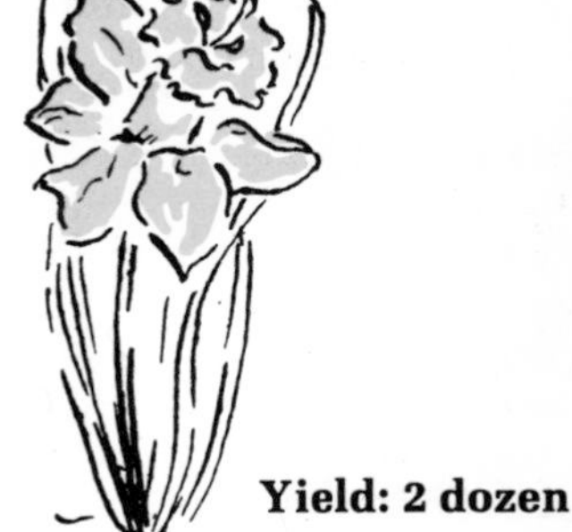

CRAZY CRACKERS

Yield: 2 dozen

24 Saltine crackers
1 stick butter, melted
2 tsp. dried dill or basil
1/2 cup grated Parmesan cheese

Fill large shallow pan with ice water. Soak a few crackers at a time for 3 minutes. Remove very carefully with slotted spatula, drain off as much water as possible and gently slide limp cracker onto cookie sheet, leaving 1″ between each. Pour 1 tsp. butter combined with herb over each cracker. Sprinkle each with 1 tsp. Parmesan. Bake at 425° for 10 minutes, reduce heat to 325° and bake 20 minutes more or until crackers are dry and crisp. Cool on racks. Store in airtight container.

This recipe doubles easily. These crackers go well with soup. Try several different herbs, coarse salt or garlic powder for flavor variations.

CHINESE FRIED WALNUTS

Yield: 4 cups

6 cups water
4 cups walnuts
1/2 cup sugar
Salad oil
1 tsp. salt

Bring water to boil, add walnuts and boil 1 minute. Pour off water. Rinse nuts in hot running water. In large bowl stir warm walnuts and sugar together with wooden spoon until sugar dissolves. Let stand 5 minutes. In deep pan heat 1" oil to 350°. Add 1/2 walnuts and fry 3-5 minutes, stirring often and watching carefully. When golden, remove with slotted spoon and place in colander to drain. Toss and sprinkle lightly with salt. Cool on paper towels. Repeat with remaining half.

These will keep for 2 weeks when stored in a tightly covered container.

CHEESE WAFERS

Yield: 5 Dozen

1/2 lb. sharp Cheddar cheese, shredded
2 sticks butter, softened
2 cups flour
1 tsp. salt
Dash Tabasco sauce
2 cups Rice Krispies

Beat together cheese and butter. Add flour, salt and Tabasco. Stir in Rice Krispies by hand. Roll in 1" balls, flatten with fork dipped in water. Bake on ungreased cookie sheet at 375° for 10 minutes or until just golden.

Flavors improve when made a few days ahead. Store in airtight container.

GRANOLA

Yield: 3 quarts

1 cup sesame seeds
1 cup coconut
1 cup slivered almonds
5 cups rolled oats
1 cup powdered milk
1 cup wheat germ
1 cup graham or soy flour
1 cup sunflower seeds
1 cup salad oil
1 cup honey
2 Tbsp. brown sugar
1 1/2 tsp. vanilla
1 cup raisins

Mix together first 8 ingredients. Combine next 4 ingredients and stir into dry ingredients. Spread on 2 cookie sheets. Bake at 250° for about 1 hour, stirring every 15 minutes. Edges will brown. Cool. Toss with raisins. It will keep weeks stored in air-tight container.

Graham or soy flour is available at health food stores. This is an excellent cereal and delicious snack.

HOMEMADE BUTTER

Yield: 1/2 cup

1 cup whipping cream
1/4 cup water
3 ice cubes

Herb Butter:
1 tsp. chopped fresh parsley
1 tsp. chopped fresh tarragon
1 tsp. chopped fresh chives

Garlic Butter:
1 clove garlic, crushed

Pour cream into blender jar and blend until whipped. Add water and ice cubes. Blend about 3 minutes. Butter particles will float on top. Pour mixture through fine sieve. Knead butter with wooden spoon to work off excess liquid. Press butter into dish or mold. For Herbed Butter: stir in ingredients before pressing into mold. For Garlic Butter: add garlic before pressing into mold.

What fun to prepare homemade biscuits and serve them with real homemade butter.

BEET RELISH

Yield: 6 cups

10 medium fresh beets
3 sweet peppers, shredded
3 large onions, shredded
1 cup sugar
1 cup water
1/2 cup vinegar
1 tsp. salt
1 tsp. mixed spices

Scrub beets and cook in water to cover for about 30 minutes or until crisp-tender. Remove skins. Shred 1/2. Julienne 1/2. Mix beets with remaining ingredients and simmer for 15 minutes. Pack in sterile jars and seal. Store 2 weeks for flavors to blend. Chill before serving.

This is a nice accompaniment for meats and can also be served as a salad.

NO-COOK BREAD AND BUTTER PICKLES

Yield: 4 pints

7 cups thinly sliced and firmly packed unpeeled cucumbers
1 cup thinly sliced onion
1 large green pepper, cut in thin strips
2 Tbsp. coarse salt
2 cups sugar
1 cup white vinegar
2 Tbsp. celery seeds

Mix together first 4 ingredients. Let stand 10 minutes. Drain, rinse lightly and drain again well. Pack vegetables tightly into jars. In small saucepan combine remaining ingredients, stir to dissolve sugar and bring to boil. Fill each jar to top with boiling liquid. Seal, cool and refrigerate. Flavors improve upon standing 3 days.

These will remain crisp and delicious for months in the refrigerator.

QUATRE SPICE PARISIENNE

Yield: 1/3 cup

2 1/2 Tbsp. ground cloves
1 1/2 Tbsp. white pepper
1 1/2 tsp. ground nutmeg
1 1/2 tsp. ground ginger

Place in small jar with tight fitting lid and shake to mix. Add to stews, raisin sauce, sweet potatoes or soups. Use in marinades or mix with salt and sprinkle over broiled meats.

This is a popular blend of spices used in French cooking, but it is difficult to find ready mixed here.

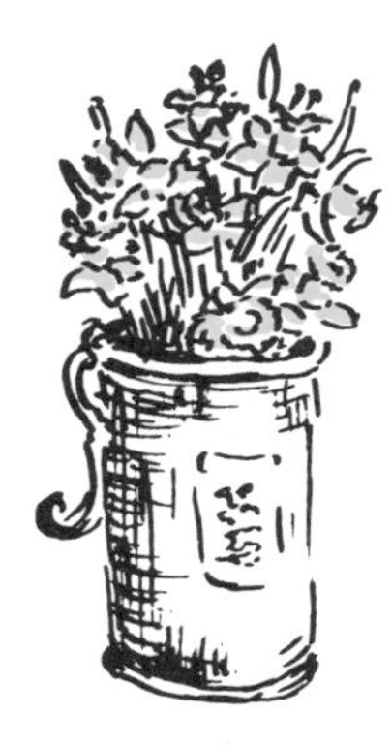

HERBED BUTTER SPREAD

Yield: 1 cup

2 sticks butter, softened
2 tsp. dried parsley
1/2 tsp. oregano
1/2 tsp. dill weed
2 cloves garlic, minced
2 Tbsp. grated Parmesan cheese
1/2 tsp. paprika

Combine all ingredients and blend well. Will keep refrigerated for weeks.

Spread this on slices of Italian bread and broil, or use to season rice, vegetables or baked or broiled fish.

RHUBARB MARMALADE **Yield: 2 1/2 cups**

5 cups 1″ slices rhubarb
3 1/2 cups sugar
1 3-oz. pkg. strawberry jello

Combine rhubarb and sugar. Simmer over medium heat 15-20 minutes, stirring occasionally. Add jello and stir until dissolved. Refrigerate.

Pour into jelly glasses and top with paraffin, if you like.

RASPBERRY JELLY **Yield: 8 cups**

6 cups beet juice
2 boxes Sure-Jell
1/2 cup lemon juice
7 cups sugar
2 6-oz. pkg. raspberry jello
Paraffin

Bring first 3 ingredients to boil. Remove from heat, stir in sugar and jello, return to heat and bring to full rolling boil. Boil 6 minutes. Skim off foam. Pour into sterilized glasses. Cover with melted paraffin.

What a surprise, for this has a very authentic raspberry flavor.

GREEN TOMATO RASPBERRY JAM **Yield: 7 cups**

5 cups green tomatoes
5 cups sugar
1 6-oz. pkg. red raspberry jello
Paraffin

Wash and core tomatoes. Grind in blender or food processor. Drain thoroughly. In large saucepan combine with sugar. Bring to boil over medium-high heat and boil rapidly, stirring frequently for 15 minutes. Remove from heat. Add jello and stir until dissolved. Pour into glasses. Cover with melted paraffin.

Another surprise!! Really tastes like raspberry preserves — seeds and all.

The Happy Ending

Cakes

APPLE CAKE **Serves: 12-16**

4 cups sliced apples
2 cups sugar
2 cups flour
1 1/2 tsp. baking soda
1 tsp. salt
2 tsp. cinnamon
2 eggs, beaten
2 tsp. vanilla
3/4 cup salad oil
1 cup chopped nuts

Mix apples and sugar and let stand ten minutes. Mix flour, soda, salt, cinnamon and stir into apples. Stir together eggs, vanilla and oil, and blend into apples. Add nuts. Spread into well greased 9″x13″ pan. Bake at 350° for about 50 minutes.

Serve plain, with whipped cream or ice cream. Freezes beautifully.

CREAM CHEESE BUTTER CAKE **Serves: 12**

1 2-layer yellow cake mix
1 stick butter, softened
2 eggs
1 8-oz. cream cheese, softened
2 eggs
1 lb. confectioners' sugar

Beat together first 3 ingredients on low until very sticky. Spread into buttered 3-qt. rectangular baking dish. Beat together cream cheese, eggs and sugar minus 1/2 cup. Spread over cake mixture. Bake at 350° for 30-40 minutes. Sift over remaining sugar. Cool. Refrigerate.

Serve plain or topped with sliced strawberries. May be cut in 1″ squares and served as cookies.

THREE-IN-ONE CAKE **Serves: 6**

Batter:
2 eggs
1 cup sugar
1 cup flour
1 tsp. baking powder
1/4 tsp. salt
1/2 cup hot milk
1 Tbsp. butter
1 tsp. vanilla

Breakfast Cake Topping:
4 Tbsp. butter, softened
2 Tbsp. cream
2/3 cup brown sugar, packed
1/8 tsp. salt
1 cup chopped walnuts

Strawberry Shortcake:
2 egg whites
1 1/2 cups sugar
5 Tbsp. water
1 1/2 tsp. white corn syrup
1 tsp. vanilla
1/2 tsp. almond extract
1 cup strawberries

Pineapple Upside-Down Cake:
4 Tbsp. butter
1/2 cup brown sugar, packed
6 pineapple slices, drained
6 maraschino cherries

For Batter: beat eggs for 5 minutes. Gradually beat in sugar until mixture is thick and pale. At low speed beat in flour, baking powder and salt. Combine hot milk, butter and vanilla. Add and stir just to blend. Batter is thin. Pour batter into greased and floured 9″ round cake pan lined with wax paper circle. Bake at 350° for 25-30 minutes. Cool 5 minutes. Remove from pan and cool on rack. For Breakfast Cake Topping: cream together first 4 ingredients. Stir in nuts. Spread topping over baked cake. Place on cookie sheet. Place under broiler until bubbly and golden brown. For Strawberry Shortcake: in top of double boiler beat together first 4 ingredients. Place over boiling water, beating until frosting stands in peaks. Blend in extracts. Ice cake. Decorate with strawberries cut in half. For Pineapple Upside-Down Cake: melt butter and brown sugar in 2-qt. rectangular baking dish. Arrange pineapple slices in dish. Place cherry in each. Pour cake batter over fruit. Bake at 350° for 30-40 minutes. Immediately invert.

Each of these cakes is delightful on its own. Double batter recipe and freeze one.

BAKED APPLE SPONGE CAKE

Serves: 10-12

3 eggs
1 3/4 cups sugar
1 cup salad oil
1 tsp. salt
2 cups flour
1 tsp. baking soda
2 cups tart apples, peeled and diced
1 cup chopped nuts

Icing:
1 1/3 cups confectioners' sugar
2 Tbsp. melted butter
1 1/2 tsp. vanilla
1-2 Tbsp. warm water

Beat eggs and sugar 5 minutes. Add oil and beat 2 minutes. Blend in combined dry ingredients. Stir in apples and nuts. Bake in greased and floured 9"x13" pan at 350° for 1 hour. If cake becomes too brown, turn temperature back to 325°. Spread icing on warm cake. For Icing: blend ingredients until smooth. Add more water if needed to spread easily.

This does not freeze well.

CHOCOLATE SUNDAE LAYER CAKE

Serves: 12

2 1/2 cups sifted cake flour
3 tsp. baking powder
1 tsp. salt
1 1/4 cups sugar
2/3 cup shortening
1 cup milk
1 1/2 tsp. vanilla
5 egg whites
1/2 cup sugar

Frosting:
4 squares unsweetened chocolate
2 1/2 cups sifted confectioners' sugar
4 Tbsp. hot water
5 egg yolks
6 Tbsp. butter
1/2 cup chopped nuts

Measure first 4 ingredients into sifter. Place shortening in bowl. Stir shortening to soften. Sift in flour mixture and add milk and vanilla and beat 2 minutes by hand or on medium speed of mixer. Beat egg whites until foamy and gradually add 1/2 cup sugar beating to form meringue. Add meringue to above mixture and beat 1 minute more. Turn into 2 9" cake pans that are greased, lined with circle of wax paper and greased again. Bake at 350° for 30 minutes. Cool on racks 10 minutes, remove from pans, peel off wax paper and cool completely. For Frosting: melt chocolate and blend with sugar and water. Add 5 egg yolks, one at a time and beat well after each. Add butter, 1 Tbsp. at a time and beat well after each. To frost; reserve 1/4 cup for decorating. Frost cake with rest. Sprinkle 1/2 cup chopped nuts over top. Add 2 tsp. hot water to 1/4 cup of frosting and dribble from teaspooon over nuts.

This made-from-the-beginning cake has a heavier texture than one from a mix.

BROWN SUGAR POUND CAKE

Serves: 16

2 sticks butter
1 stick margarine
1 lb. brown sugar
1 cup white sugar
5 eggs
3 cups flour
1/2 tsp. salt
1 tsp. baking powder
1 cup milk
1 tsp. vanilla
1 cup chopped nuts

Glaze:
1 cup confectioners' sugar
2 Tbsp. butter, softened
6 Tbsp. cream
1/2 tsp. vanilla

Cream butter, margarine, brown and white sugar until light and fluffy. Add eggs, 1 at a time, beating thoroughly after each. Sift flour, salt and baking powder and add alternately with milk in thirds. Beat well after each addition. Add vanilla and nuts. Pour batter into greased and floured 10" tube pan. Bake at 350° for 1 hour and 15 minutes or until toothpick comes out clean. Cool cake 10 minutes on rack. Remove from pan. For Glaze: Blend together ingredients and pour over warm cake.

This is one of those "round-the-clock" cakes — good anytime.

WILLIAMSBURG ORANGE CAKE

Serves: 8-12

1 1/2 cups sugar
1 1/2 tsp. baking soda
3/4 tsp. salt
1/2 cup butter, softened
1/4 cup shortening
3 eggs
1 1/2 tsp. vanilla
2 1/2 cups sifted flour
1 1/2 cups buttermilk
1 cup raisins
1/2 cup chopped nuts
1 Tbsp. grated orange peel

Williamsburg Butter Frosting:
1/2 cup butter
1 Tbsp. grated orange peel
4 1/2 cups sifted confectioners' sugar
4-5 Tbsp. orange juice

Blend sugar, soda, salt, butter and shortening. Add eggs and vanilla and mix well. Add flour and buttermilk alternately in thirds, mixing after each addition. Stir in raisins, nuts and orange peel. Pour batter into 2 greased, floured 9" cake pans. Bake at 350° for 45-50 minutes. Ice with Williamsburg Butter Frosting when cool. For Frosting: blend all ingredients well, adding enough orange juice to make a good spreading consistency.

For a special occasion, decorate the top with well drained mandarin orange sections.

CHOCOLATE DREAM CAKE

Serves: 10-12

1 stick butter, softened
1 cup sugar
4 eggs
1 cup flour
1 lb. can Hershey's syrup
1/2 tsp. vanilla

Frosting:
2 Tbsp. butter, softened
1 1/2 oz. unsweetened chocolate, melted
1 cup sifted confectioners' sugar
2 Tbsp. strong coffee
1/4 tsp. vanilla
2 tsp. marshmallow fluff

Cream butter and sugar. Add eggs 1 at a time and beat well. Add flour and syrup alternately, stirring well after each addition. Stir in vanilla. Pour into greased and floured tube or bundt pan. Bake at 350° for about 45 minutes or until toothpick comes out clean. Let stand on rack 10 minutes, turn out of pan and cool. Frost. For Frosting: beat all ingredients together well. Frosting will be thin.

There is no leavening agent in the cake, so it will not rise and will be somewhat heavy. It is moist, rich and delicious.

GREEK CHRISTMAS CAKE

Serves: 24

2 sticks butter
2 cups sugar
12 eggs, separated
1 box Zweiback crackers, crushed
2 cups finely chopped walnuts
2 tsp. baking powder
1/2 tsp. cinnamon
1/2 tsp. nutmeg
1/2 tsp. cloves

Syrup:
2 cups sugar
1 cup water
1/2 tsp. fresh lemon juice

Cream together butter and sugar until light and fluffy. Beat in egg yolks until well blended. Add next 6 ingredients. In large bowl beat egg whites until stiff. Stir 1/3 egg whites into batter. Carefully fold in remaining egg whites. Pour into large pan, 15″x10″x2″. Bake at 325° for 30-40 minutes. Slowly pour syrup over warm cake. For Syrup: combine ingredients over high heat, stirring to dissolve sugar. Boil 3 minutes. Store cake covered in refrigerator. Serve in squares topped with whipped cream or brandy sauce.

The cake keeps for several weeks in refrigerator or freezes well.

PUMPKIN CAKE ROLL

Serves: 8

Cake:
3 eggs
1 cup sugar
2/3 cup pumpkin
1 tsp. lemon juice
3/4 cup flour
1 tsp. baking powder
2 tsp. cinnamon
1 tsp. ginger
1/4 tsp. nutmeg
1/2 tsp. salt
1 cup finely chopped walnuts

Filling:
1 cup confectioners' sugar
2 3-oz. cream cheese, softened
4 Tbsp. butter, softened
1/2 tsp. vanilla

For Cake: beat eggs at high speed for 5 minutes. Gradually beat in sugar. Stir in pumpkin and lemon juice. Sift together dry ingredients. Fold into pumpkin mixture. Spread in greased and floured 15″x10″1″ jelly roll pan. Sprinkle with walnuts. Bake at 375° for 15 minutes. Turn out on tea towel sprinkled with sifted confectioners' sugar. Starting at narrow end, roll up cake and towel together. Cool.
For Filling: combine all ingredients and beat until smooth. Unroll cake. Spread with filling and roll up. Chill. Sprinkle with confectioners' sugar before serving.

This is spicy, delicious and a year-round treat.

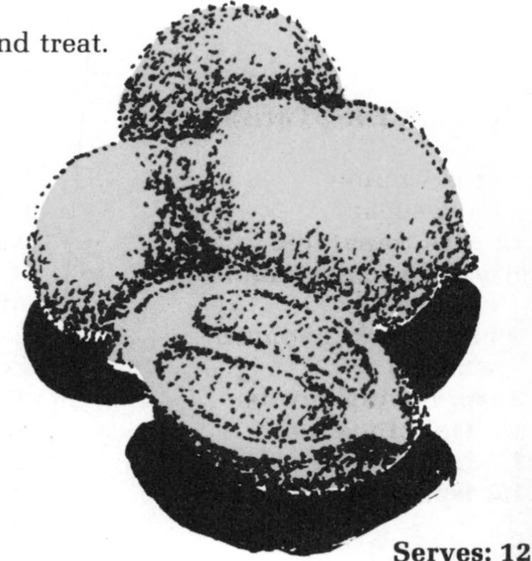

LEMON MERINGUE CAKE

Serves: 12

1 2-layer lemon cake mix
1 3 3/4-oz. pkg. lemon pudding
1 box lemon whipped frosting mix
1 4-oz. container Cool Whip, defrosted

Make cake according to directions. Pour into greased 9″x13″ pan. Bake at 350° for 30-35 minutes. Cool on rack. Make pudding as package directs. Spread over cake to within 1″ of edge. Make frosting as package directs. Stir in Cool Whip. Spread over pudding and cake, sealing edge. Refrigerate.

Betty Crocker may well take credit for this recipe.

DEVIL'S FOOD CAKE

Serves: 12

3 oz. unsweetened chocolate
3/4 cup water
1 1/2 cups sugar
1/2 cup shortening
3 eggs
1 tsp. baking soda
1 cup buttermilk
2 cups flour, less 1 Tbsp.
1 tsp. salt
1 tsp. vanilla

Whipped Cream Frosting:
1 tsp. unflavored gelatin
3 Tbsp. cold water
1 cup whipping cream
1/4 cup confectioners' sugar
1/2 tsp. vanilla

Melt chocolate in water. Cool. Cream together sugar, shortening and eggs. Add chocolate mixture. Stir soda into buttermilk. Add alternately in thirds with flour and salt. Stir in vanilla. Pour into 2 greased and floured 9″ cake pans. Bake at 350° for 25-30 minutes. Cool 5 minutes on racks. Turn out cakes. When cool, ice with whipped cream frosting. Refrigerate. For Frosting: combine gelatin and water. Dissolve over hot water 10 minutes. Cool. Slightly beat whipping cream. Add gelatin. Gradually add sugar, beating until stiff. Stir in vanilla.

This is a most marvelous combination. Consider making your favorite chocolate filling and use all of frosting on top and sides of cake.

CHOCOLATE MOUSSE CAKE

Serves: 16

Meringue:
5 egg whites, room temperature
3/4 cup sugar
1 3/4 cups confectioners' sugar
1/3 cup unsweetened cocoa
1/2 cup chopped nuts

Mousse:
13 oz. semi-sweet chocolate
7 egg whites, room temperature
3 cups whipping cream
1 1/2 tsp. vanilla
1/4 cup chopped walnuts

For Meringue: beat egg whites until stiff peaks form. Beat in sugar, 2 Tbsp. at a time until very stiff peaks form. Sift together confectioners' sugar and cocoa. Fold in with nuts. Lightly butter and flour 2 cookie sheets. Trace 2 8″ squares on one sheet, 1 8″ square on other. Divide meringue evenly among squares and spread to edges. Bake at 250° for about 1 hour. Cool on racks. For Mousse: melt chocolate. Cool. Beat egg whites until stiff peaks form. Fold chocolate into egg whites. Beat whipping cream and vanilla until stiff peaks form. Fold into chocolate mixture. To assemble, place 1 meringue in serving plate. Cover thickly with mousse. Repeat with second and third meringue. Cover sides. If desired, place some mousse in pastry bag with star tip and decorate top. Sprinkle with walnuts. Refrigerate.

This is a very elegant looking dessert and a grand finale for a special dinner. Better to make when the humidity is low.

CARROT CAKE

Serves: 10-12

1 1/4 cups salad oil
2 cups sugar
2 cups sifted flour
2 tsp. baking powder
1 tsp. baking soda
1 tsp. salt
2 tsp. ground cinnamon
4 eggs
3 cups grated raw carrots
1 cup chopped pecans

Cream Cheese Frosting:
1 8-oz. pkg. cream cheese, softened
2 sticks butter, softened
1 tsp. vanilla
1 lb. confectioners' sugar

Combine oil and sugar. Mix well. Place dry ingredients in sifter. Stir 1/2 dry ingredients into sugar mixture and blend. Sift in remaining dry ingredients alternately with eggs, adding one at a time, mixing well after each addition. Add carrots and mix well. Fold in pecans. Pour into lightly oiled 10″ tube pan. Bake at 325° for 1 hour and 10 minutes. Cool in pan upright on rack. Remove from pan. Frost with cream cheese frosting. For Frosting: beat together cheese and butter. Add vanilla and sugar. Beat until light and fluffy.

Marvelous moist cake that slices well.

COCONUT CAKE

Serves: 12

1 2-layer yellow cake mix
1 3 3/4-oz. pkg. instant vanilla pudding
1 1/3 cups water
4 eggs
1/4 cup salad oil
2 cups coconut
1 cup chopped walnuts

Topping:
4 Tbsp. butter
2 cups coconut
1 8-oz. cream cheese, softened
2 tsp. milk
3 1/2 cups confectioners' sugar
1/2 tsp. vanilla

Blend together first 5 ingredients. Beat with mixer on medium for 4 minutes. Stir in coconut and nuts. Pour into greased and floured 9″x13″ pan. Bake at 350° for 40-50 minutes. Cool on rack. Cover with topping. For Topping: melt 2 Tbsp. butter in skillet, add coconut and cook over medium heat, stirring constantly, until browned. Spread on paper towels to cool. Cream remaining butter and cheese. Stir in milk. Gradually beat in sugar. Stir in vanilla and 1 3/4 cups coconut. Spread on cake. Sprinkle with remaining coconut.

For a truly regal dessert, bake the cake in 3 layers and spread filling between each.

FRUITCAKE **Yield: 3 loaves**

8 oz. candied whole red and green cherries
4 oz. candied pineapple, cubed
1 18-oz. jar watermelon pickle, drained and cut in 1/2″ pieces
4 oz. diced candied lemon peel or citron
1 15-oz. box raisins
1 lb. walnuts
6 oz. pecan halves
1/2 cup sherry

Cake batter:
3 cups flour
1/2 tsp. baking powder
1/2 tsp. salt
1/2 tsp. nutmeg
2 sticks butter, softened
2 cups sugar
1 tsp. vanilla
6 eggs
Sherry

The day before combine fruits and nuts with sherry in large bowl. Let stand at room temperature covered, overnight. Next day prepare batter. For Batter: sift together dry ingredients. Cream butter, sugar and vanilla until smooth. Beat in eggs, one at a time until light and fluffy. Stir in flour and combine. Add batter to fruit mixture. Stir well. Pour into 3 8″x4″ loaf pans that are greased, lined with heavy brown paper and greased again, packing lightly with rubber spatula. Bake at 275° for 1 3/4 hour. Cool completely in pan on wire racks. Remove from pans, peel off paper, pour approximately 6 tablespoons sherry over all sides of each cake, wrap in plastic wrap, then in foil. Store in airtight container 3-4 weeks.

Two inch foil lined baking cups may be used. Fill each cup 3/4 full, place on baking sheet and bake at 275° for 1 hour. Carefully remove foil while still warm. Cool on racks. Pour 1 tsp. sherry over each.

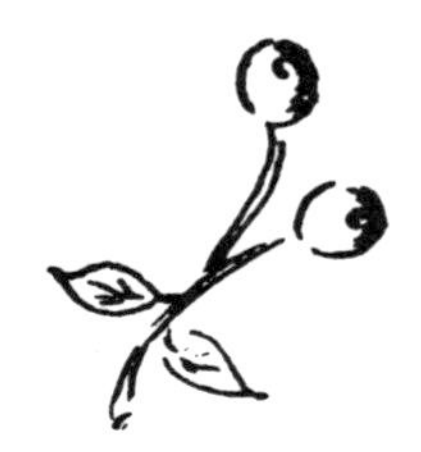

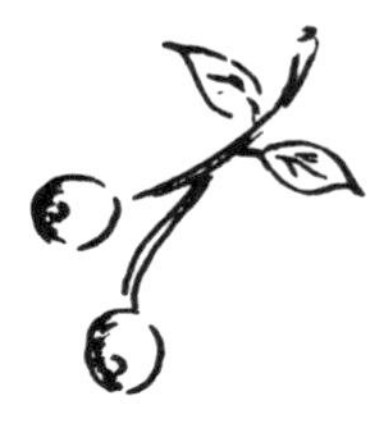

WARM PUMPKIN SPICECAKE WITH BRANDY SAUCE

Serves: 8-10

1 2/3 cups sifted flour
1 tsp. baking soda
1/2 tsp. baking powder
1 tsp. salt
1 tsp. cinnamon
1/2 tsp. nutmeg
1/2 tsp. cloves
1 cup light brown sugar, packed
1/3 cup shortening
1 cup pumpkin
1/2 cup water
1 egg
1/2 cup chopped nuts

Brandy Sauce:
1 egg white
1/8 tsp. salt
1 cup sifted confectioners' sugar
1 egg yolk
1/2 cup whipping cream
3 Tbsp. brandy

Sift together first 7 ingredients. Add next 4 ingredients. Beat at medium speed 2 minutes, scraping bowl. Add egg. Beat 2 minutes more. Fold in nuts. Turn into greased and floured 9" square pan. Bake at 350° for 40-45 minutes. Cool slightly on wire rack. Serve warm with brandy sauce. For Sauce: beat egg white and salt until foamy. Slowly add 1/2 cup sugar and beat until soft peaks form. Beat egg yolk until thick and lemon colored. Beat in remaining sugar until thick and light. Whip cream. With mixer on low, beat together all ingredients until just combined. Refrigerate. To serve, fluff with fork.

Cake may be made ahead and reheated at 300° for about 15 minutes.

RAISIN CAKE

Serves: 12

2 cups flour
1 cup sugar
1 1/2 tsp. baking soda
2/3 cup salad oil
2 eggs, beaten
1 tsp. vanilla
1 21-oz. can raisin pie filling
1/2 cup chopped nuts

Topping:
1/4 cup sugar
2 Tbsp. cornstarch
1 egg, beaten
1 cup fruit juice
1 pkg. Dream Whip

Stir together first 3 ingredients. Add remaining ingredients. Mix until well blended. Bake in greased 9"x13" pan at 350° for about 40 minutes. Cool on rack. For Topping: stir together and bring to boil first 4 ingredients. Cool. Make Dream Whip according to directions. Add to topping. Spread on cake. Refrigerate.

Cool and moist, this cake keeps well and is easily made.

CHERRY CAKE

Serves: 8-10

3/4 cup shortening
1 cup sugar
3 eggs
2 cups flour
1 cup drained sour pie cherries
1 tsp. baking soda
1/2 cup chopped nuts
4 Tbsp. milk
1 tsp. each ground cloves, allspice and cinnamon

Cream shortening and sugar. Beat in eggs, 1 at a time. Slowly add flour. Add cherries and baking soda. Stir in remaining ingredients. Batter is stiff. Spoon into greased 9″ square pan. Bake at 350° for 35-45 minutes.

Sprinkle top with cinnamon and sugar before baking. Good served hot with lemon sauce or whipped cream.

RIBBON CAKE

Serves: 12-14

1 stick butter
1 cup flour
1/2 cup chopped nuts
1 8-oz. pkg. cream cheese, softened
1 cup confectioners' sugar
2 cups Cool Whip
2 3 3/4-oz. boxes instant lemon pudding
4 cups milk
1/2 cup chopped nuts

Cut butter into flour as for pie dough. Add 1/2 cup nuts and press into 9″x13″ pan. Bake at 350° for 12-15 minutes. Cool completely. Beat together cream cheese, sugar and 1 cup Cool Whip and pour over cooled crust. Refrigerate short time until set. Mix together lemon pudding and milk, following directions on box. Pour over cream cheese. Top with second cup of Cool Whip and sprinkle with chopped nuts. Chill.

A rich and yet light dessert.

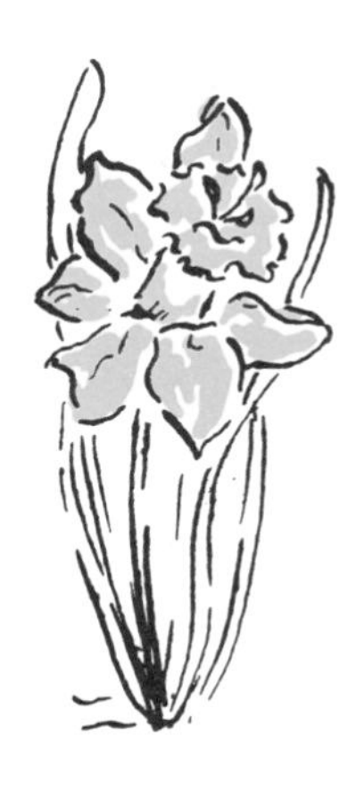

CHOCOLATE CHEESE CAKE I

Serves: 16

18 chocolate wafers
4 Tbsp. butter, melted
1/4 tsp. cinnamon
3 8-oz. cream cheese, softened
1 cup sugar
3 eggs
8 oz. semi-sweet chocolate, melted
2 tsp. cocoa
1 tsp. vanilla
2 cups sour cream
Whipped cream

Crush wafers. Combine with butter and cinnamon. Press into spring-form pan. Chill. Beat cheese until smooth and fluffy. Add sugar. Beat in eggs 1 at a time. Beat in chocolate, cocoa, and vanilla. Beat in sour cream. Pour into spring-form pan. Bake about 1 hour and 10 minutes. Cake will not be firm. Cool on wire rack. Refrigerate at least 5 hours. Serve with whipped cream.

The cake may crack but the whipped cream hides this.

CHOCOLATE CHEESE CAKE II

Serves: 16

Almond Crust:
3/4 cup graham cracker crumbs
2/3 cup slivered almonds
2 Tbsp. sugar
4 Tbsp. melted butter or margarine

Filling:
12 oz. cream cheese, softened
3/4 cup sugar
2 Tbsp. unsweetened cocoa
1/8 tsp. salt
2 eggs
1/2 tsp. vanilla
8 oz. milk chocolate bar, melted

Topping:
1/2 cup sour cream
2 Tbsp. sugar
1/2 tsp. vanilla

For crust: combine ingredients and press into bottom and on sides of 8″ spring-form pan. For filling: beat cream cheese until fluffy. Combine sugar, cocoa, salt and add. Beat in eggs and vanilla. Stir in chocolate just to blend. Pour into crust. Bake at 325° for 40 minutes. Turn oven off, do not open door. Leave cake in oven 30 minutes more. Cool on rack. For Topping: combine ingredients. Spread on cake. Chill.

This is wonderfully rich, so serve in small pieces.

NEW YORK CHEESE CAKE

Serves: 12

1 2/3 cups graham cracker crumbs
1/4 cup sugar
4 Tbsp. butter, melted
4 8-oz. pkg. cream cheese, softened
5 eggs, room temperature
1 cup sugar
2 cups whipping cream
1/2 cup milk
1 tsp. vanilla

Combine first 3 ingredients to make crust. Press firmly into bottom and on sides of 10" spring-form pan, packing tightly around bottom edge. Beat together remaining ingredients until well combined. Pour into pan. Bake at 350° for about 1 hour 15 minutes. Cool on rack. Chill.

This is so easy and just about the best cheese cake ever.

COFFEE ICE CREAM CAKE

Serves: 10-12

2 3-oz. pkg. unfilled lady-fingers
1 cup strong coffee
36 large marshmallows
2 8-oz. cartons Cool Whip
Shaved chocolate

Split ladyfingers. Stand around edge of spring-form pan and cover bottom completely. Bring coffee to boil. Add marshmallows, stirring until melted. Cool 15 minutes. Fold in 1 carton Cool Whip. Pour into spring-form pan. Freeze for 2 hours. Top with remaining carton Cool Whip. Decorate with shaved chocolate. Return to freezer. Defrost several hours in rrefrigerator before serving, or make same day and do not freeze. Refrigerate to set and serve.

For a variation, bring 2/3 cup coffee to boil, melt marshmallows and stir in 1/3 cup Kahlua.

ANGEL ALASKA

Serves: 12

1 pkg. Angel Food cake mix
1/2 gal. favorite ice cream
1 pkg. fluffy white icing mix
1/4 cup brandy

Bake cake according to directions. Cool and remove from pan. Slice 3/4" from top and set aside. Scoop out cake to form shell 1/2" thick. Place on ovenproof plate. Fill with ice cream, slightly softened. Replace top, wrap in foil and freeze. When ready to serve, heat oven to 400°. Make icing according to directions and ice cake, forming some hollows with back of spoon. Bake 3-4 minutes until just barely golden. Heat brandy, flame, and pour over cake and carry immediately to guests who should be sitting in darkened room.

Quite showy and a good dessert for its relative ease in making.

ITALIAN CREAM CAKE

Serves: 12

2 sticks butter, softened
2 cups sugar
5 eggs, separated
2 cups cake flour
1 tsp. baking soda
1 cup buttermilk
1 tsp. vanilla
1 cup shredded coconut
1 cup chopped pecans

Frosting:
2 8-oz. pkg. cream cheese, softened
1 lb. confectioners' sugar
1 tsp.vanilla
1 stick butter, softened
1/2 cup chopped pecans

Cream butter. Slowly beat in sugar. Beat in egg yolks 1 at a time. Sift flour and soda. Add alternately to creamed mixture with buttermilk. Add vanilla, coconut and 1 cup nuts. Beat egg whites until stiff and fold in. Pour into 3 greased and floured 8″ cake pans. Bake at 350° for about 25 minutes. Let stand 5 minutes, turn out of pans and cool on racks. Frost and refrigerate. For Frosting: beat together first 4 ingredients until smooth and creamy. Fold in nuts.

This delicious cake will complete any good dinner, whether of Italian, French or Oriental origin.

CHOCOLATE RUM BUNDT CAKE

Serves: 12-16

1 pkg. devil's food cake mix
1 3-oz. pkg. instant chocolate pudding
1 cup sour cream
1/2 cup salad oil
1/2 cup rum
4 eggs
1 tsp. vanilla
2 tsp. almond extract
1 1/2 cups chocolate chips
1/4 cup chopped nuts
2 tsp. flour

In large bowl combine first 8 ingredients and beat with electric mixer for 4 minutes. Dust chocolate chips and nuts with flour and carefully fold into batter with spatula. Bake in greased and floured bundt pan or angel food pan at 350° for 50-60 minutes or until done. Cool in pan 15 minutes. Turn out on plate and when cool dust with confectioner's sugar.

Wonderfully rich when iced with a chocolate frosting.

CALIFORNIA CARROT CAKE

Serves: 12-15

Cake:
1 1/2 cups whole wheat flour
1/2 cup soy flour
2 tsp. cinnamon
2 tsp. soda
1/2 tsp. salt
2 cups grated carrots
1 13-oz. can crushed pineapple, drained
1 cup coarsely chopped walnuts
3 1/2 oz. unsweetened coconut
3 eggs
3/4 cup salad oil
3/4 cup buttermilk
2 cups sugar

Sauce:
1/2 cup buttermilk
1 cup sugar
1/2 tsp. baking soda
1 tsp. corn syrup
1 stick butter

For Cake: combine flours, cinnamon, soda and salt. In another bowl mix carrots, pineapple, walnuts and coconut. In large mixer bowl beat eggs, oil, buttermilk and sugar. Add carrot mixture and combine. Stir in flour mixture and mix well. Bake in greased 9″x13″ pan at 350° for about 45 minutes. While cake is baking make sauce. For Sauce: place all ingredients in large saucepan. Stir and bring to boil. Reduce heat to medium and cook 5 minutes, watching carefully to prevent boiling over. When cake is done, poke holes in cake with large fork and pour sauce on cake. Cool on rack.

Soy flour is available at health food stores. This is extra moist and rich.

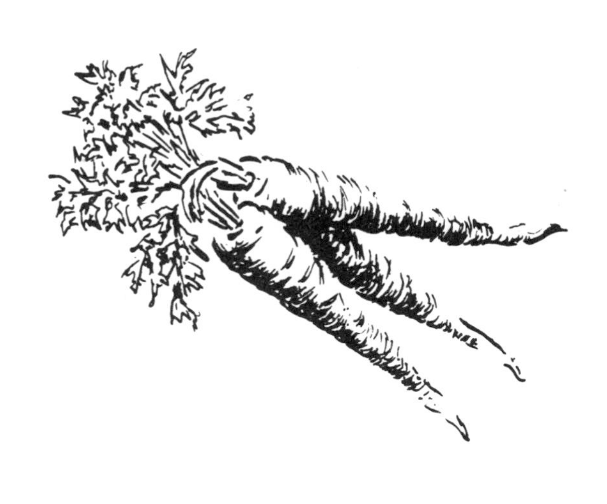

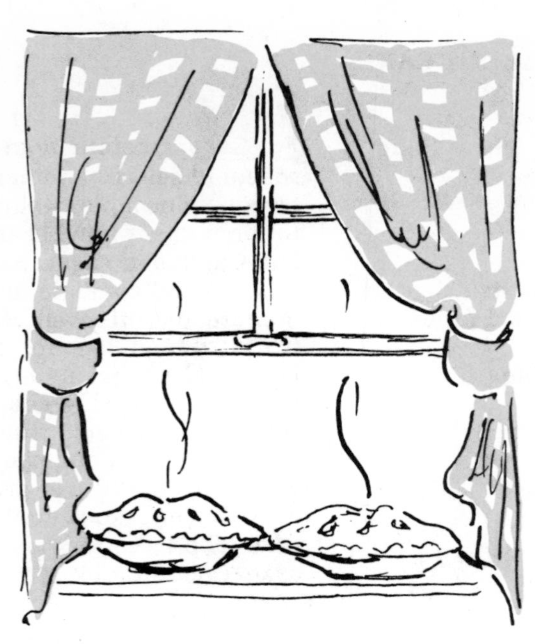

Pies

MUD PIE **Serves: 8-10**

1 1-lb. pkg. Oreo cookies
1 stick butter, melted
2 Tbsp. butter
2 oz. unsweetened chocolate
1 cup sugar
1 5 1/2-oz. can evaporated milk
2 pt. coffee ice cream, softened
Shaved semi-sweet chocolate

Scrape filling from Oreos. Crush cookies and mix with butter. Press into 9″ pie plate. Chill. Melt together 2 Tbsp. butter and chocolate. Stir in sugar and milk. Cook, stirring over medium heat until thick. Cool. Spoon 1 pt. ice cream into pie shell. Top with 1/2 fudge sauce. Freeze. Repeat. Garnish with shaved chocolate. Freeze. Remove from freezer 15 minutes before serving.

Wonderfully rich, cold and refreshing.

PINK SUNSET PARFAIT PIE **Serves: 8**

1 Tbsp. unflavored gelatin
1/2 cup pink grapefruit juice
1 pt. vanilla ice cream, softened
2 egg whites
2 Tbsp. sugar
2 cups pink grapefruit sections
1 baked 9″ pastry shell
Whipped cream

Mix gelatin and grapefruit juice. Let stand 5 minutes. Stir over low heat until mixture mounds. Beat egg whites until soft peaks form, slowly add sugar and beat until stiff. Fold egg whites and grapefruit sections into ice cream. Pour into prepared shell and chill until firm or overnight. To serve, garnish with whipped cream.

There should be 1/2 cup juice after removing 2 cups sections from fresh grapefruit.

SHAKER LEMON PIE

Serves: 6-8

2 fresh lemons
2 cups sugar
4 eggs, well beaten
Pastry for 2 crust 9″ pie
1 Tbsp. sugar

Slice lemons paper thin, rind and all. Remove seeds. Stir together with sugar. Let stand at least 2 hours. Add eggs to lemon mixture. Blend well. Line pie plate with 1/2 pastry. Pour in lemon mixture. Cover with top crust. Flute rim. Cut vents in top crust. Sprinkle with 1 Tbsp. sugar. Bake at 450° for 15 minutes. Reduce heat to 350° and bake about 30 minutes more.

Very fresh lemons must be used for this pie to be truly good.

PUMPKIN PIE

Yield: 2-9″ pies

1 1-lb. can pumpkin
1 1/2 cups sugar
1 tsp. salt
1 tsp. ginger
2 tsp. cinnamon
2 tsp. nutmeg
4 eggs, separated
1 3/4 cups milk
2 9″ unbaked pie shells

Mix together pumpkin, sugar and salt. Stir in spices. Add lightly beaten egg yolks. Beat egg whites until firm peaks form. Fold into batter. Pour into pie shells. Bake at 375° for 40 minutes, or until knife inserted near center comes out clean. To serve, top with whipped cream or dribbles of honey.

A moist layer forms on the bottom of these pies, giving an interesting texture.

PAVLOVA ANGEL PIE

Serves: 8-10

3 egg whites, room temperature
1/8 tsp. salt
1/4 tsp. cream of tartar
3/4 cup sugar
1 cup whipping cream
1 21-oz. can cherry pie filling
1/4 tsp. almond extract

Beat together first 3 ingredients until stiff. Add sugar, 2 Tbsp. at a time, beating well after each addition. Continue beating until sugar is completely dissolved. Butter 9″ pie plate. Fill with meringue. Make a well a good inch deep, pushing meringue up but not out on rim. Bake at 275° for 25 minutes. Raise heat to 300° and bake about 20 minutes more. Cool on rack. Whip cream and fill meringue. Chill overnight. A few hours before serving combine pie filling and extract and cover whipped cream. Chill again.

The whipped cream disappears into the meringue shell forming a heavenly result, hence the name.

LIME CHIFFON PIE

Serves: 8

Crust:
1 1/2 cups flour
2 tsp. sugar
1 tsp. salt
2 Tbsp. milk
1/2 cup salad oil

Filling:
1 envelope unflavored gelatin
1 cup sugar
1/4 tsp. salt
4 eggs, separated
1/2 cup fresh lime juice
1/4 cup water
1 tsp. grated lime peel
3 drops green food coloring
1 cup whipping cream

In 10″ pie plate mix together flour, sugar and salt. Stir milk into oil, add to flour mixture and stir lightly to blend. Press evenly into bottom and on sides of pie plate. Flute edges, prick all over with fork and bake at 450° for 10-12 minutes. Cool on rack. For Filling: in saucepan mix gelatin, 1/2 cup sugar and salt. Beat together egg yolks, lime juice and water and stir in. Cook, stirring constantly over medium heat until mixture boils. Remove from heat and add lime peel and food coloring. Chill until mixture mounds when dropped from spoon. Beat egg whites until foamy, gradually add 1/2 cup sugar and beat until stiff. Carefully fold into lime mixture. Whip cream and fold in. Spoon into pie shell and chill.

Buy limes when reasonably priced, squeeze and freeze juice until needed.

LEMONADE FLUFF PIE

Serves: 8

1 envelope unflavored gelatin
1/2 cup cold water
4 egg yolks, beaten
1/8 tsp. salt
1 6-oz. can frozen lemonade, defrosted
4 egg whites
1/2 cup sugar
1 cup whipping cream
1 9″ pastry shell, baked and cooled

Soften gelatin in cold water. Combine with egg yolks and salt in top of double boiler. Cook, stirring over simmering water until slightly thickened, about 5 minutes. Remove from heat, add lemonade and chill until mixture mounds on spoon. Beat egg whites until soft peaks form. Gradually add sugar, continuing to beat until stiff peaks form. Fold into lemonade mixture. Whip cream and fold in. Pile into pie shell. Chill until firm.

Can be made the day ahead. Refreshing dessert for a summer dinner.

BLACK BOTTOM RUM PIE

Serves: 6-8

1 envelope unflavored gelatin
1/4 cup cold water
1 1/2 oz. unsweetened chocolate
3 eggs, separated
3/4 cup sugar
1 Tbsp. cornstarch
1 3/4 cups milk
1/2 tsp. vanilla
1 Tbsp. rum flavoring
1/4 tsp. salt
1/4 tsp. cream of tartar
1 cup whipping cream
Chocolate curls
1 9″ graham cracker crust, baked

Soften gelatin in cold water. Melt chocolate over hot water. Beat egg yolks until light. Stir 1/2 cup sugar and cornstarch together. Slowly add to egg yolks. Scald milk. Stir a little into egg yolk mixture. Stir egg yolk mixture into milk. Cook, stirring over medium heat until thick. Blend chocolate and vanilla into 1 cup of custard. Pour into prepared pie shell. Chill. Stir gelatin into remaining custard. Refrigerate until cool. Stir in rum flavoring. Beat egg whites with salt and cream of tartar until foamy. Slowly add remaining 1/4 cup sugar beating until stiff. Fold into custard. Whip cream until soft peaks form and fold in. If thin, refrigerate to thicken. Mound on top of chocolate layer. Refrigerate 2 hours or overnight. Garnish with chocolate curls.

This makes a very high and cool-looking pie.

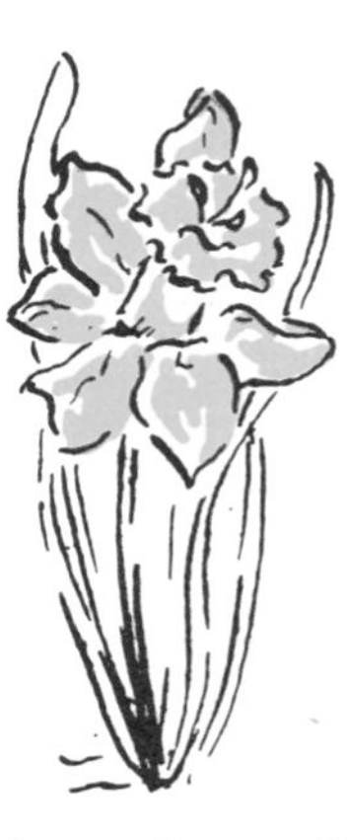

PEANUT PIE

Serves: 6

20 Ritz crackers, finely crushed
1/2 cup sugar
3/4 cup chopped roasted unsalted peanuts
3 egg whites
1/4 tsp. cream of tartar
1/2 cup sugar
1 tsp. vanilla
Whipping cream
Unsweetened chocolate curls

Combine first 3 ingredients. Beat egg whites and cream of tartar until foamy. Continue beating slowly adding sugar. Stir in vanilla. Fold in crumb mixture. Place in 9″ pie plate. Bake at 350° for about 20 minutes. Refrigerate 3 to 4 hours. To serve, top with whipped cream and curls.

Easy to make and exceptionally good.

WHOLE WHEAT PEAR PIE

Serves: 6-8

Whole Wheat Pastry:
1 1/4 cups whole wheat flour
2 Tbsp. sugar
3 Tbsp. salad oil
3 Tbsp. butter, melted
3 Tbsp. milk
1/4 tsp. salt

Filling:
5 fresh pears
1/2 cup sugar
2 Tbsp. whole wheat flour
3/4 tsp. cinnamon
1/4 tsp. nutmeg
1/8 tsp. salt
2 Tbsp. lemon juice
1/2 cup whole wheat flour
1/4 cup brown sugar, packed
1/4 tsp. cinnamon
4 Tbsp. butter, softened

For Pastry: combine ingredients. Stir well. Mixture will be crumbly. Press into 9″ pie plate to form shell. For Filling: core and slice unpeeled pears. Toss with next 6 ingredients. Place in pastry shell. Stir and cut together remaining ingredients. Sprinkle over fruit. Bake at 350° for about 50 minutes. Cool on rack.

Use this pastry shell and topping for other fresh fruits. Apples come naturally to mind.

HAWAIIAN FRUIT PIE

Serves: 6-8

1/2 cup flour
1 cup sugar
1/4 tsp. salt
2 cups milk, scalded
3 egg yolks, slightly beaten
2 Tbsp. butter
2 Tbsp. lemon juice
1 13-oz. can crushed pineapple, drained
1 cup coconut
1 9″ baked pie shell
3 egg whites
1/4 tsp. cream of tartar
6 Tbsp. sugar

Blend together first 3 ingredients in top of double boiler. Slowly stir in milk. Cook until thickened, stirring constantly. Stir small amount into egg yolks. Add egg yolks to custard and cook, stirring 3-4 minutes more. Remove from heat and add next 4 ingredients. Cool. Spoon into prepared pie shell. Beat egg whites and cream of tartar until soft peaks form. Slowly add sugar, beating until stiff peaks form. Spread over pie filling and seal against crust. Bake at 400° for 8-10 minutes. Cool on rack. Chill.

Light and refreshing, this pie is a complement to a summer supper.

LEMON CREAM PIE

Serves: 8-10

1 3 5/8-oz. pkg. lemon pudding and pie filling mix
3/4 cup sugar
2 cups water
3 egg yolks
3 Tbsp. butter
Juice of 1 lemon
3 egg whites
6 Tbsp. sugar
1 8-oz. container Cool Whip, defrosted
1 9″ pie shell, baked
Grated rind of 1 lemon

Stir together pudding mix and sugar. Add 1/4 cup water and stir until pudding mix and sugar dissolve. Stir in 3 egg yolks. Slowly add remaining 1 3/4 cups water. Cook, stirring constantly, over medium heat until mixture comes to full rolling boil. Immediately remove from heat and stir in butter and lemon juice. Cover surface with plastic wrap and chill. Beat egg whites until very soft peaks form. Continue beating, adding 6 Tbsp. sugar, 1 Tbsp. at a time to form meringue. Stir cooled pudding with spoon, fold in meringue, then 3/4 of Cool Whip. Pour into prepared pie shell. Spread top with remaining Cool Whip. Sprinkle over lemon rind. Refrigerate at least 6 hours.

A light, but satisfying, dessert.

WHITE CHRISTMAS PIE

Serves: 6-8

1/2 cup sugar
1/4 cup flour
1 envelope unflavored gelatin
1/2 tsp. salt
1 3/4 cups milk
3/4 tsp. vanilla
1/4 tsp. almond extract
3 egg whites
1/4 tsp. cream of tartar
1/2 cup sugar
1/2 cup whipping cream
1 cup shredded moist coconut
1 baked 9″ pie shell
Crushed strawberries

Combine first 4 ingredients in saucepan. Gradually add milk. Cook over medium heat stirring until mixture boils 1 minute. Cool until mixture mounds slightly. Stir in vanilla and almond extract. Beat egg whites with cream of tartar until foamy. Gradually add sugar, beating until stiff peaks form. Fold into gelatin mixture. Whip cream and fold into mixture with coconut. Mound in pie shell. Chill several hours or overnight. Serve with crushed strawberries.

This would be equally good with other fruit toppings such as pineapple, cherry or blueberry.

PEACH-BLUEBERRY PIE

Serves: 6-8

1/2 cup sugar
1 1/2 Tbsp. cornstarch
1/2 tsp. cinnamon
1 1/2 Tbsp. butter, cut up
3 cups sliced, peeled fresh peaches
2 cups fresh blueberries
1 9″ pie shell, unbaked
4 Tbsp. butter
2 Tbsp. flour
4 Tbsp. brown sugar

Mix together first 4 ingredients and toss with fruit. Spoon into pie shell. Blend remaining ingredients well and sprinkle over fruit. Bake at 425° for 15 minutes, reduce heat to 350° and bake about 35 minutes more. Cool on rack.

One-crust pies go together so quickly and seem much easier than 2-crust pies.

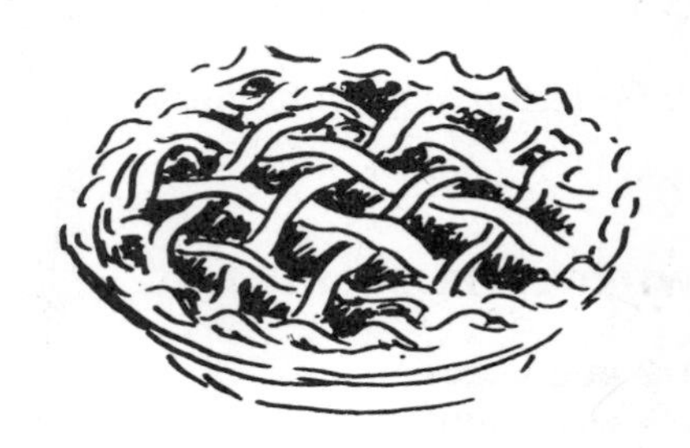

STREUSEL PEACH PIE

Serves: 6-8

8-10 barely ripe fresh peaches
1 9″ pie crust, unbaked
1/2 cup sugar
1/2 tsp. nutmeg
1/4 tsp. cinnamon
1/8 tsp. salt
1 egg
2 Tbsp. cream
1/4 cup brown sugar, packed
4 Tbsp. butter, softened
1/2 cup flour

Peel and quarter peaches. Arrange decoratively in pie crust. Combine next 4 ingredients and sprinkle over. Beat together egg and cream. Pour over peaches. Mix remaining ingredients until crumbly. Sprinkle over. Bake at 425° for 35-45 minutes. Cool on rack.

For sheer elegance serve warm topped with whipped cream or sour cream and a dash of cinnamon and sugar.

BANANA SPLIT PIE

Serves: 12

1 stick butter, melted
2 cups graham cracker crumbs
2 eggs
2 cups confectioners' sugar, sifted
1 1/2 sticks butter, softened
1 tsp. vanilla
1 20-oz. can crushed pineapple, drained
4 medium bananas, sliced
1 8-oz. carton Cool Whip
1/2 cup coarsely chopped pecans
1 4-oz. jar maraschino cherries

Combine melted butter and crumbs. Pat into bottom of 9″x13″ pan. Beat eggs at high speed 4 minutes. Add sugar, butter and vanilla. Beat 5 minutes. Spread over crumbs. Chill 30 minutes. Spread pineapple over creamed mixture. Arrange bananas over pineapple. Cover with Cool Whip. Sprinkle with nuts. Cover and refrigerate 6 hours or overnight. To serve, top each piece with a well-drained cherry.

Another good do-ahead dessert that will please those with a sweet tooth.

RAISIN NUT PIE

Serves: 8

1 1/4 cups raisins
2/3 cup broken walnuts
1 tsp. grated lemon peel
1 1/2 Tbsp. lemon juice
1 stick butter, softened
2/3 cup sugar
1/3 cup brown sugar, packed
1/2 tsp. cinnamon
1/4 tsp. salt
3 eggs
1 9″ pie shell, unbaked

Combine first 4 ingredients. Set aside. Beat butter until fluffy. Beat in sugars, cinnamon and salt. Add eggs 1 at a time, beating after each. Stir in raisin mixture. Spoon into pie shell. Bake at 400° for 15 minutes. Reduce heat to 350° and bake about 20 minutes more. Cool on rack.

This is an easily put together pie.

FUDGE PIE

Serves: 8

1 cup sugar
1 stick butter, softened
2 eggs, separated
2 oz. unsweetened chocolate, melted
1/2 cup sifted flour
1 tsp. vanilla or peppermint flavoring
1/8 tsp. salt

Sift sugar. Beat butter. Slowly add sugar. Beat until creamy. Beat in egg yolks. Add cooled chocolate. Beat in flour and flavoring. Beat egg whites and salt until stiff. Fold into batter. Pour into buttered 8″ pie plate. Bake at 325° for about 30 minutes.

This very rich pie is even more elegant when topped with vanilla ice cream.

UNUSUAL PIE

Serves: 8

3 egg whites
1 cup sugar
22 Ritz crackers, crushed
1/2 tsp. baking powder
3/4 cup finely chopped walnuts
1 tsp. vanilla
Vanilla ice cream
Chocolate sauce

Bring egg whites to room temperature and beat until stiff. Slowly fold in next 5 ingredients 1 at a time. Pour into greased 9″ pie pan and bake at 325° for 30 minutes. Cool and serve with vanilla ice cream and chocolate sauce.

Alternate choice — top with whipped cream and chopped walnuts.

BUTTERMILK PIE

Serves: 6-8

4 Tbsp. butter, softened
1 cup sugar
1 tsp. flour
3 large eggs, beaten
1/2 cup buttermilk
1/8 tsp. nutmeg
1/2 tsp. vanilla
1 8″ pie shell, unbaked

Cream together butter, sugar and flour. Slowly stir in eggs. Add remaining ingredients and pour into pie shell. Bake at 400° for 30-40 minutes or until set and golden.

Powdered buttermilk is now available, so you need not buy a whole quart of fresh to use just 1/2 cup.

PINEAPPLE CHERRY PIE

Serves: 6-8

Pastry for 2-crust 9″ pie
1 1-lb. can pitted red sour cherries, drained
1 20-oz. can pineapple chunks or crushed pineapple with syrup
1/2 cup brown sugar, packed
1/8 tsp. freshly ground nutmeg
2 Tbsp. quick-cooking tapioca

Line pie plate with 1/2 pastry. Combine remaining ingredients. Pour into shell. Cover with top crust. Flute rim. Cut vents in top crust. Bake at 425° for 40-45 minutes. Cool on rack.

Another very good fruit combination. For extra calories, top with ice cream.

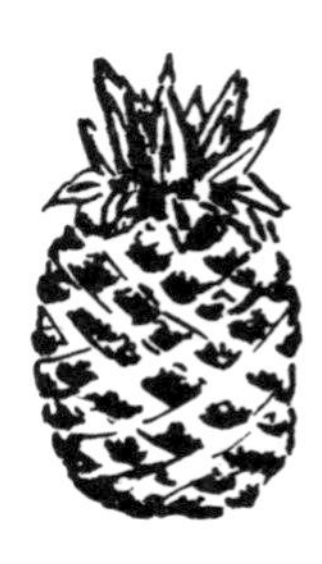

PIE CRUST MIX

Yield: 10 cups

8 cups flour
1 Tbsp. salt
5 tsp. sugar
3 cups shortening
Ice water

Stir together dry ingredients. Cut in shortening until mixture resembles coarse meal. Store in refrigerator in covered container. To use for 9″ pie pan measure out 1 1/2 cups for single crust, 2 1/2 cups for double crust. Stirring with fork add just enough ice water to hold dough together.

This mix keeps for weeks and makes pie-making easier.

Cookies and Cupcakes

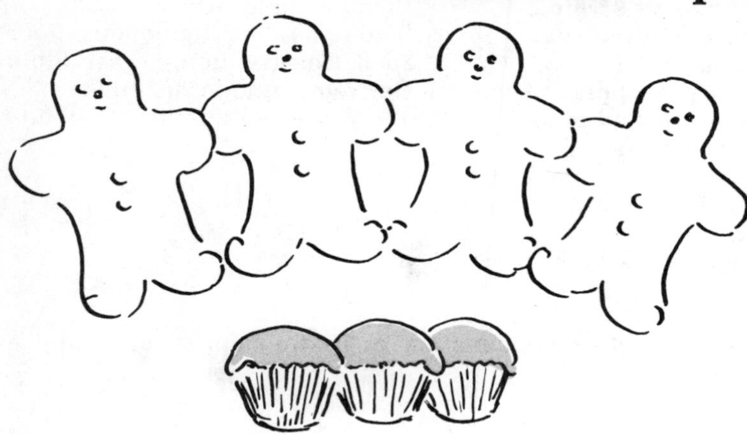

EAGLE BRAND MILK COOKIES

Yield: 4 dozen

1 14-oz. can sweetened condensed milk
1/2 cup peanut butter
1 cup raisins
1 cup Rice Krispies
1 cup shredded coconut
1 cup chopped nuts

Mix together first 2 ingredients. Add remaining ingredients and mix well. Drop by teaspoon onto ungreased cookie sheet. Bake in middle of oven at 375° for about 10 minutes.

These freeze well and recipe is easily doubled.

PIÑA COLADA COOKIES

Yield: 5 dozen

2 sticks butter, softened
1 cup sugar
1 tsp. rum flavoring
2 Tbsp. milk
2 1/2 cups sifted flour
3/4 cup chopped candied pineapple
1/2 cup chopped nuts
3/4 cup flaked coconut

Cream together butter and sugar. Stir in flavoring and milk. Add flour, pineapple and nuts. Shape into logs 8″ long and 1 1/2″ wide. Roll in coconut. Wrap and chill 2 hours or overnight. Slice 1/4″ thick. Place on ungreased cookie sheets. Bake at 375° for about 12 minutes. Cool on racks.

Will hold in the refrigerator several days, so can be baked as needed.

ITALIAN COOKIES

Yield: 16 slices

2 eggs
2/3 cup sugar
1 cup flour
1 tsp. anise flavoring

Icing:
2 cups confectioners' sugar
3 Tbsp. boiling water
1/4 tsp. anise flavoring

Beat together eggs and sugar. Stir in flour and flavoring. Pour into greased and floured loaf pan. Bake at 375° for about 25 minutes. Immediately remove from pan. Cut in 16 slices. Place on cookie sheet and lightly brown both sides under broiler. Spread with icing. For Icing: combine ingredients and beat together well.

These are very attractive sprinkled with colored nonpareils and served at holiday time.

PEANUT CRISP BARS

Yield: 2 dozen

1 cup sugar
1 cup white Karo syrup
1/8 tsp. salt
2 cups peanut butter
4 cups Rice Krispies

Icing:
4 Tbsp. butter
1/2 cup brown sugar, packed
1 Tbsp. milk
1/2 tsp. vanilla
1 1/2 cups sifted confectioners' sugar

Heat together first 3 ingredients until sugar dissolves. Blend in peanut butter. Stir in cereal. Spread in buttered 9″x13″ pan. For Icing: stir butter and brown sugar together over medium heat until butter melts. Remove from heat, add milk and vanilla. Stir in sugar and beat until smooth. Spread over cereal mixture. Chill. Cut in bars.

These are very easy and quite a child pleaser.

FORGOTTEN COOKIES

Yield: 3 1/2 dozen

2 egg whites
2/3 cup sugar
6 oz. chocolate chips
1 cup chopped nuts

Turn oven to 375°. Beat egg whites until stiff. Gradually beat in sugar. Beat until very stiff and sugar is dissolved. Add chips and nuts. Drop by teaspoonsful onto ungreased cookie sheet. Place in oven and turn oven off immediately. Leave in several hours or overnight. Do not open oven door.

Use this recipe for those leftover egg whites. These cookies are simple and good.

BLACK BOTTOM CUPS

Yield: 2 dozen

1 8-oz. pkg. cream cheese, softened
1 egg
1/3 cup sugar
1/8 tsp. salt
6 oz. semi-sweet chocolate
1 1/2 cups flour
1 cup sugar
1/4 cup cocoa
1 tsp. baking soda
1/2 tsp. salt
1 cup water
1/3 cup salad oil
1 tsp. vinegar
1 tsp. vanilla
1/2 cup chopped walnuts

Cream together first 4 ingredients. Stir in chips. Set aside. Sift together dry ingredients. Add liquids. Mix together well. Grease muffin cups or use paper liners. Fill cups 1/3 full. Top each with heaping teaspoonful cream cheese mixture. Sprinkle with walnuts. Bake at 350° for 25-35 minutes. Cool on racks.

These are scrumptious and freeze well.

SPICY OATMEAL CUPCAKES

Yield: 1 dozen

3/4 cup sifted cake flour
1/2 cup quick cooking rolled oats
6 Tbsp. brown sugar, firmly packed
4 Tbsp. sugar
1/2 tsp. baking soda
1/4 tsp. salt
1/4 tsp. cinnamon
1/8 tsp. cloves
1/8 tsp. allspice
4 Tbsp. shortening
1/2 cup milk
1 egg

Cream Cheese Icing:
1 3-oz. pkg. cream cheese, softened
2 cups sifted confectioners' sugar
3 Tbsp. honey

Combine dry ingredients. Add shortening and 6 Tbsp. milk. Beat 1/2 minute with mixer on low, then 2 minutes on high. Add remaining 2 Tbsp. milk and egg. Beat 2 minutes more. Fill paper-lined muffin cups 1/2 full. Bake at 375° for 20 minutes. Remove from pan and cool on racks. Frost with cream cheese icing. For Icing: beat cream cheese until soft. Add confectioners' sugar and honey and beat until smooth.

Frost small layer cakes or other cupcakes with this easy cream cheese icing.

DATE BARS **Yield: 2 dozen**

Batter:
1 1/2 cups flour
1/2 tsp. salt
1/2 tsp. baking soda
1 cup brown sugar, packed
1 1/2 cups rolled oats
1 cup coconut
1/2 cups chopped nuts
2 sticks butter, melted

Filling:
1 cup pitted dates
1 cup sugar
1 cup water
1 tsp. vanilla

For Batter: combine all batter ingredients and mix well. For Filling: combine dates, sugar and water and cook until thick. Cool, mash and stir in vanilla. Spread half batter in 9″x13″ pan. Spread filling over batter. Spread remaining batter over filling. Bake at 300° for 50-60 minutes.

Sweet and rich, these are the old-fashioned date squares.

PEANUT BUTTER GEMS **Yield: 4 dozen**

1/4 cup chunky style peanut butter
3/4 cup brown sugar, packed
2 1/4 tsp. corn syrup
2 1/4 tsp. hot water
2 sticks butter
3/4 cup sugar
1 egg
1 tsp. vanilla
2 1/2 cups flour
1/2 tsp. salt
1/2 tsp. baking powder

Stir together first 4 ingredients, cover and refrigerate. Cream butter and sugar until well blended. Beat in egg and vanilla. Mix dry ingredients together and stir into butter mixture. Cover and refrigerate 2 hours. Roll dough into 1″ balls and place 2″ apart on greased cooking sheet and make depression with thumb in center of each ball. Bake at 400° for 6 minutes. Remove from oven, place 1/2 tsp. peanut butter mixture in each thumb print and bake 5 minutes more. Remove to racks and cool.

Just plain peanut butter can be substituted with equally good results.

NUT HORNS

Yield: 128 cookies

1 1/2 sticks butter
1/4 cup shortening
4 cups flour
1/2 cup milk
1 pkg. active dry yeast
4 egg yolks
1 egg white
1 tsp. water

Nut Filling:
3 cups ground walnuts
3 Tbsp. melted butter
2 egg whites, beaten
1 cup sugar
2 tsp. vanilla

Cut butter and shortening into flour. Dissolve yeast in cold milk. Add egg yolks to mix and beat well. Add to flour mixture and mix. Chill dough 1 hour or up to 2 days. Divide dough into 16 pieces. Roll each piece into thin 8″ circle. Cut in 8 pie-shaped wedges. Place filling along wide end of triangle opposite point. Roll up enclosing filling, ending at point of triangle. Place on greased cookie sheet. Brush with egg white beaten with 1 tsp. cold water. Bake at 350° for 12-15 minutes. Cool on wire racks. For Nut Filling: mix ingredients well and use 3/4 tsp. in each cookie.

An all time favorite — always good.

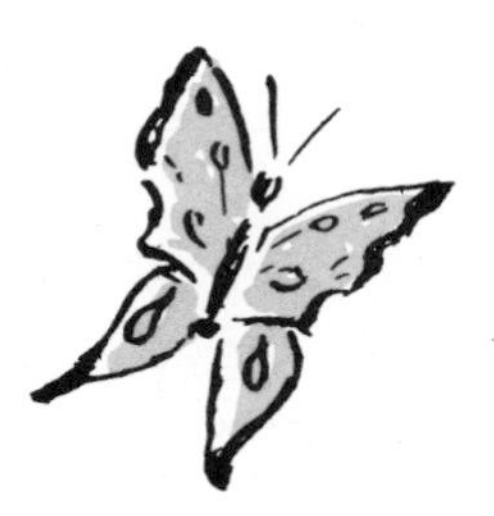

OATMEAL TRILBYS

Yield: 2 dozen

2 sticks butter, melted
2 cups rolled oats
1 cup sugar
2 cups flour
1/2 cup sour milk
1 tsp. soda

Filling:
1 lb. pitted dates, chopped
1 cup water
1 cup sugar

Pour hot butter over rolled oats. Add next 4 ingredients and mix well. Roll out on floured board or pastry cloth until very thin. Cut with round cookie cutter and place on cookie sheet. Place 1 tsp. filling on 1 cookie, top with another and finger-press edges together. Continue. Bake at 400° for 12-15 minutes or until lightly browned. For Filling: combine ingredients in saucepan and simmer, stirring until thick.

You will find this old family favorite an exceptionally good recipe.

CREAM CHEESE COOKIES

Yield: 2 dozen

4 oz. cream cheese, softened
1 stick butter, softened
1 cup flour
9 Tbsp. sugar
9 walnut halves, chopped

Cream together cheese and butter. Stir in flour, sugar and nuts. Drop by teaspoonful on ungreased cookie sheet. Wet finger and flatten until thin. Bake at 350° for 10 minutes.

These are delicious and the recipe is easily doubled.

FRUIT SALAD BARS

Yield: 3 dozen

4 Tbsp. shortening
3/4 cup sugar
2 eggs
1 tsp. vanilla
1 8 1/4-oz. can crushed pineapple, well drained
1/2 cup mashed banana
2 cups sifted flour
1 1/2 tsp. baking powder
1 tsp. salt
1/4 tsp. nutmeg
1 cup chopped walnuts
1 cup chopped dates

Lemon Glaze:
1 1/2 Tbsp. butter, melted
1 1/2 Tbsp. lemon juice
1 Tbsp. water
1/16 tsp. salt
2 cups sifted confectioners' sugar

Cream together well first 4 ingredients. Stir in pineapple and banana. Resift flour with next 3 ingredients. Beat into creamed mixture. Stir in nuts and dates. Spread in buttered 10″x15″x1″ jelly roll pan. Bake at 350° for 20-30 minutes. Cool to lukewarm. Spread with lemon glaze. When cool cut into bars. For Lemon Glaze: combine ingredients and beat until smooth.

Bananas can be frozen. Peel and leave whole or mash and freeze in measured containers for use in recipes such as this.

ANGEL CONFECTIONS

Yield: 2 1/2 dozen

1 stick butter, softened
1/2 cup sugar
8 oz. dates, chopped
1 cup chopped walnuts
1 cup Rice Krispies
1 tsp. vanilla
1/2 cup unsweetened coconut

Cream butter and sugar until light and fluffy. Add dates and cook, stirring over medium-high heat 3 minutes. Stir in nuts, cereal and vanilla. Cool. Shape into 2 1/2 dozen balls and roll in coconut.

These are sweet and could well be served as a candy.

PECAN CRISPIES

Yield: 7 dozen

1/2 cup shortening
1 stick butter
2 1/2 cups sugar
2 eggs, well beaten
2 1/2 cups flour
1/4 tsp. baking soda
1 cup chopped pecans

Cream shortening, butter and sugar thoroughly. Add eggs. Mix well. Sift flour and soda together and stir into batter. Stir in pecans. Pinch off acorn size pieces, flatten and place 2″ apart on greased cookie sheet. Bake at 350° for 12-15 minutes.

Double this and freeze some for emergencies.

SAND TARTS

Yield: 5 dozen

2 sticks butter
5 Tbsp. confectioners' sugar
2 cups flour
2 tsp. vanilla
1 1/2 cups chopped pecans

Cream butter and sugar until light. Add flour, vanilla and pecans and mix well. Form into 3/4″ balls. Bake on ungreased cookie sheets at 350° for 25-30 minutes. Remove from pans and roll in confectioners' sugar while warm. Store in airtight container.

An old-fashioned but ever good cookie.

PRINCESS BARS

Yield: 28 bars

1 1/2 cups sugar
3/4 cup shortening
2 cups cake flour
1 1/2 cups shredded coconut
1/4 tsp. salt
1 egg
1 tsp. vanilla
1 cup chopped walnuts
1 cup chopped dates
2 Tbsp. water

Combine 1 cup sugar and next 6 ingredients until well blended. Spread 1/2 mixture in 9″x13″ pan. Combine walnuts, dates, 1/2 cup sugar and water and spread over mixture in pan. Top with second half of bar mixture. Bake at 350° for 35-40 minutes. Cut into bars while warm.

This makes a very good moist bar.

SCOTCH SHORTBREAD

Yield: 32 squares

1 lb. butter, softened
1 cup sugar
4 cups flour

Cream butter. Gradually add sugar. Beat until light and fluffy. Add flour gradually. Press into 2 ungreased 8″ square pans. Prick with fork. Bake at 350° for 30-35 minutes. Cut into squares while warm.

This is a family recipe from Scotland dating back to about 1860.

CHOCOLATE DREAMS

Yield: 6 dozen

1 stick butter
1/4 cup sugar
5 Tbsp. cocoa
1 tsp. vanilla
1 egg
1/4 tsp. salt
2 cups graham cracker crumbs
1 cup finely chopped coconut
1/2 cup chopped walnuts
5 Tbsp. butter
3 Tbsp. milk
2 Tbsp. vanilla pudding mix
2 cups sifted confectioners' sugar
4 oz. semi-sweet chocolate

Combine first 6 ingredients in top of double boiler. Cook until mixture resembles custard, 5-10 minutes, stirring occasionally. Cool, then stir in next 3 ingredients. Press very firmly into 9″ square pan. Cream 4 Tbsp. butter. Stir milk and pudding mix together, add to butter and blend in sugar. Spread over chocolate base and let stand 30 minutes. Melt chocolate and remaining 1 Tbsp. butter and beat until spreading consistency. Spread over custard. Chill. Cut in squares to serve.

Another either-or recipe, cookie or candy. We are calling this a cookie.

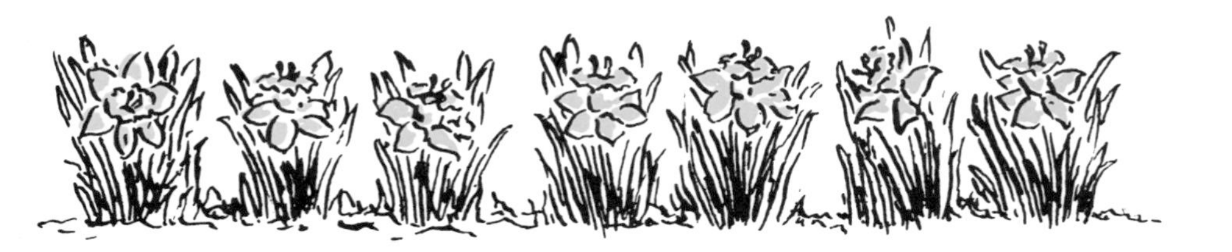

CREAM FILLED CHOCOLATE COOKIES

Yield: 5 dozen

1/2 cup shortening
2 cups sugar
1 tsp. vanilla
2 eggs
4 cups flour
1/2 tsp. baking powder
2 tsp. baking soda
1 tsp. salt
1/2 cup unsweetened cocoa
3/4 cup boiling water
1 cup buttermilk

Filling:
1 cup milk
5 Tbsp. flour
1 cup shortening
2 sticks butter
1 cup sugar
1 tsp. vanilla

Cream together shortening and sugar. Stir in vanilla and eggs. Sift dry ingredients and add in thirds alternately with water and buttermilk. Refrigerate several hours or overnight. Drop by teaspoon onto greased cookie sheet. Bake at 350° for about 15 minutes. Remove from cookie sheets. Cool on racks. Spread filling on bottom of 1 cookie. Place bottom of second cookie over filling. Repeat. For Filling: slowly stir milk into flour. Cook, stirring over medium heat until thick and bubbling. Cool. Add shortening and butter. Beat well. Slowly beat in sugar. Add vanilla.

These take a little more time to make, but are worth the effort.

PUMPKIN COOKIES

Yield: 8 dozen

3 cups brown sugar, packed
1 cup shortening
2 tsp. vanilla
4 eggs, beaten
5 cups flour
8 tsp. baking powder
1 tsp. salt
1/2 tsp. ginger
1/4 tsp. nutmeg
3/4 tsp. cinnamon
2 cups pumpkin

Icing:
4 Tbsp. butter
1/2 cup brown sugar, packed
1/8 tsp. salt
1/3 cup cream
2 cups confectioners' sugar
1/2 tsp. vanilla

Cream together sugar and shortening. Add vanilla and eggs. Sift together dry ingredients and add alternately in thirds with pumpkin. Drop by teaspoonful on greased cookie sheet. Bake at 350° for 15-20 minutes. Cool on racks. Ice. For Icing: combine first 4 ingredients over low heat until butter melts and mixture is smooth. Beat in sugar, adding more or less to make good spreading consistency. Add vanilla.

This makes a large batch and they freeze well.

PRALINE COOKIES

Yield: 5 dozen

1 Tbsp. butter
1/2 cup almonds
1/4 tsp. salt
1 stick butter
2/3 cup light brown sugar, packed
1 egg, well beaten
1 tsp. vanilla
3/4 cup flour
1/4 tsp. baking soda
1/4 cup maple syrup

Melt butter. Sauté almonds until golden. Stir in salt. Place on paper towels to cool. Chop coarsely. Cream butter. Add brown sugar. Cream well. Add egg and vanilla. Sift flour and soda. Add alternately with maple syrup. Add almonds. Drop by teaspoonsful 2″ apart on greased cookie sheet. Chill 2 hours. Bake at 350° for 8-10 minutes.

These are light, crisp and somewhat lacey.

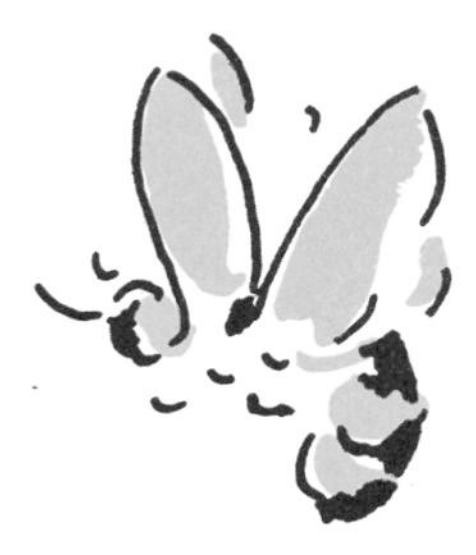

"MELT IN YOUR MOUTH" BROWNIES

Yield: 4 dozen

4 eggs, separated
2 cups sugar
2 sticks butter, melted
4 oz. unsweetened chocolate
1/2 cup hot water
2 tsp. vanilla
1 cup cake flour
Confectioners' sugar

Beat egg yolks to blend. Beat egg whites until stiff. Fold yolks into whites. Slowly stir in sugar. Add butter. Make paste of chocolate and water. Stir in. Add flour and vanilla, stirring just to mix. Pour into 9″x13″ pan. Bake at 300° for about 45 minutes. Cool on rack. If desired sprinkle with sugar.

This is the perfect name for these extra good and moist brownies. Do not double recipe.

SUGAR PLUM CUPCAKES

Yield: 16 cupcakes

1 stick butter
3/4 cup light brown sugar, firmly packed
2 eggs
1 cup sifted flour
1 tsp. baking powder
1/2 tsp. cinnamon
1/4 tsp. salt
2/3 cup graham cracker crumbs
1 cup chopped dates
1 cup chopped nuts
1 tsp. grated lemon rind
1/2 cup milk

Frosting:
4 Tbsp. butter
1 egg yolk
1 Tbsp. lemon juice
1 3/4 cups sifted confectioners' sugar
1/2 tsp. grated lemon rind
2 Tbsp. chopped nuts

Cream together butter and brown sugar. Add eggs 1 at a time and beat until fluffy. Sift together next 4 ingredients and combine with cracker crumbs, dates, nuts and rind. Fold alternately with milk into butter mixture. Divide into 16 paper-lined muffin cups. Bake at 375° for 20-25 minutes. Remove to rack and cool. Ice with frosting. For Frosting: beat together first 5 ingredients. Ice cooled cupcakes and spinkle with chopped nuts.

A treat for the holidays but good on other days as well.

SHOOFLY CUPCAKES

Yield: 3 dozen

1 Tbsp. baking soda
2 1/4 cups boiling water
1 cup molasses
1 lb. brown sugar
3/4 cup shortening
1/4 tsp. salt
4 cups flour

Add baking soda to water, stir in molasses. Set aside. Mix together brown sugar and shortening, working out any lumps. Combine salt and flour. Stir in gradually. Reserve 1 1/2 cups. Add molasses mixture to remaining flour mixture. Batter will be slightly lumpy. Fill greased muffin cups 2/3 full. Sprinkle tops with reserved crumbs. Bake at 375° for 20-25 minutes.

These remain moist for several days. They also freeze well.

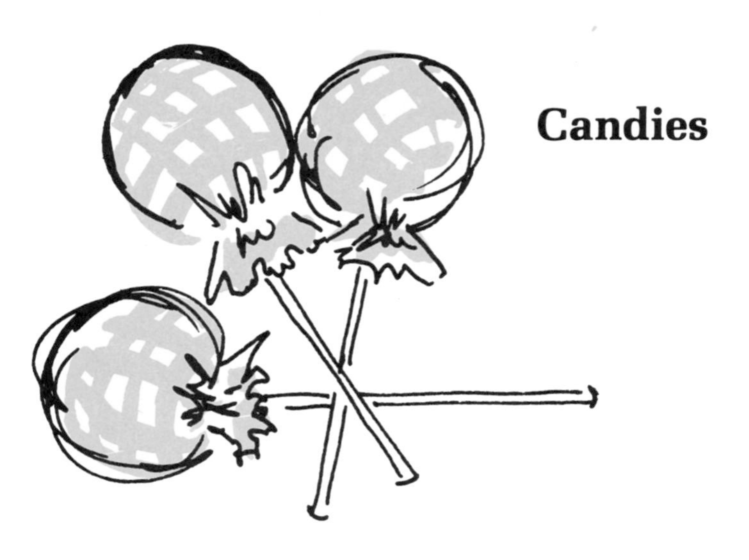

Candies

ENGLISH TOFFEE **Serves: 8**

2 sticks butter
1 cup sugar
6 oz. semi-sweet chocolate chips
1 cup chopped walnuts

Heat butter and sugar together, stirring constantly until candy thermometer registers 310°. Pour into buttered 9″ square pan. Refrigerate until hard. Melt chocolate chips. Spread 1/2 chocolate over candy. Sprinkle with 1/2 cup nuts. Refrigerate to harden. Loosen from pan and invert on waxed paper. Spread with remaining chocolate. Sprinkle with nuts. Chill again. Break candy with mallet. Age 3 days in covered container.

This is easy and can be done successfully by non-candy makers.

DIVINITY PINWHEELS **Yield: 4 dozen**

3 cups sugar
3/4 cup white Karo syrup
3/4 cup water
2 egg whites
1 tsp. vanilla
10 oz. peanut butter

Boil first 3 ingredients over medium-high heat until syrup forms a firm ball in cold water or reaches 245° on candy thermometer. Beat egg whites until stiff. Slowly pour in 1/2 syrup, beating constantly. Cook remaining syrup to crack stage or 300°. Slowly pour into egg white mixture, beating constantly. Add vanilla. Continue beating until stiff and it loses its glossy look. Spread on buttered 24″x14″ area of counter top. Cover with peanut butter. Butter hands and firmly roll up lengthwise. Cut in 1/2″ slices.

Wrap slices in plastic wrap and store in covered containers. Can be tricky for beginning candy makers.

UNCOOKED CHOCOLATE CREAM CANDY

Yield: 4 dozen

2 sticks butter, softened
3 cups confectioners' sugar
1 egg white
1/8 tsp. salt
2 tsp. vanilla
5 oz. unsweetened chocolate, melted
2 cups chopped walnuts or pecans

Cream butter and add sugar gradually. Beat in egg white, salt and vanilla. Beat in slightly cooled chocolate. Stir in nuts. Spread in buttered 9″ square pan. Chill. Cut in squares.

Fudge is good, but this is better! It actually melts in your mouth.

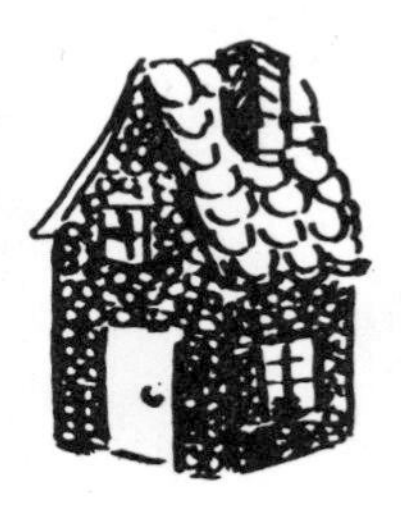

CARAMEL CORN

Serves: 6

1 stick butter
1 cup brown sugar
1/4 cup light Karo syrup
1/2 tsp. salt
1/2 tsp. baking soda
1 tsp. vanilla
3/4 cup unpopped corn

Melt butter, stir in next 3 ingredients, bring to boil, stirring constantly. Boil 5 minutes without stirring. Remove from heat and stir in baking soda and vanilla. Pop corn and stir in. Place on cookie sheet with sides and bake at 275° for about 30 minutes. Stir every 10 minutes.

Easy and fun to make, this is a treat to please all children.

PEANUT BUTTER BARS

Yield: 4 dozen

2/3 lb. graham crackers, crushed
1 lb. confectioners' sugar
1 3/4 cups butter, melted
1 cup chunky peanut butter
1/2 cake paraffin wax
1 12-oz. pkg. chocolate chips or butterscotch chips

Mix together first 4 ingredients. If dry, add more butter. Make into 1″ balls. In top of double boiler melt together wax and chips. Dip balls in mixture. Cool.

These are really delicious and can double as a cooky.

PEANUT BUTTER FUDGE

Yield: 5 dozen

2 sticks butter
1 cup creamy peanut butter
1 lb. confectioners' sugar
1 8-oz. plain or almond Hershey bar

Melt butter and peanut butter together in top of double boiler over boiling water. Remove from heat and stir in confectioners' sugar. Spread and press into an 8″ square pan. Melt chocolate bar over hot water in top of double boiler. Spread over peanut butter layer. Let set at room temperature and cut in small squares.

So easy and rich and delicious!

TOFFEE SHORTBREAD

Yield: 2 dozen

2 sticks butter, softened
6 Tbsp. sugar
1 cup flour
1 tsp. baking powder
1 Tbsp. light Karo syrup
1 14-oz. can sweetened condensed milk
4 oz. semi-sweet chocolate

Cream together 1 stick butter and 2 Tbsp. sugar. Stir in flour and baking powder. Spread in 9″ square pan. Bake at 350° for about 25 minutes or until light gold. Cool and refrigerate. In heavy saucepan combine remaining butter and sugar, syrup and milk and bring to boil. Boil slowly until mixture coats wooden spoon heavily, about 15 minutes. Stir frequently. Spread over cold shortbread. Cool. Melt chocolate and spread evenly over filling. Let layers set.

This is quite rich and exceptionally good. Is it a cookie or a candy? We tossed, and candy won.

CHOCOLATE MINT BALLS

Yield: 8 dozen

1 1/2 cups evaporated milk
4 cups sugar
1/16 tsp. salt
1 12-oz. pkg. semi-sweet chocolate chips
1 7-oz. jar marshmallow cream
1/2 tsp. peppermint extract
2 cups finely chopped nuts

Stir together milk, sugar and salt in saucepan over low heat until sugar dissolves. Bring to full boil and cook, stirring constantly, 5 minutes. Remove from heat. Beat in chocolate, marshmallow cream and extract until smooth. Cool. Form into 1″ balls and roll in nuts.

Do not worry about storing, for these candies will disappear before the need arises.

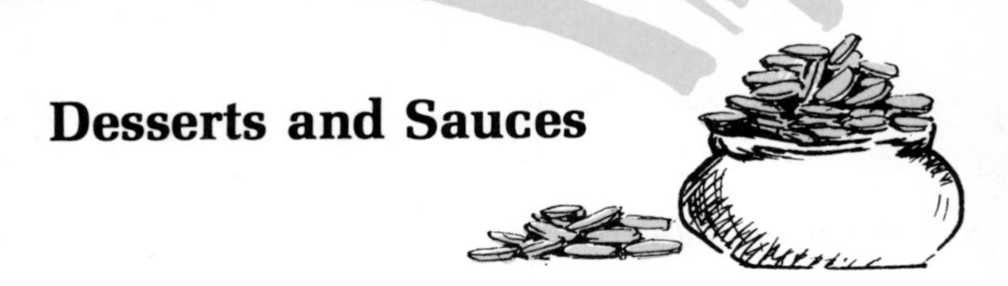

Desserts and Sauces

RHUBARB AND STRAWBERRY FLAN

Serves: 6-8

Sweet Dough Shell:
1 1/3 cups flour
1/4 cup sugar
1 tsp. grated lemon grind
3/4 tsp. ginger
1/4 tsp. mace
1 stick butter
1 egg yolk
1 cup ground nuts

Filling:
4 cups fresh strawberries
3/4 cup sugar
2 Tbsp. lemon juice
1 tsp. ginger
1 3/4 cups rhubarb
2 Tbsp. cornstarch

For Dough: combine first 5 ingredients. Cut in butter until mixture resembles small peas. Blend in egg yolk. Add ground nuts. Knead by hand in bowl until dough is smooth. Form ball, cover and refrigerate 30 minutes. Press evenly into bottom and sides of 9″ flan pan. Prick well with fork. Bake at 325° for 20-25 minutes. Cool on rack. For Filling: mash 2 cups strawberries. In saucepan combine with next 3 ingredients. Bring to boil. Add rhubarb. Simmer 5 minutes. Cool. An hour before serving remove rhubarb with slotted spoon from syrup to plate. Combine cornstarch with 3 Tbsp. syrup. Stir into syrup. Cook over medium heat, stirring constantly until boiling. Boil 1 minute. Cool. Carefully remove baked crust from pan to flat serving plate. Slice remaining strawberries. Arrange fruit by placing some sliced strawberries around outer edge of shell. Make ring with rhubarb pieces. Continue, filling center with berries. Spoon syrup over berries. Refrigerate to set glaze.

The original recipe calls for raspberries instead of strawberries. If you can find them and want to splurge, use them.

TIPSY MERINGUE SOUFFLE

Serves: 4

1/4 cup golden raisins, halved
1/4 cup chopped pecans
2 Tbsp. sherry
2 Tbsp. white rum
3 egg whites
1/2 cup sugar
Whipped cream

Stir together first 4 ingredients. Cover and let stand overnight at room temperature. Beat egg whites until soft peaks form. Slowly beat in sugar. Beat until stiff and glossy. Fold in raisin mixture. Turn into buttered 1-qt. soufflé dish. Place in pan of hot water so water comes halfway up dish. Bake at 350° for 35-40 minutes. Serve at once with whipped cream.

This doubles easily for 2-qt. soufflé dish. Extend baking time to 50-55 minutes.

BLUEBERRY BUCKLE

Serves: 8-10

3/4 cup sugar
4 Tbsp. butter
1 egg
2 cups flour
2 tsp. baking powder
1/2 tsp. salt
1/2 cup milk
2 cups blueberries
1/2 cup sugar
1/3 cup flour
1/2 tsp. cinnamon
1/4 cup butter, softened

Mix first 3 ingredients. Stir together flour, baking powder and salt. Add alternately in thirds with milk to sugar mixture. Fold in blueberries. Pour into greased and floured 9″ square pan. Cut together remaining ingredients and sprinkle over batter. Bake at 375° for about 30 minutes.

Fresh, frozen or well-drained canned blueberries may be used.

CRÈME de MÊNTHE RING

Serves: 8

8 lady fingers, split and cut in half
1 1/2 qt. lime sherbet, slightly softened
1/4 cup Crème de Mênthe
1 pt. fresh strawberries

Lightly oil bottom and sides of 6-cup ring mold. Cut wax paper to fit and lightly oil. Stand lady fingers around sides, rounded sides against mold. Stir together sherbet and Crème de Mênthe until smooth. Pour into mold. Freeze until firm. Clean and stem strawberries. To serve, unmold on large plate. Fill center with strawberries.

A refreshing and light summer dessert.

PEANUT FINGERS

Serves: 12

1 3-oz. pkg. plain lady fingers
1/3 cup jelly or preserves
1 1/2 cups confectioners' sugar
1 egg white
1 Tbsp. water
1 tsp. vanilla
4 oz. dry roasted peanuts, chopped

Split lady fingers, spread with jelly or preserves, press halves together. Beat together next 4 ingredients until smooth. Using fork, dip lady fingers in icing to coat. Let excess drip off. Roll in chopped nuts. Place on rack to set.

This fun finger food is an original recipe.

BAKED ALASKA STRAWBERRY SHORTCAKE

Serves: 8-10

1 pt. strawberry ice cream, softened
2 cups biscuit mix
3 Tbsp. sugar
1/2 cup milk
1 egg yolk
3 Tbsp. butter, melted
1 pt. fresh strawberries, sliced
4 egg whites
1/2 tsp. cream of tartar
1/2 tsp. vanilla
1/2 cup sugar

Line 8″ round pan with foil. Spoon in ice cream. Freeze. Combine biscuit mix and sugar. Beat together milk, egg yolk and butter. Stir into biscuit mix until smooth. Spread in greased 9″ round pan. Bake at 450° for 12-15 minutes. Remove from pan. Cool on rack. Place on oven-proof plate. Remove foil from ice cream. Place ice cream on shortcake. Top with fruit. Beat together next 3 ingredients until soft peaks form. Gradually add sugar. Beat until stiff peaks form. Spread over entire shortcake, sealing edges. Bake at 500° for 4 minutes.

This is easy and good enough to make in the winter using frozen strawberries.

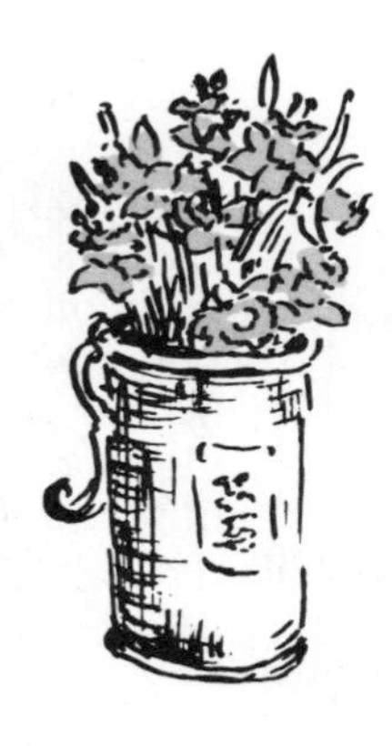

SIX LAYER TORTE

Serves: 20

12 egg yolks
1 1/2 cups sugar
9 Tbsp. cracker meal
2/3 cup ground walnuts
1/2 tsp. vanilla
12 egg whites

Chocolate Butter Cream:
1 1/2 sticks butter, softened
1 1/2 lb. confectioners' sugar, sifted
2 eggs
4 1/2 oz. unsweetened chocolate, melted
6 Tbsp. orange juice

Bring eggs to room temperature. Beat yolks until lemon colored. Gradually add sugar, beating until thickened. Stir in next 3 ingredients. Beat egg whites until stiff. Fold into batter. Grease 3 9″ cake pans. Cut foil to fit bottoms. Grease foil. Dust with extra cracker meal. Pour batter evenly into pans. Bake at 325° for 25-30 minutes. Cool on racks. Remove from pans. Remove foil. Split each layer in half to form 6 layers. Frost. For Chocolate Butter Cream: cream butter, add 1/2 lb. sugar, eggs, beat until smooth. Add chocolate. Beat in remaining sugar alternately with orange juice using slightly more or less to make good spreading consistency. Stack layers and frost sides.

Carefully cut this rich dessert into small slices.

TORTONI

Serves: 6-8

3/4 cup sugar
1/4 cup water
3 egg whites
1/8 tsp. salt
1/4 cup blanched slivered almonds
1 3/4 tsp. almond extract
1 1/2 cups whipping cream
3/4 tsp. vanilla extract
Maraschino cherries

Dissolve sugar in water in saucepan. Bring to boil and cook until syrupy, about 5 minutes. Remove from heat. Have egg whites at room temperature and beat with salt at high speed until stiff. Pour sugar syrup into egg whites slowly in thin stream, beating at high speed until very stiff and glossy. Cover and refrigerate until cool, about 30 minutes. Toast almonds on baking sheet at 400° for 10 minutes or until golden, stirring occasionally. Chop and toss with 1 1/2 tsp. almond extract. Beat cream until stiff. Add remaining 1/4 tsp. almond extract and vanilla extract. Fold cream into egg white mixture. Fold in almonds. Spoon into cup cake liners or sherbet glasses. Refrigerate or freeze. If frozen, remove from freezer at least 20 minutes before serving. Garnish with cherries at serving time.

Light, lovely and easy to prepare ahead of time.

STRAWBERRY COOKIE SHELL SUNDAES

Serves: 6

Filling:
1 pt. strawberries, sliced
1/2 cup sugar
1 qt. vanilla ice cream
1/2 cup chopped pecans

Cookie Shells:
1 egg
1/3 cup confectioners' sugar
2 Tbsp. brown sugar
1/4 tsp. vanilla
1/4 cup sifted flour
1/8 tsp. salt
2 Tbsp. butter, melted
2 Tbsp. finely chopped pecans

Combine strawberries and sugar. Set aside. For Shells: beat egg 5 minutes. Add sugars, beating until dissolved. Add vanilla. Stir in flour and salt. Blend in butter and nuts. Grease and flour 2 cookie sheets. Make 3 5″ circles on each by spreading 2 Tbsp. batter thinly for each circle. Bake, 1 sheet at a time, at 300° for about 12 minutes. Remove hot cookies with broad spatula. Place over 6 inverted 6-oz. custard cups. Cool. To serve, fill shells with ice cream and top with prepared strawberries and nuts.

Shells do not freeze. Make up to 1 week ahead and store in air-tight container.

BLUEBERRY FLIM FLAM

Serves: 12

1 2-layer yellow cake mix
2/3 cup rum
2/3 cup water
1 Tbsp. grated orange peel

Sauce:
1 qt. blueberries
1 Tbsp. lemon juice
1/2 cup water
1/8 tsp. nutmeg
1/2 cup rum
3/4 cup sugar
1/3 cup cornstarch
2 Tbsp. butter
Whipped cream

Prepare cake according to package directions using rum and water for liquid. Add orange peel. Pour into 2 greased and floured 9″ cake pans. Bake at 350° for 25-30 minutes. Cool on racks. For Sauce: combine 1/2 blueberries with next 6 ingredients. Stir over low heat until sauce thickens and bubbles. Stir in butter and remaining blueberries. Chill. Place cakes on platters. Top with blueberry sauce. Chill until serving time. Garnish with whipped cream

This is a light ending for a summer meal.

ANGEL CUSTARD CAKE

Serves: 12

4 eggs, separated
2 cups milk
1 cup sugar
2 Tbsp. flour
1/8 tsp. salt
1 envelope unflavored gelatin
1/2 cup water
3 cups whipping cream
1 large angel food cake
1/2 cup flaked coconut

In saucepan, beat egg yolks. Stir in milk. Combine sugar, flour and salt. Stir in. Cook over medium heat, stirring constantly until thick and just boiling. Dissolve gelatin in water and stir in. Cool. Whip 2 cups cream, beat egg whites until stiff and fold both into cooled custard. Tear angel food cake into pieces and fold into custard. Place in angel food cake pan with removable bottom. Cover and refrigerate overnight. To serve, remove from pan, ice with remaining cup of cream whipped and sprinkle with coconut.

A million calories but worth every bite.

STRAWBERRY DELIGHT

Serves: 8-10

1 3-oz. pkg. strawberry jello
1 1/4 cups boiling water
1 10-oz. pkg. frozen sliced strawberries, thawed
1 tsp. sugar
1/8 tsp. salt
1 cup whipping cream
1/2 10″ angel food cake, torn in pieces

Dissolve jello in water. Stir in next 3 ingredients. Cool until mixture begins to thicken. Whip cream and fold in. Cover bottom of 9″ square pan with 1/2 cake pieces. Pour 1/2 strawberry mixture over cake. Repeat. Refrigerate 4-5 hours or overnight.

This is most attractive when done in a decorative salad mold. To serve turn out and garnish with whole fresh strawberries and mint sprigs.

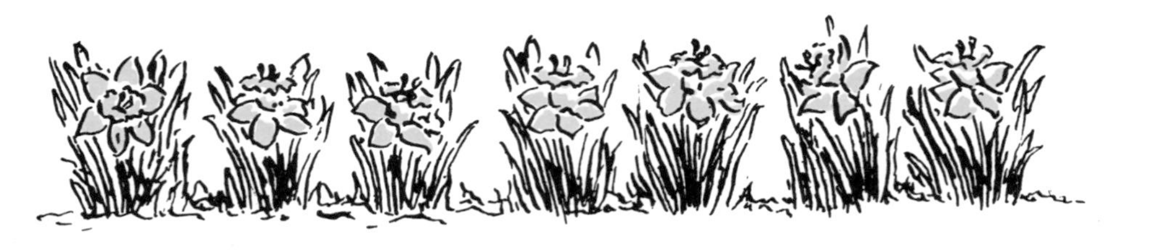

CHOCOLATE DECADENCE

Serves: 12

1 lb. dark sweet chocolate
10 Tbsp. unsalted butter
4 eggs, room temperature
1 Tbsp. sugar
1 Tbsp. flour
1 cup whipping cream
1 Tbsp. confectioners' sugar
1 tsp. vanilla or 1 Tbsp. Crème de Cacao
Shaved chocolate

Butter 8″ cake pan. Line bottom of pan with wax or parchment paper cut to fit. Butter paper. Dust with flour. Shake out excess. Melt chocolate and butter in top of double boiler over hot water. Stir to blend. Set aside. Place eggs and sugar in top of double boiler over hot water. Do not let water touch bottom of pan. Beat eggs with wire whip until sugar is dissolved and mixture is barely warm. Pour mixture into large mixer bowl. Continue beating at high speed until eggs have quadrupled and are very light, about 10 minutes. Fold flour into egg mixture. Stir 1/4 egg into chocolate, then gently fold chocolate into egg mixture. Pour into prepared pan and bake at 425° for 12-15 minutes. Cake will be liquid in center. Remove from oven. Cool, then freeze overnight in pan. Unmold by carefully dipping pan in hot water. Whip cream with confectioners' sugar and vanilla or Crème de Cacao. Frost cake or decorate with whipped cream piped through a pastry tube. Sprinkle with shaved chocolate. Refrigerate until serving time.

If one must be decadent, do it with chocolate!

TANGERINE COCONUT CUPS

Serves: 8

2 Tbsp. butter
1 3 1/2-oz. can shredded coconut, toasted
2 egg yolks, slightly beaten
2 1/2 cups milk
1 3-oz. pkg. vanilla pudding
2 tsp. finely grated tangerine peel
3-4 tangerines, peeled and sectioned
2 egg whites
1/4 cup sugar

Generously butter 8 custard cups or ramekins. Sprinkle even amounts of coconut into each. Press firmly to form shells. Chill. Combine egg yolks and milk, stir slowly into pudding and cook, stirring, over medium heat until mixture begins to bubble. Add grated peel and cool. Reserve 8 tangerine sections for garnish. Cut remaining sections in small pieces. Stir into pudding. Spoon pudding into shells. Beat egg whites until soft peaks form. Gradually add sugar beating until stiff peaks form. Swirl meringue over pudding, sealing against shells. Bake at 425° for 5-8 minutes. Cool. Garnish with reserved tangerine sections.

Tangerines are seasonal. If not available substitute fresh navel oranges.

RAISIN AND NUT PUDDING

Serves: 8

Syrup:
cup brown sugar, packed
1/3 cups water
Tbsp. butter

Batter:
Tbsp. butter
cup brown sugar, packed
/2 cup milk
tsp. vanilla
1/2 cups flour
tsp. baking powder
cup nuts
cup raisins

Combine syrup ingredients. Boil 7 minutes over medium-high heat. Pour into buttered 2-qt. rectangular dish. For Batter: stir together first 4 ingredients. Add remaining ingredients, mixing well. Drop batter by tablespoonsful into syrup. Bake at 350° for 40-45 minutes.

A rich and easy dessert that is especially good at holiday time.

APPLE TURNOVER

Serves: 12

Crust:
1/2 cups flour
cup shortening
tsp. salt
egg yolks
Milk
cups cornflakes
egg whites
Tbsp. sugar

Filling:
-10 medium apples, peeled, cored and sliced
cup sugar
tsp. cinnamon
Tbsp. flour
/2 tsp. nutmeg

For Crust: beat together first 3 ingredients. Beat egg yolks until light. Stir in enough milk to make 2/3 cup and add mix to flour until dough forms a ball. Divide in half. Roll out 1/2 to almost cover cookie sheet. Sprinkle with corn flakes. Spread filling over dough. Roll out remaining dough and cover. Seal edges. Lightly stir egg white, brush on dough and sprinkle with sugar. Bake at 400° for about 1/2 hour or until golden brown. For Filling: lightly toss together all ingredients.

One large turnover is certainly easier to make and just as good as 12 small ones!

LEMON DELIGHT

Serves: 8-10

1 1/2 cups flour
1 1/2 sticks butter
1/3 cup chopped pecans
8 oz. cream cheese, softened
1 cup confectioners' sugar
2 cups Cool Whip
3 3-oz. pkg. instant lemon pudding
4 cups milk
1/2 cup toasted coconut

Mix together flour, butter and pecans. Pat evenly into 9" × 13" pan and bake at 350° for 15-20 minutes. Cool. Beat cream cheese and sugar. Blend in 1 cup Cool Whip. Spread over baked crust. Beat pudding mix and milk 2 minutes. Spread over cheese layer. Chill to set. Spread with remaining 1 cup Cool Whip. Sprinkle with toasted coconut. Refrigerate.

This does not freeze, but it may be made a day or two ahead.

ORANGE BAVARIAN

Serves: 8

1 envelope unflavored gelatin
1/4 cup sugar
1/4 tsp. salt
2 eggs, separated
3/4 cup cold water
1 6-oz. can frozen orange juice, thawed
1/4 cup sugar
1 cup whipping cream
2 cups mandarin oranges, drained

In saucepan mix together gelatin, sugar and salt. Beat together egg yolks and water. Stir in. Cook over low heat, stirring constantly until gelatin dissolves and mixture thickens slightly, about 5 minutes. Remove from heat. Stir in undiluted orange juice. Chill until mixture molds slightly when dropped from spoon. Beat egg whites until foamy, add sugar, beating until stiff peaks form. Fold into gelatin mixture. Turn into 6-cup mold. Chill. To serve, unmold and garnish with mandarin oranges.

A light dessert that is cool in summer and refreshing in winter.

PERFECT CHOCOLATE MOUSSE

Serves: 4-6

6 oz. semi-sweet chocolate chips
5 Tbsp. boiling water
4 eggs, separated
2 Tbsp. rum
1/2 tsp. instant coffee

Place chocolate chips and water in blender. Blend 1 minute. Add egg yolks, rum and coffee. Blend 1 minute. Add egg whites. Blend 2 minutes. Pour into 4 sherbert or 6 small wine glasses. Chill.

Do not double. Make separate batches. This is so easy, foolproof and absolutely delicious.

PUMPKIN SPICED BAKED ALASKA **Serves: 8**

Sponge Cake:
2 eggs
1/2 cup sugar
3 Tbsp. water
1/2 tsp. vanilla
2/3 cup cake flour
1/2 tsp. baking powder
1/8 tsp. salt
2 Tbsp. sifted confectioners' sugar

Topping:
1 qt. vanilla ice cream
2 tsp. pumpkin pie spice
5 egg whites
1/2 tsp. cream of tartar
3/4 cup sugar
1 Tbsp. light rum

For Cake: in small mixer bowl, beat eggs 5 minutes or until thick and lemony. Pour into large mixer bowl and gradually beat in sugar. Blend in water and vanilla. Combine and add gradually next 3 ingredients, beating until batter is smooth. Pour into 9″ round pan, greased and lined with greased wax paper. Bake at 375° for 12-15 minutes. Loosen cake from sides of pan. Invert onto cake rack covered with a tea towel and sprinkled with confectioners' sugar. Carefully peel off wax paper. Trim uneven edges if necessary. Cool on rack. For Topping: soften ice cream and beat in pumpkin pie spice. Pack into 1 1/2 quart bowl that is 2-3 inches smaller in diameter than cake. Freeze until firm. Place cake right side up on ovenproof plate. Loosen ice cream from bowl by dipping quickly in hot water. Invert onto cake. Return to freezer. Beat egg whites and cream of tartar until foamy. Gradually add sugar. Continue beating until stiff and glossy. Add rum. Cover cake and ice cream completely with egg whites, sealing edges and smoothing top and sides evenly. Return to freezer. Store no more than 24 hours. To serve, preheat oven to 500°. Bake on lowest rack until light brown, 3-5 minutes. Serve immediately.

Dazzle them at Thanksgiving with this instead of pumpkin pie!

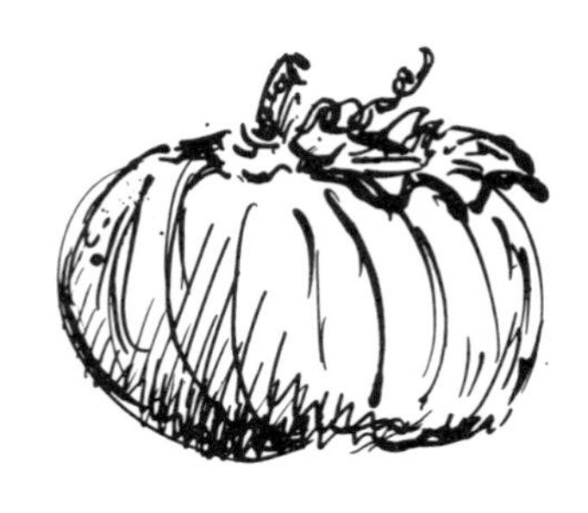

EASY CHERRIES JUBILANT

Serves: 10

2 16 1/2-oz. cans pitted dark cherries
1/2 cup sugar
3 Tbsp. cornstarch
2 Tbsp. lemon juice
1 tsp. grated orange peel
1/2 tsp. grated lemon peel
1/2 cup brandy
Vanilla ice cream

Drain cherries, adding enough water to juice to make 2 cups. In saucepan mix together sugar and cornstarch. Slowly add cherry syrup and water. Add next 3 ingredients. Cook, stirring until just boiling. Add cherries. Set aside. To serve, place over heat in chafing dish. Heat brandy, ignite and pour over cherry mixture. Ladle over ice cream.

This is always a spectacular dessert.

FROSTED CRANBERRY MOLD

Serves: 8-10

1 13 1/2-oz. can crushed pineapple
2 3-oz. pkg. lemon jello
1 7-oz. bottle ginger ale
1 1-lb. can jellied cranberry sauce
2 cups Cool Whip
1 8-oz. pkg. cream cheese, softened
1/2 cup chopped pecans
1 Tbsp. butter, melted

Drain pineapple and add enough water to juice to make 1 cup. Bring to boil, dissolve jello. Cool. Gently stir in ginger ale. Chill until partially set. Break up cranberry sauce. Fold into jello. Pour into 9″×9″ dish. Chill until firm. Blend Cool Whip and cream cheese. Spread over jello. Roast pecans in butter at 350° for 10 minutes and sprinkle on top. Chill.

This can be served as a salad to those with a very sweet tooth.

SOUFFLÉ GLACÉ GRAND MARNIER

Serves: 6-8

6 egg yolks
2 whole eggs
1 cup sugar
2 oz. Grand Marnier
2 cups heavy cream
1 Tbsp. sugar
1/4 tsp. vanilla

Combine egg yolks, eggs and sugar in mixing bowl. Place over hot water, stirring constantly, until sugar melts and mixture is very warm. Beat with mixer on high speed until thick, stiff and lemon colored, a minimum of 10-15 minutes. Fold in Grand Marnier. Whip 1 1/2 cups cream until soft peaks form and fold in. Pour into 1 1/2-qt. soufflé dish wrapped with 3″ collar. Freeze overnight. Whip remaining cream until stiff. Add sugar and vanilla. Remove collar from soufflé. Decorate with whipped cream and serve.

Garnish with mandarin oranges, if you choose. An elegant dessert!

CRANBERRY MUFFINS WITH BUTTER SAUCE

Serves: 8

Batter:
2 Tbsp. butter, softened
1/2 cup sugar
1/2 cup milk
1 cup flour
1 1/2 tsp. baking powder
1 cup fresh cranberries

Sauce:
1 cup sugar
4 Tbsp. butter
1/2 cup cream
1 tsp. vanilla

For Batter: cream butter and sugar together. Add milk. Sift together flour and baking powder. Stir in. Add cranberries. Pour into 8 greased muffin cups. Bake at 350° for 25-35 minutes. For Sauce: combine ingredients and cook over low heat until sugar dissolves and butter melts. Serve hot sauce on warm muffins.

These are delicious and the recipe easily doubled.

MINIATURE CHEESE CAKES

Yield: 4 dozen

48 midget paper cups
48 vanilla wafers
3 8-oz. pkg. cream cheese, softened
1 1/2 cups sugar
3 eggs, beaten
3 tsp. vanilla
1 1/2 tsp. lemon juice
1 21-oz. can cherry pie filling

Place paper cups in midget cupcake pans. Place vanilla wafer in each. Beat cream cheese. Add next 4 ingredients. Beat well. Divide between midget cups. Bake at 350° for 12-14 minutes. Cool. Top each cup with a cherry and filling. Chill.

These do not freeze well, but will hold 2 days in refrigerator.

LEMON FLUFF PUDDING

Serves: 4

1 cup sugar
1 Tbsp. butter
2 egg yolks
3 Tbsp. flour
Juice and grated peel of 1 lemon
1 cup milk
2 egg whites
Whipped cream

Cream sugar and butter. Add next 3 ingredients and mix thoroughly. Slowly add milk, mixing until smooth. Fold in stiffly beaten egg whites. Pour into greased 1 1/2-qt. casserole. Set casserole in pan of hot water and bake at 350° for 40-50 minutes. Cake rises to the top over smooth sauce. Serve warm or cold with whipped cream.

This may be tripled and baked in a 9″ × 13″ cake pan to serve 12.

FRENCH APPLE COBBLER

Serves: 8

5 cups peeled, sliced and cored tart apples
3/4 cup sugar
2 Tbsp. flour
1/2 tsp. cinnamon
1/4 tsp. salt
1 tsp. vanilla
1/4 cup water
1 Tbsp. butter
1/2 cup sifted flour
1/2 cup sugar
1/2 tsp. baking powder
1/4 tsp. salt
2 Tbsp. butter, softened
1 egg, slightly beaten

Combine first 7 ingredients. Spread into 9″ square pan. Dot with 1 Tbsp. butter. Beat together remaining ingredients with wooden spoon until smooth. Drop batter in 9 portions onto apples, spacing evenly. Bake at 375° for 35-40 minutes. Serve warm.

A never-fail cobbler that is even better served with rich cream or ice cream.

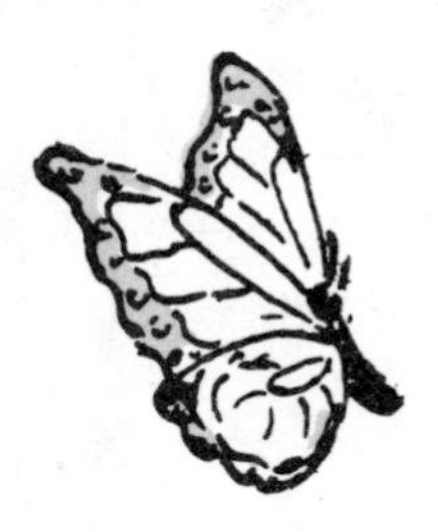

ESPRESSO FROZEN MOUSSE

Serves: 6-8

4 tsp. instant coffee
1 Tbsp. hot water
4 eggs, separated
1/2 cup sugar
1 cup whipping cream
3 Tbsp. Kahlúa
Chocolate sauce

Dissolve coffee in hot water and set aside. Beat egg whites until stiff, gradually add sugar, beating until firm glossy peaks form. Fold in coffee mixture. Beat egg yolks until thick and lemon-colored. Whip cream until stiff and blend in liqueur. Gently but thoroughly fold together egg whites, yolks and cream. Pour into glass bowl, cover and freeze. To serve, top with Chocolate Sauce found in "Dessert Sauces."

Decorate the mousse with extra whipped cream, shaved chocolate or chopped pecans.

CHILLED LEMON-RUM SOUFFLÉ

Serves: 8

6 egg yolks
1 cup sugar
1/2 cup lemon juice
1 Tbsp. finely grated lemon peel
1/8 tsp. salt
1 envelope unflavored gelatin
1/2 cup rum
8 egg whites
1 cup whipping cream

Beat egg yolks until light and fluffy. Add sugar and beat until smooth and pale. Add lemon juice, grated rind and salt. Mix well. Pour into saucepan and stir over medium heat until thickened. Do not boil. Sprinkle gelatin over rum and let dissolve. Stir into thickened custard. Cook and stir until completely dissolved and smooth. Remove from heat and cool. Beat egg whites until stiff. Whip cream to soft peaks. Fold egg whites into cooled custard, then carefully fold in whipped cream. Pour into oiled 1-qt. soufflé dish wrapped with 3″ oiled collar and chill several hours until set. May be held in refrigerator up to 24 hours. To serve, remove collar and decorate with whipped cream if desired.

Refreshing and light. Does not freeze and does not double easily. Make twice instead.

GLAZED CUSTARD

Serves: 4-6

1 cup milk
1 cup whipping cream
4 egg yolks
1 tsp. vanilla
3 Tbsp. white sugar
1 Tbsp. brown sugar

Heat milk and cream together in top of double boiler over boiling water until steaming and quite hot. Place egg yolks, vanilla and white sugar in blender. Cover and turn blender on low. Remove cover and slowly pour hot milk and cream mixture directly into center of whirling blades. Turn blender off. Pour mixture into 4 6-oz. custard cups or 1 shallow 3-cup glass casserole. Place containers into pan, add boiling water and bake at 350° for 50 minutes or until knife inserted in center of custard comes out clean. Remove from pan of water, sprinkle top with brown sugar and broil 4″ from heat for 1 minute or until brown sugar melts. Cool, then chill.

A light dessert — quite right for a rich dinner and a perfect ending for a Mexican menu.

CHOCOLATE SOUFFLÉ WITH GRAND MARNIER SAUCE

Serves: 16

3 Tbsp. butter
1/4 cup flour
1/4 tsp. salt
1 cup milk
2 oz. unsweetened chocolate, cut up
4 eggs, separated
1/2 cup sugar
1/4 tsp. cream of tartar

Sauce:
1/4 cup sugar
1 Tbsp. cornstarch
3/4 cup orange juice
1/4 cup Grand Marnier
1/4 cup slivered almonds, toasted

Melt butter in saucepan. Blend in flour and salt. Slowly add milk, cook over medium-high, stirring constantly, until mixture just comes to a boil. Remove from heat. Stir in chocolate until melted. Beat egg yolks until thick and lemon colored. Gradually beat in sugar and blend in chocolate mixture. Beat egg whites and cream of tartar until stiff peaks form. Fold whites into chocolate mixture. Pour into 5 cup soufflé dish with 2″ foil collar that is buttered and sprinkled with sugar. Bake at 325° for 1 hour-1 hour 10 minutes. Serve immediately with Grand Marnier Sauce: For Sauce: stir together and bring to boil first 3 ingredients. Remove from heat. Add Grand Marnier and almonds.

Batter could be prepared early in the day up to adding the egg whites. Complete and place in oven just before calling guests to dinner.

CHOCOLATE SILK

Serves: 20

1 cup flour
1 1/4 cups chopped pecans
1 stick butter, melted
1 8-oz. pkg. cream cheese, softened
1 cup confectioners' sugar
1 8-oz. carton Cool Whip, defrosted
1 3 3/4-oz. instant chocolate pudding
2 cups milk
1 3 3/4-oz. instant vanilla pudding
2 cups milk
Semi-sweet chocolate curls

A day ahead, combine first 3 ingredients, press into bottom of 9″×13″ pan. Bake at 350° for about 30 minutes. Refrigerate. Next day, mix together cream cheese, sugar and 1 cup Cool Whip. Spread over chilled crust. Make instant chocolate pudding according to directions. Pour over cream cheese mixture. Chill. Make instant vanilla pudding. Pour over chocolate pudding. Chill. To serve, top with remaining Cool Whip and chocolate curls. Cut in squares.

This can be prepared up to the topping and refrigerated 1 week ahead.

PINEAPPLE RITZ DESSERT

Serves: 12

72 Ritz crackers
1 stick butter, melted
2 cups sugar
8 egg yolks, beaten
1 20-oz. can crushed pineapple, drained
1 3-oz. pkg. lemon jello
8 egg whites
1 pt. whipping cream

Roll crackers finely. Add butter. Reserve 1/2 cup. Press remaining mixture firmly over bottom of 9″ × 13″ pan. Combine 1 cup sugar, egg yolks and pineapple. Cook over medium heat, stirring constantly until thick. Add lemon jello. Cool. Beat egg whites until foamy. Slowly add remaining sugar, beating until stiff peaks form. Fold into egg yolk mixture. Spread over crumbs in pan. Whip cream and spread over. Sprinkle with reserved crumbs. Refrigerate.

May be made a day ahead. Garnish with cherries or fresh strawberries.

ORANGE SAUCE FOR CAKE

Yield: 2 1/2 cups

2 eggs
1 cup sugar
3 Tbsp. lemon juice
Juice and grated rind of 1 orange
2 cups whipping cream

Beat eggs in top of double boiler. Add sugar and beat. Add lemon juice, orange juice and rind and cook until thick, stirring constantly. Chill. Whip cream and fold in. Serve over sponge or angel food cake.

Very easy and good for a quick dessert.

ZABAIONE SAUCE

Yield: 3 cups

3 egg yolks
3 Tbsp. sugar
1/2 cup dry marsala
1/2 pt. whipping cream, whipped

Blend egg yolks and sugar in top of double boiler over hot, not boiling, water. Add wine and beat constantly until mixture foams and doubles in volume. Remove and immediately place pan in large bowl of ice. Continue beating until completely cold. Fold in whipped cream. Chill.

Do not make earlier than the morning of the day sauce is to be served.

EASY FRUIT DIP

Yield: 2 1/2 cups

1 8-oz. carton Cool Whip
1 3 3/4-oz. instant vanilla pudding
1/4 cup Amaretto

Combine Cool Whip and pudding. Blend in Amaretto. Refrigerate. Stir before using.

Serve with fresh strawberries, pineapple cubes, mandarin oranges and bananas.

HOT FUDGE SAUCE I

Yield: 1 cup

1/3 cup butter
2 1/2 oz. unsweetened chocolate
1 cup confectioners' sugar
1/3 cup milk

Melt butter and chocolate in top of double boiler over simmering water. Slowly add sugar alternately with milk. Cook, stirring occasionally for 30 minutes.

Keeps for weeks in refrigerator. Reheat to use. Doubles easily.

HOT FUDGE SAUCE II

Yield: 1 1/2 cups

1 oz. unsweetened chocolate
1 14-oz. can sweetened condensed milk
1 tsp. vanilla

Melt chocolate in saucepan over low heat, watching carefully. Stir in milk and vanilla and heat until warm.

Will keep in refrigerator. Use hot or cold on ice cream or angel food cake.

BASIC LEMON SAUCE

Yield: 3 cups

2 eggs, lightly beaten
1 1/3 cups sugar
1 stick unsalted butter
2 tsp. grated lemon rind
1/3 cup + 1 Tbsp. fresh lemon juice
1 cup water

Combine all ingredients in top of double boiler and place over simmering water. Cook, stirring constantly, until sauce thickens. Serve hot, warm or cold over pudding or cake.

Leftover sauce may be frozen and then thawed at room temperature before using. Layer stale cake with sauce for a fresh dessert.

And Then We Have

Selected Recipes from Special Chefs

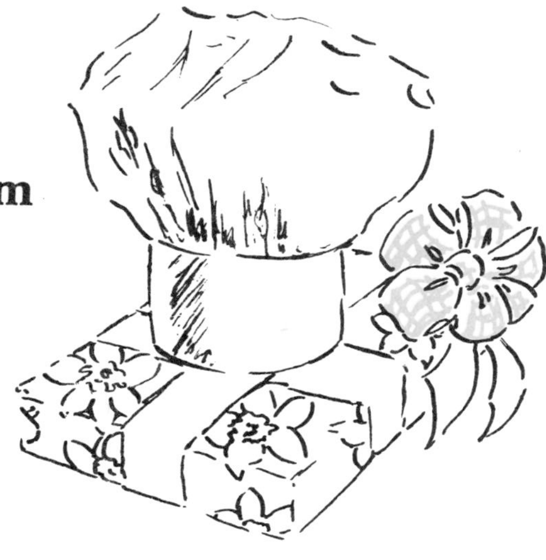

Jean-Claude Bergeret, Executive Chef
HILTON INTERNATIONAL
Tel Aviv, Israel

ICED TOMATOES SOUP

Serves: 5

6 tomatoes
1/2 cucumber
12 oz. plain yogurt
2 cups cream
5 leaves fresh mint
Salt, pepper or Cayenne pepper

Peel tomatoes, take out seeds and peel cucumber. Put tomatoes and cucumber in blender. Blend. Add yogurt and cream. Blend mixture for 2 minutes with seasoning. Leave it in refrigerator for 1 hour. Serve in glasses with 1 leaf of fresh mint on top.

ESCALOPES DE SAUMON FRAIS A LA MOUTARDE

Serves: 4

4 escalopes salmon, 150 gr. or 1/3 lb. each
6 tsp. French mustard
15 cl. fish stock or 5/8 cup
200 gr. butter or 1 stick plus 6 Tbsp.
300 gr. fresh mushrooms or 2/3 lb.
2 Tbsp. butter
Salt and pepper

Put escalopes between two sheets of wax paper, lightly oiled, and beat flat with large knife. Wash and slice mushrooms. Heat slowly mustard and fish stock in saucepan. Mix well. Add sliced mushrooms, then incorporate 1 stick plus 6 Tbsp. butter piece by piece. Mix well and season. Keep in bain-marie or double boiler. Cook salmon in fry pan with 2 Tbsp. butter, 2 minutes each side. Pour sauce in service plate and dress cooked escalopes on top. Serve hot.

Kathryn Domurot
KAY'S COOKING SCHOOL
Pittsburgh, Pennsylvania

STUFFED ONIONS

Serves: 6

6 large onions
1 pkg. smoked sausages
Garlic clove, minced
3 Tbsp. butter
Bread crumbs
Melted butter
Stock

Peel onions and in large saucepan of boiling, salted water cook onions for 10 minutes. Remove from water, drain well and let cool. Grind sausages fine and set aside. When onions are cool, hollow insides, leaving shell about 3/4″-1″ thick. Reserve shells and chop removed centers. In skillet melt 3 Tbsp. butter and stir in chopped onions and minced garlic. Sweat briefly until soft but not brown. Mix together ground sausage and onion-garlic mixture. Fill onion shells, rounding nicely on top. Sprinkle with crumbs and drizzle with melted butter. Place in shallow baking pan and add stock about 1″ up sides of onions. Bake at 400° until nicely browned.

BLANQUETTE DE PORC AUX ABRICOTS

Serves: 4-5

2 Tbsp. butter
2 Tbsp. oil, Puritan preferred
1 1/2 lb. pork, cubed, trimmed of all fat
2 ribs celery, diced
1 large onion, diced
1/4 tsp. rosemary
1 1/2 tsp. salt
1/2 tsp. white pepper
1 cup white stock, chicken or veal
1/2 cup wine
1/4 lb. dried apricots, halved
1 bay leaf

Heat butter and oil in large skillet and add pork cubes without crowding. Brown nicely on all sides. When brown remove to ovenproof casserole with cover. In same skillet lightly brown onion and celery and add these to casserole, transferring with slotted spoon to reserve shortening and brown bits in skillet. Return skillet to heat and deglaze with wine, scraping up all brown bits clinging to pan. Add white stock to skillet. Stir and taste for seasoning, then add salt, pepper and rosemary. Pour this into casserole. Add apricots, pressing down to moisten with stock. Lay 1 bay leaf on top. Place cover on casserole and set in 350° oven for 1 hour. Test meat for tenderness and if done, remove at once. Uncover and let casserole cool. When cool, re-cover and refrigerate until next day. Remove from refrigerator several hours before reheating to bring to room temperature. Reheat in 300° oven until thoroughly hot. Serve in casserole. Options: Top casserole with minced parsley. Add clove of minced garlic to celery-onion mixture. If heavier sauce is wanted, mix 1/2 tsp. arrowroot with small amount of casserole gravy, return mixture to casserole, place in oven for a few additional minutes until sauce is slightly thickened.

CÉLERI BRAISÉ MA FAÇON

Serves: 6

6 celery hearts
1 large carrot, minced
2 Tbsp. dried minced onion flakes
Chicken consommé
Salt and pepper to taste
1 1/2 tsp. arrowroot

Clean and halve celery hearts and place in saucepan. Cover with chicken consommé and bring to boil, then reduce fire so that celery simmers in broth. When celery is just tender, remove to baking dish, pour over consommé remaining in pan, add minced carrot and onion flakes and cover dish with foil. Bake at 350° for about 20 minutes or until celery is quite tender. Remove and taste for seasoning, adding salt and pepper as needed. Spoon out small amount of consommé in small dish and mix with 1 1/2 tsp. arrowroot. Blend arrowroot mixture back into baking dish and return to oven for a few minutes until sauce is slightly thickened.

René Verdon, Chef
LE TRIANON
San Francisco, California

TERRINE OF TROUT

Serves: 12

2 1/2 oz. American white bread, trimmed
3/4 cup milk
9 oz. fresh trout, boned and skinned
1 egg
1/3 cup heavy cream
Salt, pepper and nutmeg to taste

Watercress Sauce:
1 cup mayonnaise
1/2 tsp. green peppercorns
2 Tbsp. whipped cream
1/2 tsp. lemon juice
1 bunch watercress leaves, blanched
Salt to taste

Boil milk and add bread. Stir with wooden spoon over heat until smooth, about 1 minute, then cool. Using a meat grinder, grind fresh trout with bread mixture. Add this to egg in food processor and run for 1 minute. Add cream which should be half whipped. Add salt, seasoning and run 1 second. Be careful not to over-run it as it may curdle. Remove from processor and gently stir with wooden spoon. Pour into well-buttered 8″x4″ loaf pan. Cover tightly with foil. Place loaf pan into larger water-filled pan. Molded cooking time is approximately 1 hour at 350°.
For Watercress Sauce: combine all ingredients well. Serve in separate bowl.

Paul L. Chojnicki, Executive Chef
LES NUAGES RESTAURANT
Pittsburgh, Pennsylvania

COINTREAU CHEESECAKE

Serves: 8-10

Crust:
2 cups crushed graham crackers
6 Tbsp. melted butter
2 tsp. grated orange rind

Filling:
2 eggs, separated
1 1/4 tsp. unflavored gelatin
1/2 cup evaporated milk
3/4 lb. softened cream cheese
1 tsp. vanilla extract
1/4 cup sugar
2/3 cup sugar
1/4 tsp. salt
1 1/2 tsp. grated orange rind
1 1/2 Tbsp. lemon juice
4 Tbsp. Cointreau
2/3 cup cream

Mix together crushed graham crackers, orange rind and melted butter. Firmly press on bottom and sides of 9″ spring-form pan. Chill until ready to use. Combine egg yolks, sugar, gelatin, salt, evaporated milk in top of double boiler. Place over simmering water and stir constantly until mixture thickens. Stir in grated orange rind and cool. Press cream cheese through strainer and beat together with lemon juice, vanilla extract, and Cointreau. Combine cream cheese mixture and cooled custard mixture, folding gently. Beat egg whites until they form soft peaks. Slowly add sugar and continue to beat until stiff. Fold in cream cheese mixture. Whip cream until thick and gently fold into mixture. Pour into prepared crust and chill until set.

SAUCE CHOW CHOW

Serves: 4

2 Tbsp. diced onion
3 Tbsp. butter
1 cup sliced mushrooms
1 tsp. flour
3/4 tsp. salt
1/4 tsp. pepper
1/4 cup sherry
1/2 cup sour cream
2 tsp. chopped fresh parsley

In skillet sauté diced onions in butter until tender. Add mushrooms and sauté for 5 minutes. Over mushrooms sprinkle flour, salt, pepper and blend mixture well. Stir in sherry and cook sauce, stirring sauce until it is thickened. Stir in sour cream and chopped parsley and serve sauce immediately with steaks or beef roasts.

Tim Ryan, Executive Chef
LA NORMANDE
Pittsburgh, Pennsylvania

SOUPE DE POISSONS

Yield: 3 1/2 qt.

- 1 onion, diced
- 1 leek, diced
- 1 rib celery, diced
- 1/2 cup parsley, minced
- 2 carrots, peeled and diced
- 3 Tbsp. olive oil
- 6 cloves garlic, crushed with skin on
- 2 tomatoes, cut into chunks
- 3 bay leaves
- 3 lbs. fish and fish bones, such as sole, bass or snapper
- 1 pinch dried thyme
- 1 large pinch saffron
- 1 tsp. black pepper
- 1/2 cup tomato puree
- 2 cups white wine
- 3 qt. water

Heat olive oil. When hot add vegetables and herbs. Cook for 5 minutes then add garlic, tomatoes, bay leaves, fish and bones, thyme, saffron and pepper. Cook for 3 minutes. Then add remaining ingredients, bring to boil. Boil 25-30 minutes. Puree and strain. Add salt to taste. Serve with toasted croutons rubbed with olive oil.

PETONCLES AU POIREAUS AVEC PERNOD

Serves: 4-6

- 1 qt. bay scallops
- 6 Tbsp. butter
- 3 leeks, julienned
- 2 Tbsp. white wine
- 2 cups heavy cream
- 3 Tbsp. finely chopped shallots
- 2 Tbsp. Pernod or other anise-flavored liqueur

Heat 2 Tbsp. butter in skillet and add leeks. Cook, stirring often, for 2 minutes. Sprinkle with white wine and cook 1 minute. Add heavy cream and bring to a boil, reduce heat and simmer for 5 minutes. In another skillet melt 2 Tbsp. butter and add shallots. Cook 1 minute and add scallops. When scallops are cooked, deglaze with Pernod, then combine the 2 mixtures. Bring to a boil and swirl in remaining 2 Tbsp. butter. Adjust seasoning.

Art Inzinga, Executive Chef
HYEHOLDE RESTAURANT
Coraopolis, Pennsylvania

SHERRY BISQUE

Serves: 12

1 small ham hock
3/4 cup split peas
1 small bay leaf
6 cups beef stock
1/4 cup ground salt pork
3/4 cup diced onion
1/2 cup diced celery
2 1/2 Tbsp. flour
1 cup tomato puree
1 1/4 cups hot chicken stock
1/4 cup dry sherry
1/4 cup butter
Fresh ground pepper
Salt, if needed

Place ham hock, split peas, bay leaf and 4 cups beef stock into 4-qt. pot. Bring to a boil, reduce heat and simmer. In separate pan, sauté salt pork until some of the fat is rendered. Add onion and celery and cook until tender, mixing occasionally. Add flour to make roux, and cook 5-6 minutes. Add remaining beef stock gradually, and stir until slightly thickened and smooth. Combine with ham and peas mixture, and simmer until peas are soft, 1-1 1/2 hrs. Remove ham hock and puree remaining mixture in food mill. Add tomato puree and hot chicken stock. Cook over low flame. Add sherry and butter. Stir until butter is melted. Season with fresh ground black pepper and strain. If needed, add salt to taste.

VEAL ROMANO

Serves: 8

1 lb. veal cutlet cut into scallopines
Romano cheese
2 eggs
Flour
Cooking oil
3 Tbsp. butter
1/2 lemon

Pound scallopines until very thin. Blend cheese into eggs until its consistency resembles cake batter. Dredge veal with flour, then dip into egg and cheese batter. Heat oil in frying pan over moderate heat until oil is hot, add veal. Sauté veal until batter has browned slightly, then turn veal and cook other side. When veal is cooked, remove from pan and place on serving dish. Scrape out pan, then return it to fire. Add butter and when butter has melted, add juice of 1/2 lemon and pour the butter lemon sauce over veal.

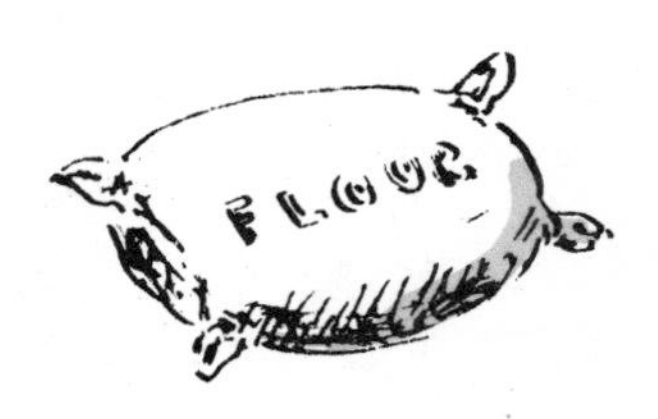

RATATOUILLE A LA NICOISE

Serves: 6

1 lb. eggplant, sliced
1 lb. zucchini, sliced
3 sweet peppers, red or green, sliced
2 onions, sliced
2 garlic cloves, chopped
1 lb. tomatoes, blanched, peeled and chopped
Salt
Pepper
Sugar
Parsley, 1 bunch, chopped

In wide pan, sauté onions and garlic until slightly browned. Add zucchini, eggplant and peppers, sauté a few minutes, then add tomatoes. Cook uncovered until vegetables are reduced to a thick stew. Season with salt, pepper and sugar. Sprinkle with chopped parsley. Ratatouille may be served hot as a side dish or served cold as an appetizer.

STRAWBERRY MOUSSE

Serves: 8

1 basket strawberries
1 1/2 cups heavy cream
6 egg whites
1 1/2 cups sugar
Vanilla, to taste

Puree strawberries in blender. Add 1/2 cup sugar. In separate bowl, whip heavy cream, 1/2 cup sugar and vanilla until stiff peaks form. In another bowl, whip egg whites and 1/2 cup sugar to stiff peaks. Fold egg white into cream. Then fold in strawberry puree. Pour into bowls and chill.

Peter Mathews, Chef
CAPRICE RESTAURANT
Penarth, South Glamorgan, Wales

VEAL CUTLETS LADY JANE

Serves: 4

1/2 oz. flour
1/2 oz. paprika
Pinch salt
4 veal cutlets, about 6 oz.
1 oz. butter
3 oz. sliced mushrooms
1 medium onion, chopped
3 oz. dry white wine
1/3 pt. cream
16 asparagus spears

Mix flour, paprika and salt. Roll cutlets in this mixture, and lightly fry cutlets in butter until lightly colored. Remove from pan and place in casserole dish. Lightly fry mushrooms and onions and add to cutlets. Swirl pan with wine and reduce by half. Add cream and bring to boil. Pour cream and wine over veal and simmer for 10 minutes. Serve in casserole garnished with plain boiled asparagus.

Craig Roth, Executive Chef
UNIVERSITY CLUB
Chicago, Illinois

JUMBO GULF SHRIMP WITH FETTUCCINE EN CASSEROLE

Serves: 6

36 jumbo shrimp, shelled and deveined
Butter
1 tsp. tarragon soaked in white wine
Salt
Freshly ground black pepper
Cayenne pepper to taste
1 oz. Pernod
3 scallions, sliced
8 oz. fettuccine, al dente
8 oz. hollandaise sauce.

Sauté shrimp in butter with tarragon and spices. Flambée with Pernod, add scallions. Sauté until tender. Serve en casserole on bed of fettuccine topped with hollandaise sauce.

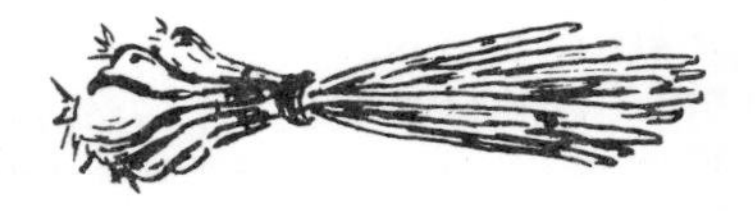

THE ENGLISH PAIR

Serves: 6

6 English muffins
7 oz. butter
7 oz. flour
1 qt. half and half
2 oz. butter
3 oz. minced onion
6 oz. sliced mushrooms
12 oz. King crabmeat, drained and chopped
2 oz. dry sherry
Salt
Pepper to taste
6 6-oz. hamburger patties
6 2-oz. slices Cheddar cheese
12 oz. Béarnaise sauce

Fork split and toast English muffins. Melt butter and add flour. Cook 2 minutes to make roux. Heat half and half, add to roux and cook mixture until thick. Stir to prevent scorching. Sauté onion and mushrooms in butter, add to cream sauce. Add King crabmeat and sherry. Salt and pepper to taste. Broil hamburger patties to desired degree of doneness. Place crabmeat mixture on 6 English muffin halves and top each with 1 slice Cheddar cheese. Run under broiler to melt cheese. Place on serving plates. Place other English muffin halves on plates with hamburger patties, each topped with 2 oz. Béarnaise sauce. Garnish with leaf lettuce and sliced tomato.

Caley Augustine, Jr., Chef
ESPRIT
Pittsburgh, Pennsylvania

NOISETTES OF LAMB PRINTANIER

Serves: 4

2 rib eye fillets from rack of lamb
12 strips bacon, blanched
2 Tbsp. clarified butter
2 Tbsp. brandy
1 cup brown stock
2 shallots
1/2 tsp. beurre manie
1 tsp. Dijon mustard
1/4 cup Chartreuse, green
4 large mushroom caps, blanched
12 asparagus spears, cut 4″
1 1/2 cup snow pea pods, stringed
3 carrots, sliced into 3″ julienne
4 artichoke bottoms

Have butcher remove two rib eye fillets from rack of lamb. Trim excess fat, cartilage and membrane. Cut each fillet into 6 noisettes. Wrap each piece with strip of blanched bacon. Secure with butcher's twine. In large skillet put 2 Tbsp. clarified butter. Sauté noisettes over medium-high heat, turning on all sides to brown exposed ends and crisp bacon, 6 minutes for very rare lamb. Reserve. Deglaze pan with 2 Tbsp. brandy and 1 cup good brown stock. Add 2 small minced shallots and reduce by 1/2. Add 1/2 tsp. beurre manie, 1 tsp. Dijon mustard and 1/4 cup Chartreuse. Flame. Garnish noisettes with blanched fresh mushroom caps and the fresh steamed spring vegetables. Brush noisettes with sauce. Serve remainder of sauce separately.

PEARS ESPRIT

Serves: 6

Pears:
1 cup burgundy
1 cup sugar
1/2 cup water
2 tsp. cinnamon
6 firm pears, Bosch preferred, peeled

Custard:
3 egg yolks
1/4 cup half and half
1 tsp. vanilla
2 Tbsp. cornstarch
1/2 cup sugar
2 cups half and half, brought to simmer

Sauce:
4 oz. bittersweet chocolate bits
2 Tbsp. brandy
2 Tbsp. whipping cream

Combine first 4 ingredients and bring to boil, add pears and simmer 20 minutes, basting pears often. Remove from heat and let pears sit in syrup an additional 15 minutes to absorb more flavor. Chill. For Custard: beat egg yolks, 1/4 cup half and half and vanilla together. Stir cornstarch and sugar together. Stir egg yolk mixture into sugar mixture. Slowly add heated half and half by drops, mixing with whisk. Heat over slow flame, stirring constantly, until mixture thickens to coat spoon. For Sauce: heat ingredients together in double boiler and whisk until smooth. In goblet, place warm custard, chilled pear, 1/2 oz. Cassis and top with warm chocolate sauce.

Peter Machamer, Wine Columnist
PITTSBURGH POST-GAZETTE
Pittsburgh, Pennsylvania

DINDÉ TRUFFE

Serves: 12

- **1 8-lb. turkey, ready for roasting and seasoned with salt and pepper in cavity**
- **3-4 truffles, canned are what's available, but fresh are preferable**
- **Glassful of sherry**
- **1 1/2 lb. pork sausage**
- **2 chicken livers, chopped**
- **1/2 cup bread crumbs**

Peel truffles and poach skins for 2 minutes in sherry. Chop peelings quite fine. Brown pork sausage and chicken livers. Mix truffle skins in sherry and meat mixture, plus 1/2 cup bread crumbs. Stuff turkey with this mixture. Slice truffles in thin slices and slip them beneath skin on breast of turkey. When turkey roasts, skin will blacken where truffles are inserted. Roast turkey in normal way, slightly covered at first, basting often. Turkey is best when stuffed and refrigerated day before using. This allows flavors to permeate bird throughout. Even stuffing early in morning before using is helpful.

SCALLOPS AU PASTIS

Serves: 4

- **16 or more medium-sized scallops, depending on whether it's a first or main course**
- **1/2 onion, chopped**
- **2 tomatoes, peeled and seeded, cut into pieces size of scallops or quartered**
- **1 clove garlic, chopped**
- **1/2 glass white wine**
- **A few drops Pastis, Pernod or Ouzo, or some non-sweet anise-flavored liqueur**
- **1 Tbsp. olive oil**
- **2-3 Tbsp. butter**
- **1/2 lemon**

Heat oil in sauté pan large enough to hold scallops. After oil is a bit hot, add butter. When it is melted and hot, add chopped onions and garlic and sauté until they are translucent. You want them to remain a bit crisp. Add scallops and sauté them until done. The time depends crucially on size of scallops. Teeny bay scallops are cooked in just over 1 1/2 minutes, while larger, thicker ones may take up to 6 minutes or so. Remove scallops to plate. Leave as much of onion in pan as you can. Add glass of white wine and reduce by 1/2. Add tomatoes. Continue reducing wine until only 1/4 remains. Sprinkle sauce with Pastis, 3 or 4 good shakes with thumb over bottle will do. Return scallops to pan and make sure they're warm. Squeeze lemon over them. Serve on warmed plates immediately. You can do this dish also with shrimp or scampi. Serve it with a full-bodied white wine. A good white Burgundy or even a Maçon will do. Another option would be a good Chardonnay from California, or a white Rhone, e.g., Hermitage.

POULET PETRUS

Serves: 3-4

1 3-lb. chicken
Butter
Olive oil
Chervil
Parsley
Fennel seeds
Salt and pepper
California Sauvignon Blanc or white Graves
4 green onions with tops
1 1-lb. can whole tomatoes, drained

Cut into pieces a fresh chicken. Remove all skin. Sauté chicken until brown in half butter and half olive oil. When browned, reduce heat. Add herbs, abundant tsp. of chervil, and 1 of parsley, if fresh use more, and then 1 large Tbsp. of fennel seeds. Add salt and pepper. Thoroughly mix herbs and spices into chicken mixture. Add good dry white wine, enough to reach half way up chicken pieces, about 1-1 1/2″ deep. Drink rest of wine while finishing the dish. Raise heat, reduce wine for about 3 minutes. Lower heat. Cover tightly, and simmer until chicken is tender, about 25 minutes. Add green onions which have been chopped into 1/4″ sections. After 10 minutes add tomatoes. Do not run out of liquid — you should not, but keep checking and add more wine if necessary. Remove the now tender chicken to warm plate. Raise heat under pan and reduce amount of wine remaining to about 1/4 amount first put in. It should begin to look a little thick because of pan drippings, etc. Stir up this sauce making sure to get in all juicy little brown bits from first frying. Pour wine mixture with onions etc. over chicken and serve immediately.

This dish is rather rich so should be served with simple accompaniments, e.g., a simple pilaff in butter, cooked in chicken stock, and say, some braised celery. The wine used in this dish should be a good one. Unlike some dishes, the quality of this dish is directly proportional to the quality of the wine. For wines to drink with, one can either drink the same wine one cooked the dish with, which is a bit of a bore since you have already downed the better part of one bottle of that while cooking, or another of the same type. Alternatively, a light fruity red wine such as a young Beaujolais or Bardolino will do nicely.

Eugene Duggan, Chef
CAPTAIN JON'S
Tahoe Vista, California

SEAFOOD CHOWDER

Serves: 4

2 stalks celery, diced
1 small onion, diced
1 medium potato, diced
2 cups fish fumé
2 cups cream
1/8 tsp. each rosemary, garlic powder, nutmeg and pepper
1/2 tsp. chopped parsley
1 Tbsp. butter

Simmer all ingredients, except butter, together until vegetables are tender. Add butter.

Edward Mauti, Chef
CONCORDIA CLUB
Pittsburgh, Pennsylvania

ESCALOPES DE VEAU ET CHAMPIGNONS SAUTES BORDELAISE

Serves: 4-6

12 slices veal scallopine, about 1 1/4 lb.
1/2 lb. mushrooms
2 Tbsp. olive oil
1/4 cup peanut, vegetable or corn oil
1/4 cup flour
Freshly ground pepper to taste
2 Tbsp. butter
1/3 cup finely chopped shallots
1/3 cup dry white wine
1/4 cup finely chopped parsley

Pound scallopine on flat surface with flat mallet. Do not break tissues. Set aside. Slice mushrooms thinly. There should be about 2 cups. Set aside. Heat olive oil in large skillet. When hot and almost smoking, add mushrooms. Cook over moderately high heat until mushrooms give up their liquid. Cook until liquid evaporates and mushrooms are browned. Set aside. Heat peanut oil in heavy skillet. Dredge scallopine in flour seasoned with pepper. Cook scallopine, a few at a time, on both sides until lightly browned, about 45-60 seconds a side. As they are cooked, transfer to warm platter. Pour off oil from skillet in which scallopine cooked. Add butter and when hot, add mushrooms. Cook briefly, shaking skillet and turning mushrooms. Add shallots and cook briefly, stirring. Add wine and cook, stirring to dissolve brown particles that cling to bottom of skillet. Pour mushrooms over veal and serve sprinkled with chopped parsley.

BREAD PUDDING

Serves: 8-10

1 lb. loaf thinly sliced white bread
1/4 cup raisins
1/4 cup glacéd fruit
10 chopped dates
1 pt. milk
1 pt. heavy cream
1/2 cup granulated sugar
1 drop vanilla
1/4 tsp. allspice
1/4 tsp. nutmeg
1/4 tsp. cinnamon
5 eggs
4 egg yolks
2 Tbsp. sugar for glaze

Trim off bread crusts and cut bread into triangles. In oval dish about 12″ long and 1 1/2″ deep, sprinkle 1/3 of fruit. Layer bread triangles around rim and then down center, overlapping slightly and making all large points face same direction. Sprinkle again with 1/3 of fruit and repeat layering. In saucepan, heat milk, cream, sugar mixed with spices and vanilla. Do not boil. In separate bowl, beat eggs and yolks, add milk gradually, mixing with each addition. Pour 1/2 custard over bread and allow it to soak in. Add remaining custard. Be sure all bread is well-coated. Sprinkle with remaining fruit and 2 Tbsp. sugar. Bake at 350° for 35-40 minutes. If more color is wanted, place dish under broiler for 30-60 seconds.

Joyce Williams, Chef
ROBAIOTTI'S GRILL ROOM
Penarth, South Glamorgan, Wales

COD CREOLE

Serves: 4

4 cod steaks or cutlets
1 1-lb. can tomatoes
2 onions, chopped
Salt
Pepper
Thyme
8 oz. American long grain rice
1 pt. stock
2 Tbsp. chopped parsley

Place steaks or cutlets in casserole. Drain tomatoes, reserving juice, and chop. Combine with onions and season to taste. Place around cod steaks and pour tomato juice over fish. Cook covered for 25 minutes at 425°. Put rice and stock into saucepan, bring to boil and stir once. Lower heat to simmer. Cover and cook for 15 minutes, or until rice is tender and liquid is absorbed. When cooked, fork in parsley and serve with cod steaks.

Peter Barber, Chef de Cuisine
ANGEL HOTEL
Cardiff, Wales

CREAMED LEEK SOUP

Serves: 8

1 1/4 lb. leeks
1/2 lb. onions
1 head celery
2 oz. butter
3 pt. mutton stock
1 oz. chopped parsley
Diced cooked mutton
5 oz. cream
Salt and pepper
Sippets

Fry vegetables, chopped roughly, in butter without browning. Add stock. Simmer for approximately 1 hour. Rub through sieve or blend in liquidiser. Stir in parsley, chopped lamb or mutton and cream. Salt and pepper to taste. Sprinkle with sippets, diced bread fried in bacon fat.

TROUT AND BACON

Serves: 1

1 rainbow trout
Pinch rosemary, thyme, parsley and sage
Butter
1 rasher of bacon

Clean fresh trout, leave on head and tail. Stuff with herbs mixed with butter. Wrap fish in rasher of bacon, enclose in foil and bake in hot oven, 375°, for approximately 25 minutes. Serve with boiled potatoes and fresh vegetables.

Thomas A. Bladel, Assistant Executive Chef
LES NUAGES RESTAURANT
Pittsburgh, Pennsylvania

FRENCH CRUMB CAKE

Serves: 6

2 cups flour
1 cup sugar
1 cup butter
2 eggs
1 cup raisins
1 cup sour milk
1/4 tsp. allspice
1/4 tsp. ground cloves
1/2 tsp. baking soda
1 1/2 tsp. baking powder
1 Tbsp. cinnamon
1/2 cup sugar

Blend first 3 ingredients like pie dough and reserve 1/2 cup. Add eggs, raisins, sour milk with allspice, cloves, soda and baking powder and mix well. Spread mixture into lightly greased tube pan. Combine reserved crumb mixture with cinnamon and sugar. Sprinkle over top and bake at 350° for 1 hour.

BEEF FILLET THOMAS

Serves: 4

2 lb. beef fillet
Salt
Dijon mustard
Fine bread crumbs
Cooking oil
Béarnaise sauce
1/2 cup brandy

Cut 1″ deep gash down length of the beef, cut from narrow end of fillet. Rub meat with salt, coat with Dijon-style mustard and roll in fine bread crumbs. Sauté fillet slowly in oil until browned on all sides and rare in center. Transfer fillet to ovenproof platter, cut into 1/2″ slices and reassemble them. Fill lengthwise gash with Béarnaise sauce. Pour 1/2 cup warm brandy over beef, ignite it, and shake platter til flame expires.

We thank Kay Domurot for her help in compiling this Special Chef's section.

Index

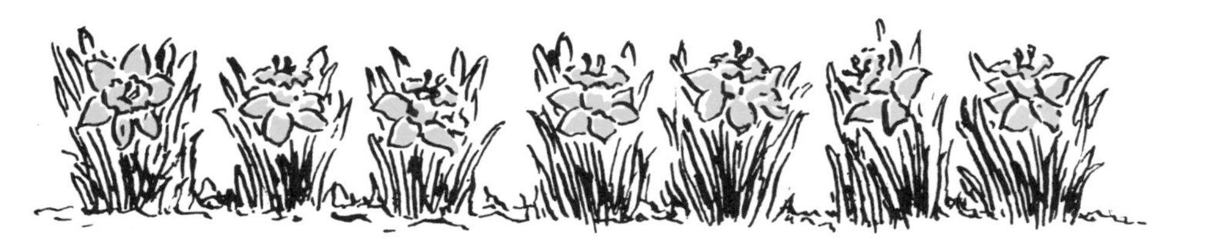

C

D

P

Q

R

S

T

U

V

W

Y

Z

NOTES

NOTES

NOTES

NOTES

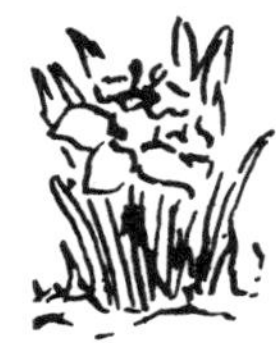

ONCE UPON A TABLE
241 Fourth Avenue
Pittsburgh, Pennsylvania 15222

________ copies of ONCE UPON A TABLE postpaid @ $9.95 ea. $____________

Tax per book for Pennsylvania residents only .54¢ ea. $____________

TOTAL ENCLOSED $____________

PLEASE PRINT

SEND TO: ____

STREET: ____

CITY: ____________________ STATE: __________ ZIP: __________

☐ Please enclose a gift card to read: ______________________________

____

Make check or money order payable to WAACS COOKBOOK
All profits realized will be given to the American Cancer Society.

ONCE UPON A TABLE
241 Fourth Avenue
Pittsburgh, Pennsylvania 15222

________ copies of ONCE UPON A TABLE postpaid @ $9.95 ea. $____________

Tax per book for Pennsylvania residents only .54¢ ea. $____________

TOTAL ENCLOSED $____________

PLEASE PRINT

SEND TO: ____

STREET: ____

CITY: ____________________ STATE: __________ ZIP: __________

☐ Please enclose a gift card to read: ______________________________

____

Make check or money order payable to WAACS COOKBOOK
All profits realized will be given to the American Cancer Society.

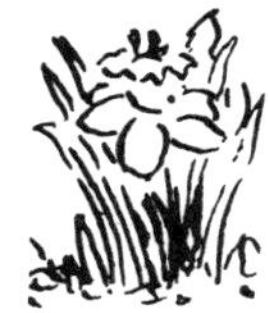

ONCE UPON A TABLE
241 Fourth Avenue
Pittsburgh, Pennsylvania 15222

______ copies of ONCE UPON A TABLE postpaid @ $9.95 ea. $__________

Tax per book for Pennsylvania residents only .54¢ ea. $__________

TOTAL ENCLOSED $__________

PLEASE PRINT

END TO: ______________________________

TREET: ______________________________

ITY: ______________ STATE: ________ ZIP: ________

☐ Please enclose a gift card to read: ____________________

____

Make check or money order payable to WAACS COOKBOOK
All profits realized will be given to the American Cancer Society.

ONCE UPON A TABLE
241 Fourth Avenue
Pittsburgh, Pennsylvania 15222

______ copies of ONCE UPON A TABLE postpaid @ $9.95 ea. $__________

Tax per book for Pennsylvania residents only .54¢ ea. $__________

TOTAL ENCLOSED $__________

PLEASE PRINT

END TO: ______________________________

TREET: ______________________________

ITY: ______________ STATE: ________ ZIP: ________

Please enclose a gift card to read: ____________________

____

Make check or money order payable to WAACS COOKBOOK
All profits realized will be given to the American Cancer Society.

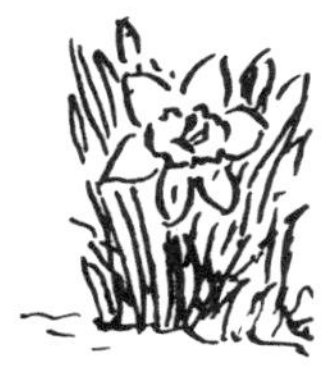

ONCE UPON A TABLE
241 Fourth Avenue
Pittsburgh, Pennsylvania 15222

________ copies of ONCE UPON A TABLE postpaid @ $9.95 ea. $________

Tax per book for Pennsylvania residents only .54¢ ea. $________

TOTAL ENCLOSED $________

PLEASE PRINT

SEND TO: ________

STREET: ________

CITY: ________ STATE: ________ ZIP: ________

☐ Please enclose a gift card to read: ________

____

Make check or money order payable to WAACS COOKBOOK
All profits realized will be given to the American Cancer Society.

- -

ONCE UPON A TABLE
241 Fourth Avenue
Pittsburgh, Pennsylvania 15222

________ copies of ONCE UPON A TABLE postpaid @ $9.95 ea. $________

Tax per book for Pennsylvania residents only .54¢ ea. $________

TOTAL ENCLOSED $________

PLEASE PRINT

SEND TO: ________

STREET: ________

CITY: ________ STATE: ________ ZIP: ________

☐ Please enclose a gift card to read: ________

____

Make check or money order payable to WAACS COOKBOOK
All profits realized will be given to the American Cancer Society.